Biotribology

Emerging Materials and Technologies
Series Editor
Boris I. Kharissov

Recycled Ceramics in Sustainable Concrete: Properties and Performance
Kwok Wei Shah and Ghasan Fahim Huseien

Photo-Electrochemical Ammonia Synthesis: Nanocatalyst Discovery, Reactor Design, and Advanced Spectroscopy
Mohammadreza Nazemi and Mostafa A. El-Sayed

Fire-Resistant Paper: Materials, Technologies, and Applications
Ying-Jie Zhu

Sensors for Stretchable Electronics in Nanotechnology
Kaushik Pal

Polymer-Based Composites: Design, Manufacturing, and Applications
V. Arumugaprabu, R. Deepak Joel Johnson, M. Uthayakumar, and P. Sivaranjana

Nanomaterials in Bionanotechnology: Fundamentals and Applications
Ravindra Pratap Singh and Kshitij RB Singh

Biomaterials and Materials for Medicine: Innovations in Research, Devices, and Applications
Jingan Li

Advanced Materials and Technologies for Wastewater Treatment
Sreedevi Upadhyayula and Amita Chaudhary

Green Tribology: Emerging Technologies and Applications
T V V L N Rao, Salmiah Binti Kasolang, Xie Guoxin, Jitendra Kumar Katiyar, and Ahmad Majdi Abdul Rani

Biotribology: Emerging Technologies and Applications
T V V L N Rao, Salmiah Binti Kasolang, Xie Guoxin, Jitendra Kumar Katiyar, and Ahmad Majdi Abdul Rani

Bioengineering and Biomaterials in Ventricular Assist Devices
Eduardo Guy Perpétuo Bock

Semiconducting Black Phosphorus: From 2D Nanomaterial to Emerging 3D Architecture
Han Zhang, Nasir Mahmood Abbasi, Bing Wang

Biotribology
Emerging Technologies and Applications

Edited by
T. V. V. L. N. Rao
Salmiah Binti Kasolang
Xie Guoxin
Jitendra Kumar Katiyar
Ahmad Majdi Abdul Rani

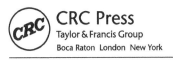

CRC Press
Taylor & Francis Group
Boca Raton London New York

CRC Press is an imprint of the
Taylor & Francis Group, an **informa** business

First edition published 2022
by CRC Press
6000 Broken Sound Parkway NW, Suite 300, Boca Raton, FL 33487-2742

and by CRC Press
2 Park Square, Milton Park, Abingdon, Oxon, OX14 4RN

© 2022 Taylor & Francis Group, LLC

CRC Press is an imprint of Taylor & Francis Group, LLC

Reasonable efforts have been made to publish reliable data and information, but the author and publisher cannot assume responsibility for the validity of all materials or the consequences of their use. The authors and publishers have attempted to trace the copyright holders of all material reproduced in this publication and apologize to copyright holders if permission to publish in this form has not been obtained. If any copyright material has not been acknowledged please write and let us know so we may rectify in any future reprint.

Except as permitted under U.S. Copyright Law, no part of this book may be reprinted, reproduced, transmitted, or utilized in any form by any electronic, mechanical, or other means, now known or hereafter invented, including photocopying, microfilming, and recording, or in any information storage or retrieval system, without written permission from the publishers.

For permission to photocopy or use material electronically from this work, access www.copyright.com or contact the Copyright Clearance Center, Inc. (CCC), 222 Rosewood Drive, Danvers, MA 01923, 978-750-8400. For works that are not available on CCC please contact mpkbookspermissions@tandf.co.uk

Trademark notice: Product or corporate names may be trademarks or registered trademarks and are used only for identification and explanation without intent to infringe.

ISBN: 978-0-367-68785-4 (hbk)
ISBN: 978-0-367-68840-0 (pbk)
ISBN: 978-1-003-13927-0 (ebk)

DOI: 10.1201/9781003139270

Typeset in Times
by SPi Technologies India Pvt Ltd (Straive)

Contents

Preface vii
Editors ix
Contributors xi

Chapter 1 Recent Developments in Biotribology 1

*T. V. V. L. N. Rao, Salmiah Kasolang, Guoxin Xie,
Jitendra Kumar Katiyar and Ahmad Majdi Abdul Rani*

Chapter 2 Lubrication of Hip and Knee Joint Replacements:
The Contribution of Experiments and Numerical Modeling 33

D. Nečas, M. Marian and Y. Sawae

Chapter 3 Computational Modeling of Biotribology on
Artificial Knee Joints 63

Liming Shu, Xijin Hua and Naohiko Sugita

Chapter 4 Development of a Multibody Biomechanical Model of
the Human Upper Limb 91

Alessandro Ruggiero and Alessandro Sicilia

Chapter 5 Metal-Organic Frameworks-Polymer Composites for
Practical Applications: Compatibility, Processability,
and Biotribology Studies 123

*J. A. Sánchez-Fernández, Rodrigo Cué-Sampedro and
Domingo Ricardo Flores-Hernandez*

Chapter 6 The Use of C.P. Titanium in Medical Friction Pairs 147

S. Ye. Sheykin, I. M. Pohrelyuk and O. V. Tkachuk

Chapter 7 Electrochemical Techniques Applied to the Tribocorrosion
Tests: Advantages and Limitations of Stationary and
Non-Stationary Methods 179

J. A. C. Ponciano Gomes and C. D. R. Barros

Chapter 8 Future Outlooks in Biotribology 231

*T. V. V. L. N. Rao, Salmiah Kasolang, Guoxin Xie,
Jitendra Kumar Katiyar and Ahmad Majdi Abdul Rani*

Index 235

Preface

Biotribology includes tribological phenomena of natural and implant surface interactions under relative motion in human body. With the theme of "Emerging Technologies and Applications in Biotribology," this book disseminates ideas and research trends in the field of Biotribology. The aim of the book is to present pioneering recent research advances impacting the field of Biotribology. The book focuses on the role of mathematics, chemistry, physics, materials and mechanical engineering on the recent advancements and developments in Biotribology. The scope of the book includes recent developments and future outlooks to the emerging technologies and applications in Biotribology. The state of the art and future technological developments impacting Biotribology are provided. An overview of the recent developments in Biotribology in the areas of lubrication characteristics of artificial joints, biotribological characteristics of textured surfaces, and tribological characteristics of implants are also presented. The book chapters discuss tribological design, mechanisms and characterizations of artificial joints, computational and multibody biomechanical modeling, tribological characteristics, wear analysis and tribocorrosion behavior of metallic implants. The challenges and opportunities for Biotribology are discussed. Biotribology is an important growing field, and topics covered in the book are of great interest to the international tribology community.

Editors

Dr. T. V. V. L. N. Rao received his PhD in Tribology of Fluid Film Bearings from the Indian Institute of Technology Delhi in 2000, and MTech in Mechanical Manufacturing Technology from the National Institute of Technology (formerly known as Regional Engineering College) Calicut in 1994. Rao's current research interests are in Bearings, Lubrication, and Tribology. He has authored (and co-authored) over 120 publications to date. He has secured (as PI and Co-PI) several research grants from the Ministry of Higher Education, Malaysia and a research grant from The Sumitomo Foundation, Japan. Rao is a member of the editorial board (2022) of *Tribology & Lubrication Technology* (TLT). He is a guest associate editor for the *Journal of Engineering Tribology, Industrial Lubrication and Tribology, Tribology – Materials, Surfaces & Interfaces*, and the *Arabian Journal for Science and Engineering*. Rao is an executive member (2015–2021) of the Malaysian Tribology Society. He is a member of the Society of Tribologists and Lubrication Engineers, Malaysian Tribology Society, and Tribology Society of India. Rao is currently professor in the Department of Mechanical Engineering at Madanapalle Institute of Technology & Science. Prior to joining MITS, he served as research associate professor at SRMIST (2017–2020), visiting faculty at LNMIIT (2016–2017), associate professor at Universiti Teknologi PETRONAS (2010–2016), and assistant professor in BITS Pilani at Pilani (2000–2004, 2007–2010) and Dubai (2004–2007) campuses.

Prof. Dr. Salmiah Binti Kasolang is currently the rector of Universiti Teknologi MARA (UiTM) Pulau Pinang Branch. Her research interest is in Tribology, and specifically hydrodynamic lubrication. She graduated from the University of Wisconsin-Madison in 1992 and later pursued her master's degree in Manufacturing System Engineering at Universiti Putra Malaysia UPM. She did her PhD in the University of Sheffield under the supervision of Prof. Rob Dwyer-Joyce. She has an administrative experience of 10 years as the deputy dean (7 years from 2009 to 2015) and dean (3 years from 2015 to 2017) at Universiti Teknologi MARA (UiTM). She is actively leading a Tribology research group in UiTM with more than 100 indexed publications. Her engagement with MYTRIBOS has enabled her to connect with other tribologists in Malaysia. Currently, she is the president of the Malaysian Tribology Society (MYTRIBOS). She is also the president of President of Society of Mechanical Engineering Liveliness SOMEL, which promotes many aspects of engineering including but not limited to education, research, industry-community engagement, engineering art, and engineering lifestyle.

Dr. Xie Guoxin received his doctoral degree at Tsinghua University, China in 2010, majoring in Mechanical Engineering. After that, he spent two years at State Key Laboratory of Tribology, Tsinghua University, China for postdoctoral research. From 2012 to 2014, he worked at Royal Institute of Technology, Sweden, for another two years' postdoctoral research. Since 2014, he has worked at Tsinghua University as a tenure associate professor. His research interests include solid lubrication, electric contact lubrication, thin film lubrication, etc. He has published more than 80 referred papers in international journals. He won several important academic awards, such as Chinese Thousands of Young Talents, the Excellent Doctoral Dissertation Award of China, and Ragnar Holm Plaque from KTH, Sweden. He is currently an associate editor of *Friction*, and he will be the director of Young Committee of Chinese Tribology Institution.

Dr. Jitendra Kumar Katiyar is presently working as a Research Assistant Professor, in Department of Mechanical Engineering, SRM Institute of Science and Technology Kattankulathur Chennai, India. His research interests include tribology of carbon materials, polymer composites, self-lubricating polymers, lubrication tribology, modern manufacturing techniques and coatings for advanced technologies. He obtained his bachelor's degree from UPTU Lucknow, graduating with Honors in 2007. He obtained his master's from the Indian Institute of Technology Kanpur, India in 2010 and a PhD from the same institution in 2017. He is the life member of Tribology Society of India, Malaysian Society of Tribology, Institute of Engineers, India, and The Indian Society for Technical Education (ISTE) etc. He has authored/co-authored/published more than 25 articles in reputed journals, 30+ articles in international/national conferences, 12+ book chapters, two books published such as, *Automotive Tribology and Tribology in Materials and Application* (Springer) and *Engineering Thermodynamics* for UG level (Khanna Publications). He has served as a guest editor for a special issue of *Tribology Materials, Surfaces and Interfaces*, *Journal of Engineering Tribology Part J*, *Arabian Journal for Science and Engineering*, and the *Industrial Lubrication and Tribology*. He is also an active reviewer in various reputed journals related to materials and tribology. He has delivered more than 30+ invited talks on various research fields related to tribology, composite materials, surface engineering, and machining. He has received research grants from various government organizations such as MHRD, SERB. He has also organized 5+ FDP/short-term courses in tribology and the International Tribology Research Symposium.

AP Dr. Ahmad Majdi Abdul Rani received his PhD in Mechanical & Manufacturing Engineering from Loughborough University, UK, MSc in Industrial Engineering and a BSc in Manufacturing from Northern Illinois University, USA. His research interests are in BioMedical Engineering, Mechanical & Manufacturing Engineering and Tribology. He has supervised and currently supervising more than 20 postgraduate (PhD and MSc) students. He recently received the Leadership in Innovation Fellowship – Newton Award, UK. He has secured three patents and won more than 15 gold awards in exhibitions such as ITEX, MaGRIs (MOSTI), MARS, PENCIPTA, IME, SPDEC, CoRIC, etc. He has authored over 150 publications to date. He has secured (as PI and Co-PI) several research grants from the Ministry of Higher Education, Malaysia (FRGS, PRGS, ERGS, MyBrain) and Universiti Teknologi PETRONAS (YUTP, I-GEN, STIRF). He has been associated with the Department of Mechanical Engineering at Universiti Teknologi PETRONAS since 1998. He has been head of the Department of Mechanical Engineering at Universiti Teknologi PETRONAS from 2009 to 2011.

Contributors

C. D. R. Barros
Federal University of Rio de Janeiro
Rio de Janeiro, Brazil

Rodrigo Cué-Sampedro
Tecnologico de Monterrey
Escuela de Ingeniería y Ciencias
Monterrey, México

Domingo Ricardo Flores-Hernandez
Tecnologico de Monterrey
Escuela de Ingeniería y Ciencias
Monterrey, México

J. A. C. Ponciano Gomes
Federal University of Rio de Janeiro
Rio de Janeiro, Brazil

Xijin Hua
Institute for Manufacturing
University of Cambridge
Cambridge, United Kingdom

Salmiah Kasolang
Universiti Teknologi MARA
Shah Alam, Malaysia

Jitendra Kumar Katiyar
SRM Institute of Science and Technology
Chennai, India

M. Marian
Friedrich-Alexander-University Erlangen-Nuremberg
Erlangen, Germany

D. Nečas
Brno University of Technology
Brno, Czechia

I. M. Pohrelyuk
Karpenko Physico-Mechanical Institute of the National Academy of Sciences of Ukraine
Kiev, Ukraine

Ahmad Majdi Abdul Rani
Universiti Teknologi PETRONAS
Seri Iskandar, Malaysia

T. V. V. L. N. Rao
Madanapalle Institute of Technology & Science
Madanapalle, India

Alessandro Ruggiero
Department of Industrial Engineering
University of Salerno
Fisciano, Italy

J. A. Sánchez-Fernández
Centro de Investigación en Química Aplicada
Saltillo, México

Y. Sawae
Kyushu University
Fukuoka, Japan

S. Ye. Sheykin
V. Bakul Institute for Superhard Materials of the National Academy of Sciences of Ukraine
Kiev, Ukraine

Liming Shu
Department of Mechanical Engineering
School of Engineering
The University of Tokyo
Tokyo, Japan

Alessandro Sicilia
Department of Industrial Engineering
University of Salerno
Fisciano, Italy

Naohiko Sugita
Department of Mechanical Engineering
School of Engineering
The University of Tokyo
Tokyo, Japan

O. V. Tkachuk
Karpenko Physico-Mechanical Institute
 of the National Academy of
 Sciences of Ukraine
Kiev, Ukraine

Guoxin Xie
Tsinghua University
Beijing, China

1 Recent Developments in Biotribology

T. V. V. L. N. Rao
Madanapalle Institute of Technology & Science, Madanapalle, India

Salmiah Kasolang
Universiti Teknologi MARA, Shah Alam, Malaysia

Guoxin Xie
Tsinghua University, Beijing, China

Jitendra Kumar Katiyar
SRM Institute of Science and Technology, Chennai, India

Ahmad Majdi Abdul Rani
Universiti Teknologi PETRONAS, Seri Iskandar, Malaysia

CONTENTS

1.1 Introduction 1
1.2 Lubrication Characteristics of Artificial Joints 2
    1.2.1 Squeeze Film/Elastohydrodynamic Lubrication 3
    1.2.2 Layered Surfaces 5
    1.2.3 Hydrogels 8
1.3 Biotribological Characteristics of Textured Surfaces 11
    1.3.1 Micro-Dimple Surfaces 12
    1.3.2 Micro Pattern Surfaces 13
    1.3.3 Bionic Surfaces 15
1.4 Tribological Characteristics of Implants 16
    1.4.1 Coatings 17
    1.4.2 Surfaces 18
    1.4.3 Composites 20
1.5 Conclusions and Further Outlook 24
References 24

1.1 INTRODUCTION

Biotribology covers all characteristics of tribology involved with biological systems. The biotribological characteristics cover a widespread range of tribological mechanisms recognized from biological systems which offer important perceptions of

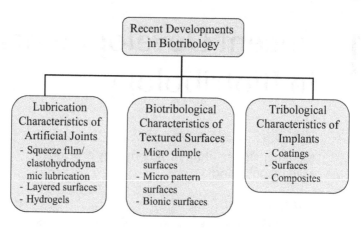

FIGURE 1.1 An overview of recent developments in biotribology.

means and methods for developing biotribology research. The most exclusive and vital concerns in biological systems deal with the medical interventions to be employed for combating diseases to make an influence on enhancement in quality of life. The fundamental theories, design and fabrications have been undertaken driven by the enhancement of life quality and stimulated by natural biological and tribological systems [1]. The natural association particularly develops between tribology, mechanics, and biology because many biological systems rely on adhesion, lubrication, and motion [2].

An overview of the recent developments in biotribology presented in Figure 1.1 is in the areas of: lubrication characteristics of artificial joints, biotribological characteristics of textured surfaces, and tribological characteristics of implants.

1.2 LUBRICATION CHARACTERISTICS OF ARTIFICIAL JOINTS

The squeeze film and elastohydrodynamic lubrication of bearing surfaces play a dominant role in the complex lubrication of artificial joints. There is an emphasis on the efficient numerical tools to predict the lubricant film considering the bearing surface geometry and deformation of artificial hip joints. The importance of lubricant film prediction is further enriched with the transient elastohydrodynamic lubrication process considering the bearing surface geometry and deformation of artificial hip joints [3]. It has been observed that there is an extremely efficient friction reducing effect in synovial joints arising from the presence of charged macromolecules (brush-like) at the superficial lubricated zone of synovial cartilage surface [4]. The coefficient of friction response of lubricated cartilage surface with interstitial synovial fluid pressurization is lower for potentially higher load under steady or transient mechanisms [5]. The investigations on friction-reducing behavior of synovial joints reveal that the boundary lubrication play a major role in contributing to the superior tribological properties of the cartilage surface. The lubricating properties of the synovial fluid, the chemical properties of the surface as well as the mechanical properties of the surface/structure contribute to the friction reducing behavior between the sliding surfaces [6]. The geometric and material parameters of implants facilitate in the progress of lubrication and wear models for extended life and superior performance of synovial joints [7].

TABLE 1.1
Recent Developments in Lubrication Characteristics of Artificial Joints

Lubrication Characteristics of Artificial Joints	Authors
Emphasized the need of efficient numerical tools to solve complex artificial hip joints lubrication	Jin [3]
Highlighted the synovial joints cartilage surface lubrication models	Klein [4]
Emphasis on the cartilage surface interstitial synovial fluid pressurization	Ateshian [5]
Investigated synovial joints cartilage surface boundary lubrication	Crockett [6]
Explored lubrication and wear models of hip implants for extended life and superior performance	Mattei et al. [7]
Examined the synovia constituents and cartilage surface conditions	Murakami et al. [8]
Bearing designs for in-vivo contacts in knee joint prostheses	Kennedy et al. [9]
Investigated film interfacial formation in the contact inlet zone by synovial fluid protein aggregates	Myant & Cann [10]
Modeling and simulation of total knee replacement	Shu et al. [11]

The lubrication and wear behavior is a significant concern for the success of artificial joints, as undesirable wear debris initiates loosening and malfunctioning of joints. The artificial joint's ability to resist tissue loosening and failure due to wear debris is a crucial concern for the successful tribological performance. The lubrication and wear are portrayed overlooking each other while new cutting-edge models embracing both features could be useful. The lubricating and wear models in mixed and boundary lubrication regimes considering surface topography, deformation, wear, and asperity contact determine the superior performance of synovial artificial joints [7]. The soft-on-hard and the hard-on-hard implants are modeled considering elastic deformation as well as wear. The effective lubrication mechanisms of articular cartilage surface and synovial fluid offer extremely low friction and minimal wear in natural synovial joints. The complex structure of cartilage surface (composed of collagen and proteoglycan with high water content) and synovial fluid (composed of phospholipid, protein, and hyaluronic acid) play an important role in friction/lubrication mechanisms with contribution to high load capacity [8]. The customary knee joint prostheses materials are femoral component of cobalt–chrome–molybdenum in contact with tibial bearing of ultra-high molecular weight polyethylene (UHMWPE). The wear of tibial bearings is most acute where contact pressure is maximum and lubricant film thickness is minimum [9]. The knee joint contact interface is in the mixed lubrication regime mostly due to the thin lubricating film, and at sometimes falls into the boundary lubrication regime. The interfacial film formation of high viscosity in the contact inlet zone is driven by the synovial fluid protein aggregates in shear flow [10]. The outcomes of modeling and simulation of joint replacement during the design process of the implant are widely used to undertake in-vitro and in-vivo testing to provide insights into the implant performance [11].

The recent developments in lubrication characteristics of artificial joints are presented in Table 1.1.

1.2.1 Squeeze Film/Elastohydrodynamic Lubrication

The squeeze film/elastohydrodynamic lubrication is of significance to biological systems. There has been substantial progress made in the theoretical/numerical/

experimental studies in squeeze film/elastohydrodynamic lubrication of artificial joints. The eventual target of artificial joints lubrication is to present design guidelines for wear particles reduction. The synovial fluids in joints containing long-chain hyaluronic acid molecules are governed by micropolar fluid film lubrication theory with an increase in the effective viscosity near the cartilage porous structure [12]. The poroelastic rough cartilage considerations with couple stress synovial fluid are important in the analysis of squeeze film behavior of synovial joints [13]. The sliding surfaces conformity play an important role on the ability and mechanism of squeeze film lubrication in synovial joints [14]. The considerable elastic deformation of the sliding contacts combined with compliant tissues is accountable for lubrication at the biological surface interfaces [15]. The sliding surfaces are safeguarded by the dominant influence of micro-elastohydrodynamic lubrication in smoothing out surface asperities on the biological surfaces. The elastohydrodynamic lubrication studies should comprise a more reasonable representation of the surface roughness and synovial fluid rheology which are significant for UHMWPE/metal-on-metal artificial implants [3]. The surface topography factors may indicate likelihoods of nano-textures to improve lubrication and reduce wear, in particular for metal-on-metal implants. A number of assumptions such as no-slip/slip boundary conditions are required for analysis of artificial joints lubrication. The no-slip conditions are used for hydrophilic (metallic and ceramic) sliding surfaces, while slip conditions are used for hydrophobic (UHMWPE) sliding surfaces. It is indicated that if the lubrication regime in an artificial joint is predominantly boundary, which exists in UHMWPE-on-metal hip joints, and then the fluid film lubrication investigations are no longer pertinent. The average film thickness obtained from steady state lubrication analysis based on the average load often presents a useful estimate to the transient walking cycle [3]. The salient tribological properties of cartilage are closely linked to the musculoskeletal system properties and the lubrication regimes in cartilage spread outside the fluid film or boundary lubrication [16]. The fluid film lubrication influences the joint conformity conditions during the walking stance in knee replacements [17].

The squeeze film effects in transient elastohydrodynamic non-Newtonian lubrication of artificial knee joints helps prevent the reducing film thickness with declining surface relative velocity [18]. The minimum film thickness attained for a non-Newtonian fluid (shear thinning) is lower compared to a Newtonian fluid. The film thickness (elastohydrodynamic) increases with increasing contact area and decreasing film pressure in the artificial knee joints using ultra-high molecular weight polyethylene (UHMWPE) against metal component [18]. The minimum film thickness is larger for softer surfaces, higher viscosity, smaller load, and greater relative surface velocity during walking cycle. The analytical model permits the closed form synovial fluid film force and film thickness under the considerations of hydrodynamic squeeze motion, Darcy's permeability model, Newtonian synovial fluid [19] and non-Newtonian couple stress synovial fluid [20]. The closed form synovial fluid film force is assessed based on the synovial pressure field for the articular joints depicting the synovial fluid motion through the porous cartilage. The finite element model predictions on time dependent response of biphasic cartilage layers are influenced by the cartilage modulus and clearance, permeability, and thickness in hip joint [21]. The fluid film retention in metal-on-metal (CoCrMo balls and cups) hip prosthesis is necessary to extend lubrication ability, long term reliability and to avoid severe wear in prosthesis due to metal-to-metal contact [22]. The radial clearance is also a vital parameter as lower radial clearance enhances squeeze film retention, while a too low radial clearance induces severe contact. The articular rough cartilage influences the hydrodynamic lubrication performance of synovial knee joint throughout the gait cycle [23]. The squeeze film load of partial bearing is significantly influenced by three-layered film and couple stress fluid lubrication [24]. The novel design of squeeze-film hip implant utilizing low modulus elastic structure with high modulus metallic coatings exhibited likely alternative to conventional artificial hip implant designs [25]. The 'tribological rehydration' or fluid recovery mechanism is due to pressurization of elastohydrodynamic films and subsequently causes tissue thickening and friction reduction [26]. The articular cartilage interstitial fluid effusion is suppressed in wedge just ahead cartilage contact region that increases biphasic lubrication ability of articular cartilage [27]. The articular cartilage interstitial fluid effusion is even more suppressed near the contact region periphery at higher sliding speeds which improves cartilage lubrication due to higher interstitial fluid pressurization. The fluid pressurization generated by squeeze flow at lower speeds increases fluid load support on the biphasic lubrication of articular cartilage [28]. The effect of fluid pressurization generated by the squeeze flow pressure reduces with increasing compressive load and increases with increasing speed. The lubricated hip joint (hard metallic femoral head and polymeric acetabular cup) is analyzed in unsteady state based on mixed elastohydrodynamic lubrication with non-Newtonian fluids [29]. The wear volume in lubricated hip joint (hard metallic femoral head and polymeric acetabular cup) is evaluated by a modified Archard's model over a single gait cycle. The wear volume in lubricated hip joint (ceramic on polyethylene hip) using a lubrication-contact model (hydrodynamic-boundary) is evaluated by a modified Archard's model over a single gait cycle [30].

The recent developments in squeeze film/elastohydrodynamic lubrication are presented in Table 1.2.

1.2.2 Layered Surfaces

Synovial fluid lubrication is reliant on the formation of protein films protecting the joint surfaces. The frictional response of cartilage is regulated by the surface porosities which play a role in the interstitial pressurization of fluid inside cartilage during loading of joints [31]. The boundary friction models are formulated to theoretically explain the experimental frictional response of cartilage. The lubricant comprising only albumin (a large amount of α-helix structure) exhibited low friction in comparison to the lubricant comprising only γ-globulin (a large amount of β-sheet structure) [32]. Hence to lower both friction and wear, it is vital to apply the layered structure of γ-globulin (tight layer) at the bottom topped with albumin (layer with low shearing strength) and γ-globulin. The protein boundary layer film mainly composed of γ-globulin is enhanced by adsorption of hyaluronic acid (HA) on surface which contributes to the establishment of a stable boundary film [33]. The contribution to friction reduction is due to a gel like layer which is created due to the inclusion of hydrophilic HA molecules into boundary film. The phospholipids loss in

TABLE 1.2
Recent Developments in Squeeze Film/Elastohydrodynamic Lubrication

Squeeze Film/Elastohydrodynamic Lubrication	Authors
Synovial micropolar fluid film lubrication theory in joints	Sinha et al. [12]
Squeeze film effects of poroelastic rough cartilage with couple stress synovial fluid	Bujurke & Kudenatti [13]
Sliding surfaces conformity on the squeeze film lubrication mechanism	Mabuchi et al. [14]
Elastohydrodynamic lubrication applications in biology	Jin & Dowson [15]
Elastohydrodynamic lubrication analysis of hip implants	Jin [3]
Friction and wear of articular cartilages	Ateshian & Hung [16]
Joint conformity conditions during the walking stance	Pascau et al. [17]
Transient elastohydrodynamic non-Newtonian lubrication of artificial knee joints	Mongkolwongrojn et al. [18]
Squeeze film lubrication analytical model of the porous cartilage ankle joint with Newtonian and non-Newtonian synovial fluid	Ruggiero et al. [19], Ruggiero et al. [20]
Finite element model of biphasic cartilage layers response in natural hip joint	Li et al. [21]
Lubrication ability of the CoCrMo balls and cups specimens	Tanaka et al. [22]
Articular rough cartilage of synovial knee joint under hydrodynamic lubrication	Abdullah et al. [23]
Squeeze film load of three-layered partial bearing under couple stress fluid lubrication	Rao et al. [24]
Wear in a novel design of squeeze-film hip implant	Boedo & Coots [25]
Friction reduction attributed to fluid film rehydration	Burris & Moore [26]
Friction coefficient and load capacity of poroelastic model with biphasic synovial fluid lubrication	Horibata et al. [27], Horibata et al. [28]
Wear in lubricated hip replacements with contact models	Ruggiero et al. [29], Ruggiero & Sicilia [30]

osteoarthritis joints has consequence to hydrophobicity deficiency. The lower coefficient of friction is attained on a surface comprising phospholipid bilayer with higher wettability [34]. The lubrication mechanism of the joint is influenced by the lubricant's pH and interfacial energy with a consequent influence on coefficient of friction. The synovial joint cartilage integrity is due to secretion of phospholipid multibilayer surface coating on the cartilage surface as solid lubricant delivering hydration boundary lubrication [35]. The ultra-high molecular weight polythene (UHMWPE) plate surface grafted with a polymer membrane extends the useful lifespan of artificial joints. The large water-retaining ability of the porous hydrophilic 2-methacryloyloxyethyl phosphorylcholine (MPC) graft-polymerized membrane with finely porous inner structure provides lubrication and serves to reduce wear in the UHMWPE component [36]. The main factors to enhance hydrodynamic lubrication performance and to reduce the dry contact in metal-on-metal hip bearing implant surfaces are diametral clearance and diameter. An aspherical 'alpharabola' metal-on-metal hip-bearing implant surface generates a thicker lubricant film thickness when compared to a spherical conventional hip bearing implant surface [37]. A significant decrease in the dry contact is attained in an aspherical metal-on-metal hip-bearing implant surface with appropriate selection of geometric parameters.

The proteins increase the film thickness with time (rolling distance) for a metal ball compared to a ceramic ball under pure rolling conditions [38]. The proteins increase the film thickness swiftly with time (rolling/sliding distance) and the film thickness starts to dip by a few nanometers after the maximum film thickness is attained under rolling/sliding conditions. The mechanism of surface film development under static conditions is through adsorption, while the film development under dynamic conditions occurs through protein aggregation. The film thickness increases with increasing adsorption mass and adsorption rate under rolling conditions [39]. The adsorption mass, adsorption rate, and film thickness are reduced due to increasing pH. In the comparison of lubricants macromolecular solutions (HA, mucin, or lubricin), the mucin shows improved performance compared to the HA or lubricin [40]. The signs of wear or changes in topography are not noticed by utilizing mucin for lubrication of the cartilage surfaces. The synergistic combination of various lubrication modes (boundary, gel, biphasic, and hydration) from the boundary to film lubrication appears to promote the superior tribological characteristics in natural synovial joints [41]. The synovial constituent albumin plays a leading role in pure rolling thus enhancing the film thickness [42]. The albumin and γ-globulin enhance the film thickness at lower speeds, while the effect of γ-globulin is not significant at higher speeds. The synovial constituents albumin, γ-globulin, phospholipids, and HA, play a leading role in noticeably influencing the lubricant boundary film [43]. The γ-globulin jointly with HA form a comparatively thin stable boundary film allowing the improved adsorption of albumin, and thus enhancing the lubricant boundary film. The albumin and γ-globulin proteins in interface between the femoral knee implant metal and real polymer insert are examined to be of importance [44]. A better tribological performance is achieved by supplementing organic constituents to the surface-lubricant contacts which have influencing roles on the frictional and material volume loss [45]. The principal mechanism of lubrication influencing the protection of surfaces during rubbing is the formation of denatured insoluble protein films [46]. The denatured insoluble protein lubricating films are induced into the contact region due to inlet shear. The long-life design of artificial joints essentially requires accomplishment of effective biolubrication. The structural integrity of small unilamellar vesicles adsorbed on the silicon nitride (Si3N4) surfaces is linked effectively with exceptional lubrication abilities of liposomes with longer carbon chain length [47]. The exceptional lubrication abilities of liposomes are also due to the boundary layer formed due to the synergistic interface of liposomes and biocompatible negative-charged polymer. The friction and wear of ultra-high molecular weight polyethylene (UHMWPE) surface adsorbed with proteins is increased due to the change in the predominant abrasive to adhesive wear mechanism [48]. However, the wear of ultra-high molecular weight polyethylene (UHMWPE) surface is increased when mixing proteins with phospholipids and HA, due to the enhanced the entrainment of the proteins in the contact area. The friction is increased with phospholipids while the friction is reduced with HA with increasing lubricants' viscosity. Phospholipids bilayers in cartilage boundary can reduce friction by means of hydration lubrication [49].

TABLE 1.3
Recent Developments in Biotribology of Layered Surfaces

Layered Surfaces	Authors
Friction model for articular cartilage boundary	Ateshian et al. [31]
Albumin or γ-globulin in natural synovial fluid	Nakashima et al. [32]
Lubricant composition on proteins adsorption and stability	Yarimitsu et al. [33]
Mechanisms of lubrication of phospholipids-bilayer of cartilage	Pawlak et al. [34], Pawlak et al. [35]
Grafted polymer membrane onto UHMWPE plate	Sawano et al. [36]
Aspherical metal-on-metal hip bearing implant surface	Meng et al. [37]
Proteins effect on film formation	Vrbka et al. [38]
Mechanisms of film formation of proteins in synovial fluids	Parkes et al. [39]
Lubricants macromolecular solutions comparison	Boettcher et al. [40]
Boundary, biphasic, gel, and hydration lubrication modes	Murakami et al. [41]
Mechanisms of lubrication of protein film in ceramic femoral heads	Nečas et al. [42]
Mechanisms of lubrication in hard-on-soft hip artificial joints	Nečas et al. [43]
In situ lubricant development in knee joint replacements	Nečas et al. [44]
Protein-metal interactions on tribofilm formation	Taufiqurrakhman et al. [45]
Artificial joint lubrication with bovine calf serum and human synovial fluid	Stevenson et al. [46]
Lubrication mechanisms between biomimetic surfaces	Wang et al. [47]
In-vivo tribology of implant joint prostheses	Shinmori et al. [48]
Phospholipids in lubrication of cartilage boundary	Cao et al. [49]

The recent developments in biotribology of layered surfaces are presented in Table 1.3.

1.2.3 Hydrogels

Hydrogels with suitable properties are potential materials for cartilage repair. Synthetic hydrogels have potential applications for articular cartilage as well as a developing cartilage in a damaged joint. The wear of synthesized poly(2-hydroxyethyl) methacrylate (polyHEMA) hydrogels increases with increasing applied load and hydration, while the wear of hydrogels decreases with increasing cross-link density [50]. The friction and wear of poly (vinyl alcohol) hydrogel for artificial cartilage depends on protein contents in lubricants. The friction properties of bovine serum albumin comprising the α-helix structure is lower compared to human gamma globulin comprising the β-sheet structure in mixed/boundary lubrication regime [32]. The β-sheet structure is strongly adsorbed on poly (vinyl alcohol) hydrogel, while the α-helix structure lacks adsorption ability (as the α-helix structure is easily released from surfaces due to low cohesive strength of formed shear layer). Lower friction artificial cartilage is maintained with a layered structure of a blend of various proteins. Soft biomaterials are frequently employed in applications that include contact of biological tissues. In the investigations of friction coefficients of soft hydrogel biomaterials, the lower friction coefficients were noted on undamaged cells and higher friction coefficients were noted on damaged cells [51]. The salient parameters to establish the wear performance of hydrogels are cross-link density and hydration. The wear phenomena in most compliant hydrogels is adhesive wear, while the wear phenomena with increasing cross-linking density and reducing water absorption capacity of hydrogels, is abrasive wear [52].

The low friction and wear in artificial cartilage interface contacts is maintained by adsorbed film formation (at micro/nano levels) in mixed/boundary lubrication regime [53]. The presence of albumin and γ-globulin constituents exhibited the lowest friction in the mixed regime of lubrication. The low friction and wear in the articular cartilage are maintained by proteoglycan gel film as a consequence of hydration lubrication mechanism even after removal of adsorbed layer [54]. The hydration lubrication with protein adsorbed film is effectual when restarted under loading. The friction and wear characteristics of articular cartilage in mixed/boundary lubrication regime are significantly influenced by adsorbed layer formed on a gel film at articular cartilage in synovial joints. In the absence of adsorbed layer, the proteoglycan gel film is likely to maintain low friction and wear of bulk articular cartilage with an efficient hydration mechanism of lubrication. The friction in articular cartilage is lowered by the mechanism of biphasic lubrication [55]. The larger friction coefficients for the hydrogels considering elastic effects are recognized as the outcome of the greater interface of the intra/inter-polymer chains generated by the higher degree of polymerization and saponification value [56]. The larger friction coefficients for the hydrogels under hydrodynamic lubrication are recognized as the outcome of the lower hydrophilicity of the poly(vinyl alcohol) hydrogels with lower saponification value at relatively lower load and higher velocity. The exceptionally low friction and wear in natural synovial joints are maintained by their outstanding lubricating capability which appears to be a synergistic blend of multimode mechanisms such as boundary, gel film, hydration, biphasic, and/or fluid film lubrication [57]. However, in artificial joints comprised of ultra-high molecular weight polyethylene against metal/ceramic material, contact of interfaces in boundary and/or mixed lubrication mechanism generates high friction and wear. The improvement in friction and wear characteristics through artificial biomimetic hydrogel cartilage, such as poly(vinyl alcohol) hydrogel, is required to prolong the durability and life of an artificial joint [57]. The wear resistance of ultra-high molecular weight polyethylene for total joint prostheses has been enhanced with recent developments of material technologies. The artificial hydrogel cartilage with identical properties to natural articular cartilage is expected to solve the friction and wear problems by enhancement of lubrication mechanism with excellent tribological behaviors. The tribological behaviors of artificial cartilage material, ellipsoidal poly(vinyl alcohol) hydrogel, evaluated against glass plate in saline solution are as follows [58]: hybrid (CD on FT) method < cast-drying (CD) method < freeze-thawing (FT) method < hybrid (FT on CD) method. PVA hydrogels prepared by the hybrid (CD on FT) method displayed exceptionally low friction and wear. The tribological behaviors of ideal artificial cartilage material, poly (vinyl alcohol) (PVA) hydrogel, evaluated in ultra-pure water are as follows [59]. PVA hydrogels prepared by (i) FT method exhibited high friction coefficient and wear, (ii) CD method exhibited low friction coefficient with scratches, and (iii) hybrid method (i and ii) exhibited the lowest friction coefficient and minimum wear.

Polyvinyl alcohol (PVA) hydrogels display outstanding tribological characteristics and are opted as potential biomaterials to replace damaged articular cartilage due to their low coefficient of friction and wear, high permeability, and superior biocompatibility [60]. The surface characteristic of alloys plays a significant role in friction coefficient reduction, and the alloys are grouped according to the surface oxide compositions as Ti-oxide-surface alloys and Fe/Cr-oxide-surface alloys [61]. Based on the wettability test, Ti-oxide-surface alloys show higher polar components of surface free energy than Fe/Cr-oxide-surface alloys. The elastic friction coefficients are governed by the hydrogel polymer adsorption, and Ti-oxide-surface alloys show lower friction coefficients than those of Fe/Cr-oxide-surface alloys [61]. The mechanical rigidity and strength of the structural hydrogel materials are taken into account for diverse biotribological applications. The structural hydrogel materials originate with low polymer mesh size and high polymer concentrations, that causes high friction coefficients under aqueous environments [62]. The large mesh size, flexible and soft polyhydroxyethylmethacrylate (pHEMA) hydrogels will be able to deliver ultra-low friction, but at the loss of mechanical strength. The entangled networks of polymer will be able to deliver reduced coefficient of friction. The swift reinstatement of biotribological and biomechanical functions endures a noteworthy test for articular cartilage restoration. The poly (vinyl alcohol) (PVA) hydrogel is considered as a prospective articular cartilage substitute for its low friction and fair strength [63]. The coefficient of friction decreased with adding up of ploy (lactic-co-glycolic acid) (PLGA) content. The low friction coefficient of the composite hydrogel on the UHMWPE surface under biphasic lubrication is due to its porous configuration with sizable water content [64]. The friction and drag at the interface are effectively reduced due to the shear of the hydrogel surface which is caused by the structural changes related to the surface chains alignment [65]. The phospholipid is a hydrophilic membrane with a negatively charged surface (-PO4−) formed by adsorption of articular cartilage surface-active phospholipid (SAPL) molecules to negatively charged proteoglycan matrix [66]. The friction in Gemini hydrogel configurations made from polyacrylamide (PAAm) formulations under direct sliding contact increases with increasing viscosity and decreasing mesh size with decreasing temperature [67]. The fiber-reinforced structure is potential biomimetic articular synovial cartilage materials that take part a vital role in enhancing the fluid load support and frictional properties. The fiber-reinforced poly(vinyl alcohol) (PVA) hydrogel reinforced with surface PVA fiber layers have a low friction coefficient [68]. The friction characteristics of hydrogel brushy surfaces are reliant on the interface contacts and surface hydration intensity. The friction characteristics of acrylamide hydrogels in sliding at low pressure contacts is due to the mechanism of interfacial shearing of the liquid film, rather than viscoelastic or poroelastic dissipation [69]. The mechanism of deformation induced poro-elastic flow is substantial at high pressure contacts. The double-network physically cross-linked poly (vinyl alcohol)-(nano-hydroxyapatite)/(2-hydroxypropyltrimethyl ammonium chloride chitosan) hydrogel with presence of nano-hydroxyapatite (HA) displayed lower coefficient of friction and wear properties, and exceptional cytocompatibility [70].

The recent developments in biotribology on hydrogels are presented in Table 1.4.

TABLE 1.4
Recent Developments in Biotribology on Hydrogels

Hydrogels	Authors
Poly(2-hydroxyethyl) methacrylate hydrogels	Freeman et al. [50]
Investigations of proteins on friction	Nakashima et al. [32]
Soft hydrogel biomaterial surfaces investigations	Dunn et al. [51]
Tribological properties of synthetic hydrogels	Bavaresco et al. [52]
In situ examination of adsorption behavior of proteins	Murakami et al. [53]
Adsorbed layer and gel film on articular cartilage	Murakami et al. [54]
Biphasic and hydration lubrication mechanism	Murakami et al. [55]
Poly(vinyl alcohol) hydrogel	Mamada et al. [56], Murakami et al. [57], Murakami et al. [58], Yarimitsu et al. [59], Sardinha et al. [60]
Tribology of medical devices in contact with soft tissue	Kosukegawa et al. [61]
Polyhydroxyethylmethacrylate (pHEMA) hydrogel	Pitenis et al. [62]
Semi-degradable porous hydrogel	Cao et al. [63]
Composite hydrogel on the UHMWPE surface	Chen et al. [64]
Structural change effects/local dehydration	Kim & Dunn [65]
Articular cartilage hydrophilic surfaces	Mreła & Pawlak [66]
Polyacrylamide Gemini configurations	McGhee et al. [67]
Poly(vinyl alcohol) (PVA) hydrogel with PVA fibers	Sakai et al. [68]
Polyacrylamide hydrogel lubrication	Simič et al. [69]
Dual physically cross-linked hydrogels with double-network	Gan et al. [70]

1.3 BIOTRIBOLOGICAL CHARACTERISTICS OF TEXTURED SURFACES

Owing to the advances in surface preparation/modification/coating techniques, surface texture designs have been employed to take advantage of tribological performance. The surface texturing has prospects of improving the tribological behavior of metal-on-metal hip joint replacements or smooth ultra-high molecular weight polyethylene (UHMWPE) total joint replacements. Micro-textures and diamond-like carbon coatings are prominent surface preparation/modification/coating techniques for biotribological orthopedic implants in order to lower friction and wear.

Biomimetic approaches embracing tribology (friction, wear, and lubrication), mimic the lessons learned from the fascinating biological and tribological features of natural systems [71]. The prospects of application of biomimetic approaches in tribology have been impressive, with closer association between biomimetics and biotribology. The bionic surfaces are in great demand to realize or exceed specific functionalities of creatures in nature with superb tribological designs [72] such as: the anisotropic friction design (e.g. claws of animals), adhesion due to van der Waals forces (e.g. gecko), super hydrophobic surfaces (e.g. lotus leaf), composite structures (e.g. pangolin), lubricious mucus (e.g. fish) and wedge-shaped scales (e.g. sharks). Understanding tribology of biological systems is very crucial to generate bionic surfaces with similar or exceeding tribological behavior. The computer modeling and

TABLE 1.5
Recent Developments in Biotribology of Textured Surfaces in Implants

Textured Surfaces in Implants	Authors
Biotribological fascinating features	Dowson & Neville [71]
Creatures with tribological designs	Liu et al. [72]
	Tang & Zhang [73]
Bio-inspired nanofunctionalized surfaces	Xie [74]
Biocompatibility in the design of soft medical implants	Pitenis & Sawyer [75]
Orthopedic textured biomaterial surfaces	Allen & Raeymaekers [76]

simulations of interface and surface interactions will lay foundation for developments of bio-surface/bio-interface applications [73].

The potential way out to resolve the clinical complications related to biomaterials is provided by nanofunctionalization approaches to fabricate. The biomaterials with bio-inspired nanofunctionalized surfaces imitate not only the physical constructions, but also the chemical compositions in nature, which can be used successfully in the areas of cartilage repair and bone regeneration [74]. The implant biocompatibility should be taken into consideration in the design of roughness and texturing of soft medical implants [75]. The innovative methods to reduce wear to the bearing surfaces are to add a microtexture patterns, coatings, and highly cross-linked polyethylene materials [76]. The microtexture pattern features on orthopedic implant biomaterial surfaces are viable with advances in manufacturing.

The recent developments in biotribology of textured surfaces in implants are presented in Table 1.5.

1.3.1 MICRO-DIMPLE SURFACES

The micro-dimple surfaces have a potential beneficial influence on the reduction of asperity contacts in implants, predominantly under boundary lubrication regimes. The dimples on the metal femoral head fabricated using electrical discharge etching lower the polyethylene wear in hip implants [77]. The primary source of UHMWPE wear/scratch marks is the Co–Cr–Mo alloy particles in sliding interface. A micro-dimpled UHMWPE sliding surfaces inhibits the wear/scratch marks by entrapping the wear particles in dimples [78]. The dimple configurations assist in lowering of polyethylene wear in hip implants by decreasing abrasive wear and enhancing lubricant supply. The dimple surfaces in metal-on-metal hip implants under the mixed elastohydrodynamic lubrication conditions significantly influence the asperity contacts and film thickness [79]. In comparison to plain/dimpled artificial implants, the micro-dimple implant surfaces coated with diamond-like carbon (DLC) under an osteoarthritis-oriented synovial fluid (OASF) lubrication generated lower coefficient of friction and wear [80]. The micro-dimple implant surfaces coated with DLC displayed a lower rate of increasing friction coefficient with increasing load due to the development of graphite transfer film (graphitization) on the coated surfaces. The tribological performance of micro-dimple implant surfaces are significantly

TABLE 1.6
Recent Developments in Biotribology on Micro-Dimpled Surfaces

Micro-Dimpled Surfaces	Authors
Dimples on metal femoral head	Ito et al. [77]
Micro-dimples to reduce UHMWPE wear	Sawano et al. [78]
Dimples in metal-on-metal hip prosthesis	Gao et al. [79]
DLC coated micro-dimples	Ghosh et al. [80]
Micro-dimples in ceramic-on-ceramic hip prosthesis	Roy et al. [81]
DLC coated micro-dimples against ceramic cups	Choudhury et al. [82]
Cr-coated glass disk against micro-dimples on steel ball	Choudhury et al. [83]
Micro-dimples on femoral heads	Choudhury et al. [84]
Micro-dimples on CrCoMo femoral heads in hip joint	Choudhury et al. [85]

influenced by surface wettability and lubricant viscosity. The ceramic-on-ceramic hip prosthesis with micro-dimples of large diameter and high density under bovine serum lubrication exhibited substantial decrease in coefficient of friction and wear [81]. The micro-dimpled DLC coated prosthesis heads against ceramic cups enhanced the tribological behavior of artificial hip joints [82]. The micro-dimpled DLC coating yielded an insignificant change in surface roughness and decreased abrasive third body wear rate against ceramic cups. A substantial reduction in coefficient of friction of the micro-dimpled DLC coated heads against ceramic cups is revealed compared to a micro-dimpled metal (CoCr) heads against ceramic cups. The micro-dimples maintain lubrication resulting in minimization of wear [83]. The DLC promotes scuffing-free surfaces with lower friction coefficient but with minor lubricant film formation (boundary lubrication under the nonconformal contact). The combination of micro-dimples and DLC should be taken into account to maximize tribological performance (reduced friction and wear). The metallic micro-dimpled femoral heads against a metallic cup yielded significantly lower coefficient of friction, while the metallic micro-dimpled femoral heads increased the coefficient of friction against a polyethylene cup [84]. The mechanism of improved film formation in micro-dimpled arrays influenced the friction reduction. The lubricant film thickness in artificial hip joints with micro-dimples on CrCoMo femoral heads is appreciably higher than the contact interface roughness indicating hydrodynamic lubrication [85].

The recent developments in biotribology on micro-dimple surfaces are presented in Table 1.6.

1.3.2 MICRO PATTERN SURFACES

The prosthetic joints surfaces with texture pattern designs mimic the natural articular cartilage which exhibits microtexture surfaces with shallow indentations. The honed surface textures demonstrate lower coefficients of friction in comparison to non-textured surfaces due to enhanced lubricant film thickness and reduced third body abrasive wear [86]. The width, depth, and number of grooves of honed surface textures affect the coefficient of friction and wear rate in metal-on-metal hip joints using a lubricant with viscosity similar to that of pseudo-synovial fluid. The honed surface textures demonstrate lower coefficients of friction during transient walking cycles proving their potential application in metal-on-metal hip joints for improved hip implant longevity [87]. The surface wettability behaviors of laser textured specimens are attained in the range of superhydrophobic to superhydrophilic. The surface wettability behaviors of laser textured Co–Cr–Mo specimens have excellent wear resistance in bovine serum albumin (BSA) solution [88]. The wear of textured surfaces with wettability is lesser than that of the untextured surfaces. The microtexture patterns on the femoral component of a prosthetic knee joint enhances the bearing load and film thickness, thus ensuing decreased friction between the knee bearing surfaces [89]. The microtexture designs on a femoral component also revealed that the friction in a prosthetic knee joint is decreased taking into account of the polyethylene tibial insert deformation.

The texturing design, based on the two-dimensional solution of transient Reynolds equation, can be successfully employed to enhance lubrication effects of UHMWPE surfaces [90]. The coefficient of friction is appreciably influenced by the surface texture (of the harder counterpart) and the transfer film development in sliding of ultra-high molecular weight polyethylene (UHMWPE) pins against steel plates [91]. The textured surfaces deliver lowered coefficient of friction of carbon-fiber-reinforced polyether ether ketone (CFR-PEEK) compared to the plain surfaces, which is apt for the advancement of acetabular cup designs [92]. Surface texture reduces friction and increases load of mechanical seals, as well as brings about the denatured protein accumulations on the sealing surface. The lower (and stable) frictional properties assuring a higher critical load are achieved in the mechanical seals in ventricular devices by surface texture pattern designs followed by DLC coating [93]. The benefits from surface texture pattern designs on sliding wear of lateral contact area of the polyethylene soft surface (tibial insert) in metal-on-UHMWP knee joint is evaluated using mixed elastohydrodynamic lubrication model [94]. The micro-texture patterns are designed based on elastohydrodynamic lubrication model to increase hydrodynamic pressure and lubricant film thickness in a hard-on-soft bearing [95].

The recent developments in biotribology on micro-pattern surfaces are presented in Table 1.7.

TABLE 1.7
Recent Developments in Biotribology on Micro-Pattern Surfaces

Micro Pattern Surfaces	Authors
Honed surface textures in metal-on-metal hip joints	Choudhury et al. [86], Choudhury et al. [87]
Wettability of textured Co–Cr–Mo surfaces	Qin et al. [88]
Micro-textures in deformed polyethylene tibial insert	Qiu et al. [89]
Texture designs on UHMWPE surfaces	Zhang et al. [90]
Texture and roughness effects on UHMWPE surfaces	Menezes & Kailas [91]
Surface textures on CFR-PEEK for acetabular cups	Wyatt et al. [92]
Surface texture designs of seals with DLC coating	Kanda et al. [93]
Texture designs of metal-on-UHMWP knee joint	Gao et al. [94]
Microtexture patterns in a hard-on-soft bearing	Allen & Raeymaekers [95]

1.3.3 Bionic Surfaces

The amazing properties of biological systems in nature are a significant foundation of motivation to advance artificial techniques of textured surfaces that can accommodate lubricant as well as trim down the frictional area of contact. The design of biomimetic textured surface with shark skin, body, and rib morphology provides good frictional performance and lubrication characteristics [96]. The lubrication theory models are established to evaluate the influence of geometric parameters of biomimetic surfaces on tribological behavior. The prospects of bionic design stem from the multi-scale dental anti-wear mechanism produced by the exclusive hierarchical structure, self-repair process, salivary pellicle lubrication and hydration proteins [97]. Bionic texturing improves the nanohardness of the modified surface layer biotribological properties. Bionic texturing on Ti6Al4V alloy reduces the friction coefficient and increases wear resistance of the surface modified layers [98].

The geometrical characteristics of hexagonal textures modeled using "X" shaped cells have a significance impact on the tribological performance. The hexagonal texture density has noteworthy influence in the friction coefficient reduction under full film lubrication regime [99]. The concept of blending diverse bionic features within a sample is based on rigorous examinations of some species that have disclosed microstructure properties of adhesion on surfaces [100]. The blending diverse biomimetic microstructure features, such as micro-shaped (mushroom and wall), are based on the optimized properties of adhesion on surfaces. The optimized surfaces with diverse bionic features achieved enhanced friction and adhesion performance in comparison to those comprised with the non-optimized/same surface features [100]. The high reciprocating velocity piston pair with superior frictional performance is attained with the various parametric arrangements of mimicking fish scale texture [101]. A representative mathematical model of mimicking fish scale texture is formed on the understanding of characteristic function approximation and coordinate transformation. The fish scale texture effects with superior frictional performance on the high reciprocating velocity piston pair are obtained using experimental design and simulations. The microrectangular pocket pad bearing together with fish scale texture design yields significant increase in minimum film thickness and decline in friction coefficient as assessed against the other pad designs [102].

The recent developments in biotribology on bionic surfaces are presented in Table 1.8.

TABLE 1.8
Recent Developments in Biotribology on Bionic Surfaces

Bionic Surfaces	Authors
Biomimetic surface of shark skin, body, and rib morphology	Lu et al. [96]
Bionic design prospects of dental anti-wear performance	Zhou et al. [97]
Bionic texturing for modified surface layers	Wang [98]
Hexagonal textured surfaces	Zhong et al. [99]
Biomimetic adhesive microstructure combinations	Badler & Kasem [100]
Piston model with fish scale texture	Quan et al. [101]
Fish scale texture microrectangular pocket pad design	Atwal and Pandey [102]

1.4 TRIBOLOGICAL CHARACTERISTICS OF IMPLANTS

There is significant attention in decreasing the severe wear through the use of enhanced materials and alternate designs of total replacements joints [103]. The polyethylene wear debris has been related to the tribological process in implants of the metal-on-polymer arrangement. The advancements of in-vitro models are vital to be familiar with the tribological characteristics, substitution, and treatments of cartilage [104]. The graphene-materials (graphene-oxide and reduced graphene-oxide) and graphene-nanocomposites have invited great attention with promising tribological, mechanical and biocompatibility properties [105]. In addition to the implant design and material selection, there are numerous important biotribological parameters that can significantly influence the wear of articulating surfaces with large joint replacements and total disk replacements [106]. The mechanism of tribological phenomena of biomaterials comprising alloys, ceramics and polymers necessarily emphasized in order to fabricate artificial biomaterials to replace the damaged tissues in human body [107]. The biotribological tests of thermally oxidized titanium alloy revealed potential applications in artificial joints with improved friction and wear performance characteristics [108].

The changes in translational (anterior–posterior) and rotational motion (internal–external) limits the tibio-femoral knee joint kinematics and wear behavior of a mobile bearing posterior stabilized knee design [109]. The hip joint models for the dry and lubricated revolute joints are employed for the interaction of kinematic and dynamic response of femur head inside the hip bone or acetabulum [110]. The intrajoint force peaks observed with the dry hip model are related to the multiple impacts of the femur head and the cup. The hip joint system's response has a tendency to be smoother in the presence of the lubricant, due to the synovial fluid damping mechanism.

Surface roughness of knee prostheses has been proposed as the mechanism for premature tribological prosthesis failure in total knee joint replacement performance. The roughness of tibial ultra-high molecular weight polyethylene of retrieved knee implants is characterized to assess the tribological failure in knee joint replacements [111]. The roughness dissimilarities are quantified between medial and lateral condyles taking into consideration the load experience differences of the two condyles. The biotribological performance of the hip implants recovered from patients after implantation is assessed by metal transfer characterization on the ceramic femoral head bearing surfaces [112]. The reactivity at the surface structure of the metal interface in artificial hip joints is improved by surface interaction due to friction. The formation of the tribofilms developed by surface interactions can be categorized by various arrangements of organic layers and oxide films [113]. The formation of surface reaction tribolayer establishes a way to minimize wear of CoCrMo for metal-on-metal hip implants.

The recent developments in biotribology of orthopedic implants are presented in Table 1.9.

TABLE 1.9
Recent Developments in Biotribology of Orthopedic Implants

Orthopedic Implants	Authors
Metal-on-polymer wear in joints	Dowson [103]
Articular cartilage biotribology	Katta et al. [104]
Graphene-materials and graphene-nanocomposites	Dong & Qi [105]
Biological articulating surfaces wear	Harper et al. [106]
Biomaterials of alloys, ceramics, and polymers	E et al. [107]
Wear resistance of titanium alloy by thermal oxidation	Luo et al. [108]
Mobile bearing posterior stabilized knee design	Grupp et al. [109]
Femur head interaction inside the hip bone	Costa et al. [110]
Roughness characterization of retrieved knee implants	Ruggiero et al. [111]
Metal transfer characterization on ceramic femoral heads	Affatato [112]
Metal-on-metal hip joint in-vitro and in-vivo studies	Espallargas et al. [113]

1.4.1 Coatings

The tribological behaviors of the bioceramics are enhanced against ultra-high molecular weight polyethylene (UHMWPE) in human plasma lubrication [114]. The lower wear rate of UHMWPE in human plasma lubrication is due to the protein deposited on the surfaces. The bioceramic compositions of sintered HA/yttria-partially-stabilized zirconia composite against UHMWPE in human plasma lubrication yield an optimum minimum friction coefficient and wear rate and maximum hardness. Bioceramic coatings are utilized to enhance the wear, mechanical and biological characteristics of bone implants [115]. The benefits of HAp-TiO2 compact coatings, with less amorphous phase contributes to lower wear rates and higher friction coefficients for better implant fixation, and thus ensures the integrity of the bioceramic coating. A wear-resistant formulation of silicon nitride and silicon carbon nitride coatings for hard-bearing implants surfaces can potentially extend the implant lifetime [116]. The wear resistance of silicon nitride coatings is similar to that of bulk silicon nitride (hardness of silicon nitride coatings is similar to that of sintered silicon nitride) and significantly higher than that of cobalt chromium (elastic modulus of silicon nitride coatings is similar to that of cobalt chromium). The multilayer surface zirconium nitride coating with carbon-fiber-reinforced poly-ether-ether-ketone (CFR-PEEK) is used to enhance the wear performance of knee joint system [117]. The biotribological performance of CFR-PEEK/ZrN multilayer surface coating in a knee joint system yielded low wear and negligible surface fatigue. The DLC is a potential material to improve wear resistance characteristics in orthopedic implant treatments. The hydrogenated amorphous carbon (a-C:H) has moderate elastic modulus and high hardness with relatively high hardness/elasticity ratio which enables the film to conform well with the substrate [118]. The a-C:H coated pin against counterface (a-C:H coated) showed low coefficient of friction due to the transfer film formation which is attributed to degree of graphitization with increasing applied load. The a-C:H coated surface also displays hydrophilic features for protein absorption. Significantly low friction coefficient and good wear resistance (good adhesion between the substrate and coating) of the coated layer against the alumina counterface is observed [118]. The DLC-layered coatings with improved surface/material properties (ratio of hardness vs elasticity) and absorbed protein portrayed a very important role in the tribological characteristics appropriate for orthopedics implants [119]. The layered coatings acquired columnar and very fine-grained microstructures with micro-cracks of very low inter-columnar density. The DLC (a-C:H) layers are noticed to produce outstanding tribological characteristics at "DLC on Polyethylene/ DLC" sliding pairs under hip joint simulated circumstances. The DLC coatings with interlayers (Zr and ZrN (Zr:ZrN) sublayers, Zr and DLC (Zr:DLC) and N-doped DLC layer) on titanium alloy (Ti-6Al-4V) are employed for advancing the biotribological functioning of orthopedic implants [120]. The Zr:ZrN layer is intended for augmenting load capacity and corrosion resistance; the Zr:DLC layer is aimed for gradual stress transition and enhancing layer adhesion thus reducing DLC delamination from the substrates; and the N-doped DLC layer is for reducing friction and wear. The hydroxyapatite (Fe-HA) in tooth enamel is comprised of iron and thus displays good hardness and high wear resistance [121]. The Fe-HA ceramics exhibited better wear resistance when compared with the pure HA ceramics. The iron content has a considerable effect on the crystal structure and morphology of Fe-HA powders. Titanium alloys are extensively used in the clinical purpose of artificial joints, and their wear resistance is improved with the deposition of DLC film on titanium alloy surface. The wear mechanisms of DLC films on Ti6Al4V alloy surface involved fatigue, abrasive, and adhesive wear [122]. The chitosan coating surface under several sliding speeds displayed lower friction coefficient in comparison with the uncoated surface [123]. The culturing of coated super hydrophilic surface with osteoblast cells favored adhesion and good proliferation of cells. The multi-walled carbon nanotubes (MWCNTs) generated microstructural amendments in plasma electrolytic oxidation coating yielded low friction and reduced wear damage [124]. The MWCNTs' enhanced coating tailors surface properties such as dense barrier layer and irregular porosities and reinforcement that reduce the coefficient of friction and wear in comparison to a MWCNT-free coating.

The recent developments in biotribology on implant coatings are presented in Table 1.10.

1.4.2 Surfaces

Metal-on-metal (MOM) hip joint bearings have established low wear rates, nevertheless, wear of MOM joints is apprehensive due to the biological reaction and toxicity of wear debris. The DLC and PVD coatings guards the femoral heads lowering wear in comparison to the MOM femoral heads [125]. The stem–cement interface debonding arises certainly for all stem designs under physiological loading. The wear debris produced at the stem–cement interface reveals an increasing importance in the mechanical failure of cemented total hip replacements [126]. The friction coefficient is dependent on the surface finish, with a low value obtained for the polished contacting surfaces. The proteins from the calf serum are found to

TABLE 1.10
Recent Developments in Biotribology on Implant Coatings

Implant Coatings	Authors
Hydroxyapatite (HA) nanoparticles synthesis	Wang et al. [114]
Compact coatings integrity with less amorphous phase	Melero et al. [115]
Silicon nitride and silicon carbon nitride coatings for hard bearing implants surfaces	Pettersson et al. [116]
Zirconium nitride multilayer surface coating with carbon-fiber-reinforced poly-ether-ether-ketone	Grupp et al. [117]
Hydrogenated amorphous carbon (a-C:H) on alumina	Hee et al. [118]
Diamond-like carbon coatings (DLC) on orthopedic implants	Choudhury et al. [119]
DLC coatings with interlayers of zirconium on titanium alloy	Choudhury et al. [120]
Influence of iron on wear resistance of nano-hydroxyapatite	Han et al. [121]
Deposition of DLC film on Ti6Al4V alloy surface	Xu et al. [122]
Layer-by-layer deposition on CoCrMo alloy with grafting	Qin et al. [123]
Coating structure with tailoring surface properties using multi-walled carbon nanotubes (MWCNTs)	Daavari et al. [124]

adsorb onto both the bone cement surfaces and femoral stem. The wear at the stem–cement interface may be improved by tailoring physicochemical properties of the femoral components to promote protein adsorption. The effect of bovine calf serum (BCS) and human synovial fluid (HSF) fluid compositions are assessed for friction and wear of cobalt chromium molybdenum (CoCrMo) materials. The cobalt chromium molybdenum (CoCrMo) material pairs recorded higher wear for the HSF samples compared to BCS fluid compositions [127]. The wear scar size on the CoCrMo material is dependent on protein content which reduced appreciably for higher BCS concentration. The protein deposits are adherent which established the significance of proteins in determination of CoCrMo wear [127]. The anterior–posterior translation and internal–external rotation influences the wear of knee implants. The two wear models, contact pressure independent and dependent models, are employed in conjunction with finite element numerical model for wear prediction. The contact pressure independent model shows decreased wear during forward movement of the tibial insert in flexion, while the contact pressure dependent model shows increased wear [128]. The results predicted by the contact pressure dependent model are consistent with those of reported experimental wear trends. The precise quantification of bearing material deficiency from MOM retrieved hip replacement implants is fundamental to identifying their failure. The geometrical methods are the viable approaches to assess volumetric wear (material loss) from the retrieved bearing hip implants [129]. The key concern influencing joint prosthesis is wear, bringing about loosening and implant failure. The joint load distributions have presented important understanding that the knee loading configurations, exhibiting different contact joint loads in medial and lateral condyles [130]. The surface roughness is not appreciably dissimilar relating medial and lateral sides, nevertheless, surface damage is higher in the lateral condyles than in the medial condyles. The implant surface roughness affects the early wear and metal transfer surface area. Based on the roughness factors taken into account on the articular surface, the metal transfer regions were rougher than the

TABLE 1.11
Recent Developments in Biotribology on Implant Surfaces

Implant surfaces	Authors
Hip prostheses with thin hard coated metallic heads	Ortega-Saenz et al. [125]
Biotribological stem–cement interface properties	Zhang et al. [126]
Hip implants under reciprocating sliding conditions	Stevenson et al. [127]
Anterior–posterior translation and internal–external rotation influence on the knee implants wear	Zhang et al. [128]
Volumetric wear estimation from hip implant bearing	Bergiers [129]
Implant surface roughness influences the metal transfer surface area and premature wear	Affatato et al. [130], Affatato [112]
Total knee arthroplasty medial and lateral wear	Affatato et al. [131]
Ceramic-on-ceramic hip implant	de Villiers & Collins [132]

non-metal transfer regions [112]. The material properties, surface topography, and prosthetic components movements impact the wear mechanisms, steady damage patterns, and implant failures in total knee arthroplasty. The increasing femoral component's surface roughness of total knee prostheses may be a contributing factor to accelerated scratches (wear) observed in the anterior/posterior (AP) direction of all the femoral components and ultimately prosthesis failure [131].

The ceramic-on-ceramic hip implant of the zirconia toughened alumina ceramics is an appropriate replacement material with biocompatibility and low wear. The ceramic-on-ceramic hip implant presents a bone preserving treatment without the metal ion related issues linked with MOM devices [132].

The recent developments in biotribology on implant surfaces are presented in Table 1.11.

1.4.3 Composites

The wear and lubrication of artificial joints are vital concerns for their endurance, durability, and long life. The failure of tibial bearings generally made from ultra-high molecular weight polyethylene (UHMWPE) is due to subsurface fatigue crack commencement and propagation. The fatigue cracks originated in the embrittled oxidized layer in UHMWPE specimens is an unfavorable consequence from sterilization of the tibial bearings [133]. The number of cycles required for fatigue cracks commencement is dependent on the intensity of oxidation and on the contact stress. The implant loosening and ensuing failure leads to vital parameters in the biological response (osteolysis) to the wear debris as shape, size, and number of particles. The clinical hip replacement studies with highly cross-linked polyethylene (XLPE) cups have shown greatly reduced wear (and XLPE wear debris particles) compared with conventional polyethylene (PE) [134]. The reduced wear rate of XLPE should reduce the osteolytic potential, but the reduced debris size may have the possibility to build up the biological activity. The decreased debris size due to cross-linking of UHMWPE can result in greater osteolysis with appropriately large number of generated particles. The capability to provide improved evaluation in-vivo requires an increased understanding of the osteolysis and associated biological processes [134].

The lowest wear rate and friction coefficient of UHMWPE are achieved under human plasma lubrication [135]. The wear mechanism of UHMWPE under (i) dry friction is plastic deformation and adhesive wear, (ii) water lubrication is fatigue fracture wear and severe plowing, and (iii) human plasma lubrication is plastic deformation and fine plowing. The protein serum deposition occurred on worn surface of UHMWPE as the nitrogen content in worn surface areas is much higher than that in unworn surface areas. The main reason for failure of total joint replacements in the long period is the wear of ultra-high molecular weight polyethylene (UHMWPE). The addition of bovine bone hydroxyapatite (BHA) to the UHMWPE composites increases the biocompatibility and wear resistance vital for high quality artificial joints. The BHA/UHMWPE composites under human plasma lubrication conditions reduced the friction coefficient and wear rate, and enhanced the hardness and modulus of elasticity [136]. The ultra-high molecular weight polyethylene (UHMWPE) substrate is treated to augment the adhesion of the hydrogen-containing carbon (HCC) coating [137]. The HCC coating has enhanced wear resistance as a sizable amount of HCC coating remained with the deposited substrate as compared with the polished substrate. The total joint replacements encompass formulation between a metal/alloy and UHMWPE in orthopedic applications. The addition of micro-sized zirconium particles in compression molded ultra-high molecular weight polyethylene (UHMWPE) composites have shown outstanding biocompatibility and substantial reduction in wear compared to conventional UHMWPE [138]. The cross-linking decreases the wear rate of UHMWPE, but brings about reduction in impact toughness. The ultra-high molecular weight polyethylene (UHMWPE) biomaterial is employed as the acetabular cup in artificial hip joints. The main cause of long-term failure of hip joints is the wear debris generation of UHMWPE in human body after their replacements which have demonstrated to induce osteolysis and implant loosening. The natural coral (NC) particles addition in UHMWPE resulted in the enhancement of micro-hardness and scratch resistance of the NC/UHMWPE composites [139]. The NC/UHMWPE composites wear resistance increased with the increasing contents of NC particles. The NC/UHMWPE composites wear mechanism is mainly due to adhesive wear and the NC constituents in UHMWPE altered the adhesive wear severity. The bovine bone hydroxyapatite (BHA) filler is a suitable component to enhance the wear resistance of BHA/UHMWPE composites for biotribological applications [140].

The BHA/UHMWPE composites acetabular cups (obtained by hot pressing formation method) against CoCrMo alloy femoral heads under bovine synovial lubrication can increase the hardness and decrease the wear rates. The principal wear mechanisms for UHMWPE and its composites are adhesive wear, fatigue, and plowing. The major long-term failure identified for metal-on-UHMWPE is implant loosening due to wear generation. The wear progression is simulated taking into consideration Archard's wear model with the finite element simulation of femoral head and acetabular cup [141]. The bearing surface generated under the influence of wear would be beneficial to the hip implant replacement by enhancing the lubricant film and reducing wear. The ultra-high molecular weight polyethylene (UHMWPE) cross-linking without stabilization has potential for the use in biomedical applications with increased bearing wear resistance, yet reduce degradation in stiffness and oxidation resistance [142]. The UHMWPE cross-linking without stabilization revealed a substantial increase in wear resistance yielding a reasonable drop in elastic modulus thus retaining a sizable share of the crystalline polymer original stiffness. The cross-linking followed by thermal stabilization substantially decreased the elastic modulus of UHMWPE, while the thermal stabilization decreased crystallinity more than that obtained without stabilization. The lamellae (crystalline) play an important role in the wear mechanisms and deformation of ultra-high molecular weight polyethylene (UHMWPE) in artificial knee joints [143]. The lamellae (crystalline) under tribologically loaded conditions assemble similar to the alignment of collagen fibrils in natural cartilage. The proposed tribologically loaded UHMWPE model reflects the different depth zones deformations. The stresses which are most influential in modifying the microstructure and are therefore most detrimental to generate wear particles are close by the surfaces subjected to the application of collective large normal loads with high relative velocity. The MWCNT/UHMWPE nanocomposites signify an alluring substitute for the conventional UHMWPE used as bearing surfaces in joint prostheses. The addition of multi-walled carbon nanotubes (MWCNTs) to conventional ultra-high molecular weight polyethylene (UHMWPE) led to a substantial decrease in wear rate in orthopedic applications [144]. The biocompatibility of wear particles from the MWCNT/UHMWPE nanocomposites have been related to decreased implant loosening and osteolysis in comparison to those generated from the conventional UHMWPE. The third-body particle effect on artificially aged vitamin E stabilized polyethylene is a constant wear behavior with effectiveness in oxidation prevention under prolonged artificial aging [109]. The highly cross-linked polyethylene (remelted) has a higher oxidation resistance, whereas standard polyethylene shows oxidative degradation and subsequently increased wear. The highly cross-linked (HXL) UHMWPE blended with vitamin E has superior wear characteristics than that of highly cross-linked (HXL)/conventional UHMWPE (acetabular cups) counterfaced with CoCrMo alloy (femoral head) [145]. The tribological testing of the (i) highly cross-linked (HXL) UHMWPE blended with vitamin E produces surface layer abrasion, (ii) highly cross-linked (HXL) UHMWPE produces surface layer abrasion and flaking facture, and (iii) conventional UHMWPE produces accumulated plastic flow and yielding. The highly cross-linked (HXL) UHMWPE blended with vitamin E can prevent oxidative degradation along with decreasing the surface layer flaking facture occurrence. The Ti6Al4V material comprises an alternate selection to the metal-polymers for total hip arthroplasty (THA) due to high load capacity and good biocompatibility. The Ti6Al4V material contact surfaces display superior levels of preservation and bone transfer by adhesion. The Ti6Al4V material with hydroxyapatite (HAp) and tricalcium phosphate (TCP) is used as metal prostheses coatings owing to the stability of the implants [146]. The biocomposite implant design based on polished surfaces of Ti6Al4V material with hydroxyapatite (HAp) and tricalcium phosphate (TCP) leads to an enhanced primary implant stability. The secondary stability is enhanced due to the adhesion between bone and biocomposite implant, increasing on the whole implant stability [146]. Friction in polyethylene/metal contact pair is significantly affected by protein concentration and sliding speed. The protein content and sliding conditions of polyethylene/metal (UHMWPE/CoCrMo) contact pair have a certain effect on both the structure of the adsorbed molecules and adsorbed film formation and hence

Recent Developments in Biotribology

affect the friction coefficient [147]. The proteins undergo significant changes in their initial structure complemented by the development of protein film with an increase of friction coefficient. The retrieved UHMWPE tibial implants lead to a key role of third body layer in tribological analysis [148]. The formation of a third body layer composed of a synovial fluid (a Gel-IN calf serum and a calf serum) and UHMWPE wear particles mixture in the implant leads to good tribological performance with a lower wear rate. The Gel-IN calf serum yielded the formation of a third body layer on the UHMWPE surface owing to protein and lipid adsorption which led a lower friction factor [148]. However, the calf serum is unable to attach to the UHMWPE surface which led to a high friction factor. Polyether ether ketone (PEEK) is utilized in arthroplasty along with its composites due of their superior nature. The tribological characteristics of tibia and femur prosthesis contact mode simulation of PEEK against the CoCrMo alloy in torsion under calf serum solution are as follows [149]: (i) the coefficient of friction decreases with increasing torsional angle, and (ii) the wear depth is extended, the wear width is expanded, and wear scars are stretched with an increasing normal load. The PEEK wear mechanism in the central region is plastic deformation, while in the marginal region is mostly due to fatigue and abrasive wear. The ceramic-on-UHMWPE hip replacement implant design enhancement is carried out based on the wear maps displaying the progress of the structure and position of the wear damage [150].

The recent developments in biotribology on implant composites are presented in Table 1.12.

TABLE 1.12
Recent Developments in Biotribology on Implant Composites

Implant composites	Authors
Surface pitting and fatigue cracks in UHMWPE	Kennedy et al. [133]
XLPE implant wear and particles debris	Williams et al. [134]
Tribological behavior of femoral bone against UHMWPE	Wang et al. [135]
BHA filled UHMWPE composites	Liu et al. [136]
HCC coating adhesion enhancement to UHMWPE	Takeichi et al. [137]
Zirconium reinforcement filler particles into UHMWPE	Plumlee et al. [138]
NC reinforcement filler particles into UHMWPE	Ge et al. [139]
BHA/UHMWPE acetabular cups with CoCrMo femoral heads	Wang et al. [140]
Wear simulation prediction of hip joint replacement	Harun et al. [141]
UHMWPE with increased bearing wear resistance	Schwartz & Bahadur [142]
Modeling deformation zones in the UHMWPE sample	Galetz & Glatzel [143]
Tribological behavior of nanocomposite MWCNT/UHMWPE	Suñer et al. [144]
Tribological behavior of artificially aged vitamin E stabilized polyethylene	Grupp et al. [109]
Tribological properties of HXL-UHMWPE/CoCrMo pair	Chen et al. [145]
Tribological properties of metal matrix bioactive composite	Dantas et al. [146]
Adsorbed protein film effect on UHMWPE/ CoCrMo pair	Nečas et al. [147]
Tribological analysis of layered medial knee implants	Sava et al. [148]
Tibia and femur prosthesis contact mode simulation	Liu et al. [149]
Ceramic-on-UHMWPE hip replacements wear map	Mattei et al. [150]

1.5 CONCLUSIONS AND FURTHER OUTLOOK

This chapter highlights the significance of biotribology in biological systems. This chapter reviews developments based on the recent literature on lubrication characteristics of artificial joints, biotribological characteristics of textured surfaces, and tribological characteristics of implants. The significant progresses in biotribology on lubrication enhancement, friction, and wear reduction are elaborated. Further outlooks will be toward enhancement in quality of life with developments in biotribology.

REFERENCES

1. Zhou Z.R., Jin Z.M. 2015. Biotribology: recent progresses and future perspectives, *Biosurface and Biotribology*, 1(1), 3–24.
2. Smyth P.A., Green I. 2018. Storage and loss characteristics of coupled poroviscoelastic and hydrodynamic systems for biomimetic applications, *The Journal of Tribology*, 140(4), 041703.
3. Jin Z.M. 2006. Theoretical studies of elastohydrodynamic lubrication of artificial hip joints. *Proceedings of the IMechE Journal of Engineering Tribology*, 220, 719–727.
4. Klein J. 2006. Molecular mechanisms of synovial joint lubrication, *Proceedings of the Institution of Mechanical Engineers, Part J: Journal of Engineering Tribology*, 220(8), 691–710.
5. Ateshian G.A. 2009. The role of interstitial fluid pressurization in articular cartilage lubrication, *Journal of Biomechanics*, 42(9), 1163–1176.
6. Crockett R. 2009. Boundary lubrication in natural articular joints. *Tribology Letters*, 35, 77–84.
7. Mattei L., DiPuccio F., Piccigallo B., Ciulli E. 2011. Lubrication and wear modelling of artificial hip joints: A review, *Tribology International*, 44, 532–549.
8. Murakami T., Yarimitsu S., Nakashima K., et al. 2013. Influence of synovia constituents on tribological behaviors of articular cartilage. *Friction*, 1, 150–162.
9. Kennedy F.E., Wongseedakaew K., McHugh D.J., Currier J.H. 2013. Tribological conditions in mobile bearing total knee prostheses, *Tribology International* 63, 78–88.
10. Myant C., Cann P. 2014. On the matter of synovial fluid lubrication: implications for metal-on-metal hip tribology, *Journal of the Mechanical Behavior of Biomedical Materials* 34, 338–348.
11. Liming S., Shihao L., Naohiko S. 2020. Systematic review of computational modelling for biomechanics analysis of total knee replacement, *Biosurface and Biotribology*, 6(1), 3–11.
12. Sinha P., Singh C., Prasad K.R. 1982. Lubrication of human joints – a microcontinuum approach, *Wear* 80, 159–181.
13. Bujurke N.M., Kudenatti R.B. 2006. An analysis of rough poroealstic bearings with reference to lubrication mechanism of synovial joints, *Applied Mathematics and Computation*, 178, 309–320.
14. Mabuchi K., Ujihira M., Sasada T. 1998. Relationship between the conformity and the lubricating ability of synovial joints, *Clinical Biomechanics*, 13(4–5), 250–255.
15. Jin Z.M., Dowson D. 2005. Elastohydrodynamic lubrication in biological systems, *Proceedings of the Institution of Mechanical Engineers, Part J: Journal of Engineering Tribology*, 219(5), 367–380.

16. Ateshian G.A., Hung C.T. 2006. The natural synovial joint: Properties of cartilage, *Proceedings of the Institution of Mechanical Engineers, Part J: Journal of Engineering Tribology*, 220(8), 657–670.
17. Pascau A., Guardia B., Puertolas J.A., Gómez-Barrena E. 2009. Knee model of hydrodynamic lubrication during the gait cycle and the influence of prosthetic joint conformity, *Journal of Orthopaedic Science*, 14, 68–75.
18. Mongkolwongrojn M., Wongseedakaew K., Kennedy F.E. 2010. Transient elastohydrodynamic lubrication artificial knee joint with non-Newtonian fluids, *Tribology International*, 43, 1017–1026.
19. Ruggiero A., Gòmez E., D'Amato R. 2011. Approximate Analytical Model for the Squeeze-Film Lubrication of the Human Ankle Joint with Synovial Fluid Filtrated by Articular Cartilage, *Tribology Letters*, 41, 337–343.
20. Ruggiero A., Gòmez E., D'Amato R. 2013. Approximate closed form solution of the synovial fluid film force in the human anke joint with non-Newtonian lubricant, *Tribology International*, 57, 156–161.
21. Li J., Stewart T.D., Jin Z., Wilcox R.K., Fishera J. 2013. The influence of size, clearance, cartilage properties, thickness and hemiarthroplasty on the contact mechanics of the hip joint with biphasic layers, *The Journal of Biomechanics*, 46(10), 1641–1647.
22. Tanaka K., Uchijima D., Hasegawa K., Katori T., Sakai R., Mabuchi K. 2013. Limitation of the lubricating ability of total hip prostheses with hard on hard sliding material, *Tribology*, 8(5), 272–277.
23. Abdullah E.Y., Edan N.M., Kadhim A.N. 2017. Study Surface Roughness and Friction of Synovial Human Knee Joint with Using Mathematical Model, Special Issue: 1st Scientific International Conference, College of Science, Al-Nahrain University, November, 21–22, Part I, pp. 109–118.
24. Rao T.V.V.L.N., Rani A.M.A., Manivasagam G. 2019. Squeeze film bearing characteristics for synovial joint applications. In: Bains P., Sidhu S., Bahraminasab M., Prakash C. (eds) *Biomaterials in Orthopaedics and Bone Regeneration. Materials Horizons: From Nature to Nanomaterials*. Springer, Singapore.
25. Boedo S., Coots S.A. 2017. Wear chacteristics of conventional and squeeze-film artificial hip joints, *Journal of Tribology*, 139, 031603.
26. Burris D.L., Moore A.C. 2017. Cartilage and joint lubrication: new insights into the role of hydrodynamics, *Biotribology*, 12, 8–14.
27. Horibata S., Yarimitsu S., Fujie H. 2018. Influence of synovial fluid pressure on biphasic lubrication property in articular cartilage, *Tribology*, 13(3), 172–177.
28. Horibata S., Yarimitsu S., Fujie H. 2019. Effect of synovial fluid pressurization on the biphasic lubrication property of articular cartilage, *Biotribology*, 19, 100098.
29. Ruggiero A., Sicilia A., Affatato S. 2020. In silico total hip replacement wear testing in the framework of ISO 14242-3 accounting for mixed elasto-hydrodynamic lubrication effects, *Wear*, 460–461, 203420.
30. Ruggiero A., Sicilia A. Lubrication modeling and wear calculation in artificial hip joint during the gait, *Tribology International* 142, 2020, 105993.
31. Ateshian G.A., Wang H., Lai W.M. 1998. The role of interstitial fluid pressurization and surface porosities on the boundary friction of articular cartilage, *Journal of Tribology*, 120(2), 241–248.
32. Nakashima K., Sawae Y., Murakami T. 2007. Effect of conformational changes and differences of proteins on frictional properties of poly(vinyl alcohol) hydrogel, *Tribology International*, 40(10–12), 1423–1427.

33. Yarimitsu S., Nakashima K., Sawae Y., Murakami T. 2009. Influences of lubricant composition on forming boundary film composed of synovia constituents, *Tribology International*, 42(11–12), 1615–1623.
34. Pawlak Z., Figaszewski Z.A., Gadomski A., Urbaniak W., Oloyede A. 2010. The ultra-low friction of the articular surface is pH-dependent and is built on a hydrophobic underlay including a hypothesis on joint lubrication mechanism, *Tribology International*, 43, 1719–1725.
35. Pawlak Z., Yusuf K.Q., Pai R., Urbaniak W. 2017. Repulsive surfaces and lamellar lubrication of synovial joints, *Archives of Biochemistry and Biophysics*, 623–624, 42–48.
36. Sawano H., Warisawa S.I., Ishihara S. 2010. Study on wear reduction mechanism of artificial joints grafted with hydrophilic polymer membranes, *Wear* 268, 233–240.
37. Meng Q., Gao L., Liu F., Yang P., Fisher J., Jin Z. 2010. Contact mechanics and elastohydrodynamic lubrication in a novel metal-on-metal hip implant with an aspherical bearing surface, *Journal of Biomechanics*, 43, 849–857.
38. Vrbka M., Návrat T., Křupka I., Hartl M., Šperka P., Gallo J. 2013. Study of film formation in bovine serum lubricated contacts under rolling/sliding conditions, *Proceedings of the Institution of Mechanical Engineers, Part J: Journal of Engineering Tribology*, 227(5), 459–475.
39. Parkes M., Myant C., Cann P.M., Wong J.S.S. 2015. Synovial fluid lubrication: the effect of protein interactions on adsorbed and lubricating films, *Biotribology*, 1–2, 51–60.
40. Boettcher K., Winkeljann B., Schmidt T.A., Lieleg O. 2017. Quantification of cartilage wear morphologies in unidirectional sliding experiments: Influence of different macromolecular lubricants, *Biotribology*, 12, 43–51.
41. Murakami T., Yarimitsu S., Sakai N., Nakashima K., Yamaguchi T., Sawae Y. 2017. Importance of adaptive multimode lubrication mechanism in natural synovial joints, *Tribology International*, 113, 306–315.
42. Nečas D., Vrbka M., Křupka I., Hartl M., Galandáková A. 2016. Lubrication within hip replacements – Implication for ceramic-on-hard bearing couples, *Journal of the Mechanical Behavior of Biomedical Materials*, 61, 371–383.
43. Nečas D., Vrbka M., Galandáková A., Křupka I., Hartl M. 2019. On the observation of lubrication mechanisms within hip joint replacements. Part I: Hard-on-soft bearing pairs, *Journal of the Mechanical Behavior of Biomedical Materials*, 89, 237–248.
44. Nečas D., Sadecká K., Vrbka M., Gall J., Galandáková A., Křupka A., Hartl M. 2019. Observation of lubrication mechanisms in knee replacement: a pilot study, *Biotribology*, 17, 1–7.
45. Taufiqurrakhman M., Bryant M.G., Neville A. 2019. Tribofilms on CoCrMo alloys: Understanding the role of the lubricant, *Biotribology*, 19, 100104.
46. Stevenson H., Jaggard M., Akhbari P., Vaghela U., Gupte C., Cann P. 2019. The role of denatured synovial fluid proteins in the lubrication of artificial joints, *Biotribology*, 17, 49–63.
47. Wang Z., Li J., Ge X., Liu Y., Luo J., Chetwynd D., Mao K. 2019. Investigation of the lubrication properties and synergistic interaction of biocompatible liposome-polymer complexes applicable to artificial joints, *Colloids and Surfaces B: Biointerfaces*, 178, 469–478.
48. Shinmori H., Kubota M., Morita T., Yamaguchi T., Sawae Y. 2020. Effects of synovial fluid constituents on friction between UHMWPE and CoCrMo, *Tribology*, 15(4), 283–292.

49. Cao Y., Kampf N., Kosinska M.K., Steinmeyer J., Klein J. 2021. Interactions between bilayers of phospholipids extracted from human osteoarthritic synovial fluid, *Biotribology*, 25, 100157.
50. Freeman M.E., Furey M.J., Love B.J., Hampton J.M. 2000. Friction, wear, and lubrication of hydrogels as synthetic articular cartilage, *Wear*, 241(2), 129–135.
51. Dunn A.C., Cobb J.A., Kantzios A.N., et al. 2008. Friction coefficient measurement of hydrogel materials on living epithelial cells. *Tribology Letters*, 30, 13.
52. Bavaresco V.P., Zavaglia C.A.C., Reis M.C., Gomes J.R. 2008. Study on the tribological properties of pHEMA hydrogels for use in artificial articular cartilage, *Wear*, 265(3–4), 269–277.
53. Murakami T., Sawae Y., Nakashima K., Yarimitsu S., Sato T. 2007. Micro- and nanoscopic biotribological behaviours in natural synovial joints and artificial joints, *Proceedings of the Institution of Mechanical Engineers, Part J: Journal of Engineering Tribology*, 221(3), 237–245.
54. Murakami T., Nakashima K., Sawae Y., Sakai N., Hosoda N. 2009. Roles of adsorbed film and gel layer in hydration lubrication for articular cartilage, *Proceedings of the Institution of Mechanical Engineers, Part J: Journal of Engineering Tribology*, 223(3), 287–295.
55. Murakami T., Nakashima K., Yarimitsu S., Sawae Y., Sakai N. 2011. Effectiveness of adsorbed film and gel layer in hydration lubrication as adaptive multimode lubrication mechanism for articular cartilage, *Proceedings of the Institution of Mechanical Engineers, Part J: Journal of Engineering Tribology*, 225(12), 1174–1185.
56. Mamada K., Fridrici V., Kosukegawa H., et al. 2011. Friction properties of poly(vinyl alcohol) hydrogel: effects of degree of polymerization and saponification value. *Tribol Lett* 42, 241–251.
57. Murakami T., Yarimitsu S., Nakashima K., Yamaguchi T., Sawae Y., Sakai N., Suzuki A. 2014. Superior lubricity in articular cartilage and artificial hydrogel cartilage, *Proceedings of the Institution of Mechanical Engineers, Part J: Journal of Engineering Tribology*, 228(10), 1099–1111.
58. Murakami T., Yarimitsu S., Sakai N., Nakashima K., Yamaguchi T., Sawae Y., Suzuki A. 2017. Superior lubrication mechanism in poly(vinyl alcohol) hybrid gel as artificial cartilage, *Proceedings of the Institution of Mechanical Engineers, Part J: Journal of Engineering Tribology*, 231(9), 1160–1170.
59. Yarimitsu S., Sasaki S., Murakami T., Suzuki A. 2016. Evaluation of lubrication properties of hydrogel artificial cartilage materials for joint prosthesis, *Biosurface and Biotribology*, 2(1), 40–47.
60. Sardinha V.M., Lima L.L., Belangero W.D., Zavaglia C.A., Bavaresco V.P., Gomes J.R. 2013. Tribological characterization of polyvinyl alcohol hydrogel as substitute of articular cartilage, *Wear*, 301(1–2), 218–225.
61. Kosukegawa, H., Fridrici, V., Kapsa, P. et al. 2013. Friction properties of medical metallic alloys on soft tissue–mimicking poly(vinyl alcohol) hydrogel biomodel. *Tribology Letters*, 51, 311–321.
62. Pitenis A.A., Urueña J.M., Nixon R.M., Bhattacharjee T., Krick B.A., Dunn A.C., Angelini T.E., Sawyer W.G. 2016. Lubricity from entangled polymer networks on hydrogels, *The Journal of Tribology*, 138(4), 042102.
63. Cao Y., Xiong D., Wang K., Niu Y. 2017. Semi-degradable porous poly (vinyl alcohol) hydrogel scaffold for cartilage repair: Evaluation of the initial and cell-cultured tribological properties, *The Journal of the Mechanical Behavior of Biomedical Materials*, 68, 163–172.

64. Chen K., Yang X., Zhang D., Xu L., Zhang X., Wang Q. 2017. Biotribology behavior and fluid load support of PVA/HA composite hydrogel as artificial cartilage, *Wear*, 376–377(Part A), 329–336.
65. Kim J., Dunn A.C. 2018. Thixotropic mechanics in soft hydrated sliding interfaces. *Tribology Letters*, 66, 102.
66. Mreła A., Pawlak Z. 2019. Articular cartilage. Strong adsorption and cohesion of phospholipids with the quaternary ammonium cations providing satisfactory lubrication of natural joints, *Biosystems*, 176, 27–31.
67. McGhee E.O., Urueña J.M., Pitenis A.A., et al. 2019. Temperature-dependent friction of gemini hydrogels. *Tribology Letters*, 67,117.
68. Sakai N., Yarimitsu S., Sawae Y., Komori M., Murakami T. 2019. Biomimetic artificial cartilage: fibre-reinforcement of PVA hydrogel to promote biphasic lubrication mechanism, *Biosurface and Biotribology*, 5(1), 13–19.
69. Simič R., Yetkin M., Zhang K., et al. 2020. Importance of hydration and surface structure for friction of acrylamide hydrogels. *Tribology Letters*, 68, 64.
70. Gan S., Lin W., Zou Y., Xu B., Zhang X., Zhao J., Rong J. 2020. Nano-hydroxyapatite enhanced double network hydrogels with excellent mechanical properties for potential application in cartilage repair, *Carbohydrate Polymers*, 229, 115523.
71. Dowson D., Neville A. 2006. Bio-tribology and bio-mimetics in the operating environment, 220(3), 109–123.
72. Liu Z., Yin W., Tao D., Tian Y. 2015. A glimpse of superb tribological designs in nature, *Biotribology*, 1–2, 11–23.
73. Tang Y.H., Zhang H.P. 2016. Theoretical understanding of bio-interfaces/bio-surfaces by simulation: A mini review, *Biosurface and Biotribology*, 2(4), 151–161.
74. Xie C. 2019. Bio-inspired nanofunctionalisation of biomaterial surfaces: a review, *Biosurface and Biotribology*, 5(3), 83–92.
75. Pitenis A.A., Sawyer W.G. 2020. Soft textured implants: roughness, friction, and the complications, *Biotribology*, 22, 100127.
76. Allen Q., Raeymaekers B. 2021. Surface texturing of prosthetic hip implant bearing surfaces: a review, *The Journal of Tribology*, 143(4), 040801.
77. Ito H., Kaneda K., Yuhta K., Nishimura I., Yasuda K., Matsuno K. 2000. Reduction of polyethylene wear by concave dimples on the frictional surface in artificial hip joints, *The Journal of Arthroplasty*, 15(3), 332–338.
78. Sawano H., Warisawa S., Ishihara S. 2009. Study on long life of artificial joints by investigating optimal sliding surface geometry for improvement in wear resistance, *Precision Engineering* 33, 492–498.
79. Gao L., Yang P., Dymond I., Fisher J., Jin Z. 2010. Effect of surface texturing on the elastohydrodynamic lubrication analysis of metal-on-metal hip implants. *Tribology International*, 43, 1851–1860.
80. Ghosh S., Choudhury D., Roy T., Mamat A.B., Masjuki H.H., Pingguan-Murphy B. 2015. Tribological investigation of diamond-like carbon coated micro-dimpled surface under bovine serum and osteoarthritis oriented synovial fluid, *Science and Technology of Advanced Materials*, 16, 035002.
81. Roy T., Choudhury D., Ghosha S., Mamatd A.B., Pingguan-Murphy B. 2015. Improved friction and wear performance of micro dimpled ceramic-on-ceramic interface for hip joint arthroplasty, *Ceramics International*, 141, 681–690.
82. Choudhury D., Urbana F., Vrbka M., Hartla M., Krupkaa I. 2015. A novel tribological study on DLC-coated micro-dimpled orthopedics implant interface, *Journal of the Mechanical Behavior of Biomedical Materials*, 45, 121–131.

83. Choudhury D., Ghosh S., Ali F., Vrbka M., Hartl M., Krupka I. 2016. The influence of surface modification on friction and lubrication mechanism under a bovine serum–lubricated condition, *Tribology Transactions*, 59(2), 316–322.
84. Choudhury D., Vrbka M., Mamat A.B., Stavness I., Roy C.K., Mootanah R., Krupka I. 2017. The impact of surface and geometry on coefficient of friction of artificial hip joints, *Journal of the Mechanical Behavior of Biomedical Materials*, 72, 192–199.
85. Choudhury D., Rebenda D., Sasaki S., Hekrle P., Vrbka M., Zou M. 2018. Enhanced lubricant film formation through micro-dimpled hard-on-hard artificial hip joint: An in-situ observation of dimple shape effects, *Journal of the Mechanical Behavior of Biomedical Materials*, 81, 120–129.
86. Choudhury D., Walker R., Roy T., Paul S., Mootanah R. 2013. Performance of honed surface profiles to artificial hip joints: an experimental investigation, *International Journal of Precision Engineering and Manufacturing* 14(10), 1847–1853.
87. Choudhury D., Walker R., Shirvani A., Mootanah R. 2013. The influence of honed surfaces on metal-on-metal hip joints, *Tribology*, 8(3), 195–202.
88. Qin L., Lin P., Zhang Y., Dong G., Zeng Q. 2013. Influence of surface wettability on the tribological properties of laser textured Co–Cr–Mo alloy in aqueous bovine serum albumin solution, *Applied Surface Science* 268, 79–86.
89. Qiu M., Chyr A., Sanders A.P., Raeymaekers B. 2014. Designing prosthetic knee joints with bio-inspired bearing surfaces, *Tribology International*, 77, 106–110.
90. Zhang Y.L., Zhang X.G., Matsoukas G. 2015. Numerical study of surface texturing for improving tribological properties of ultra-high molecular weight polyethylene, *Biosurface and Biotribology*, 1(4), 270–277.
91. Menezes P.L., Kailas S.V. 2016. Role of surface texture and roughness parameters on friction and transfer film formation when UHMWPE sliding against steel, *Biosurface and Biotribology*, 2(1), 1–10.
92. Wyatt H., Elliott M., Revill P., Clarke A. 2016. The effect of engineered surface topography on the tribology of CFR-PEEK for novel hip implant materials, *Biotribology*, 7, 22–30.
93. Kanda K., Sato H., Kinoshita H., Miyakoshi T., Kanebako H., Adachi K. 2016. Influence of surface texture on friction properties of mechanical seals for blood-design concept of sealing surface of mechanical seal for ventricular assist device, *Tribology*, 11(2), 366–375.
94. Gao L., Hua Z., Hewson R., Andersen M.S., Jin Z. 2018. Elastohydrodynamic lubrication and wear modelling of the knee joint replacements with surface topography, *Biosurface and Biotribology*, 4(1), 18–23.
95. Allen Q., Raeymaekers B. 2020. Maximizing the lubricant film thickness between a rigid microtextured and a smooth deformable surface in relative motion, using a soft elasto-hydrodynamic lubrication model, *The Journal of Tribology*, 142(7), 071802.
96. Lu Y., Hua M., Liu Z. 2014. The biomimetic shark skin optimization design method for improving lubrication effect of engineering surface, *The Journal of Tribology*, 136(3), 031703.
97. Zhou Z.R., Gong W., Zheng J. 2017. Bionic design perspectives based on the formation echanism of dental anti-wear function, *Biosurface and Biotribology*, 3(4), 238–244.
98. Wang Y. 2018. Effect of the bionic morphologies on bio-tribological properties of surface-modified layers on Ti6Al4V with Ni+/N+ implantation, *Industrial Lubrication and Tribology*, 70(2), 325–330.
99. Zhong Y., Zheng L., Gao Y., Liu Z. 2019. Numerical simulation and experimental investigation of tribological performance on bionic hexagonal textured surface, *Tribology International*, 129, 151–161.

100. Badler D., Kasem H. 2020. Synergetic effect of the simultaneous use of different biomimetic adhesive micro-structures on tribological performances, *Biotribology*, 22, 100124.
101. Quan S., Yong G., Jun G., Liu X., Yongping J., Shuyi Y. 2019. Effect of fish scale texture on friction performance for reciprocating pair with high velocity, *Industrial Lubrication and Tribology*, 72(4), 497–502.
102. Atwal J.C., Pandey R.K. 2020. Performance analysis of thrust pad bearing using microrectangular pocket and bionic texture, *Proceedings of the Institution of Mechanical Engineers, Part J: Journal of Engineering Tribology*, 235(6), 1232–1250.
103. Dowson D. 1995. A comparative study of the performance of metallic and ceramic femoral head components in total replacement hip joints, *Wear*, 190(2), 171–183.
104. Katta J., Jin Z., Ingham E., Fisher J. 2008. Biotribology of articular cartilage—A review of the recent advances, *Medical Engineering & Physics*, 30(10), 1349–1363.
105. Dong H.S., Qi S.J. 2015. Realising the potential of graphene-based materials for biosurfaces – a future perspective, *Biosurface and Biotribology*, 1(4), 229–248.
106. Harper M.L., Dooris A., Paré P.E. 2009. The fundamentals of biotribology and its application to spine arthroplasty, *SAS Journal*, 3(4), 125–132.
107. Shi S.F.E.L., Guo Z.G., Liu W.M. 2015. The recent progress of tribological biomaterials, *Biosurface and Biotribology*, 1(2), 81–97.
108. Luo Y., Chen W., Tian M., Teng S. 2015. Thermal oxidation of Ti6Al4V alloy and its biotribological properties under serum lubrication, *Tribology International*, 89, 67–71.
109. Grupp T.M., Holderied M., Mulliez M.A., Streller R., Jäger M., Blömer W., Utzschneider S. 2014. Biotribology of a vitamin E-stabilized polyethylene for hip arthroplasty – Influence of artificial ageing and third-body particles on wear, *Acta Biomaterialia*, 10(7), 3068–3078.
110. Costa J., Peixoto J., Moreira P., Souto A.P., Flores P., Lankarani H.M. 2016. Influence of the hip joint modeling approaches on the kinematics of human gait, *The Journal of Tribology*, 138(3), 031201.
111. Ruggiero A., Merola M., Affatato S. 2017. On the biotribology of total knee replacement: a new roughness measurements protocol on in vivo condyles considering the dynamic loading from musculoskeletal multibody model, *Measurement*, 112, 22–28.
112. Affatato S., Ruggiero A., Merola M., Logozzo S. 2017. Does metal transfer differ on retrieved Biolox® Delta composites femoral heads? Surface investigation on three Biolox® generations from a biotribological point of view, *Composites Part B: Engineering*, 113, 164–173.
113. Espallargas N., Fischer A., Igual Muñoz A., Mischler S., Wimmer M.A. 2017. In-situ generated tribomaterial in metal/metal contacts: Current understanding and future implications for implants, *Biotribology*, 10, 42–50.
114. Wang Q., Ge S., Zhang D. 2005. Nano-mechanical properties and biotribological behaviors of nanosized HA/partially-stabilized zirconia composites, *Wear*, 259(7–12), 952–957.
115. Melero H., Torrell M., Fernández J., Gomes J.R., Guilemany J.M. 2013. Tribological characterization of biocompatible HAp-TiO2 coatings obtained by high velocity oxy-fuel spray, *Wear*, 305(1–2), 8–13.
116. Pettersson M., Tkachenko S., Schmidt S., Berlind T., Jacobson S., Hultman L., Engqvist H., Persson C. 2013. Mechanical and tribological behavior of silicon nitride and silicon carbon nitride coatings for total joint replacements, *Journal of the Mechanical Behavior of Biomedical Materials*, 25, 41–47.
117. Grupp T.M., Giurea A., Miehlke R.K., Hintner M., Gaisser M., Schilling C., Schwiesau J., Kaddick C. 2013. Biotribology of a new bearing material combination in a rotating hinge knee articulation, *Acta Biomaterialia*, 9(6), 7054–7063.

118. Hee A.C., Zhao Y., Choudhury D., Ghosh S., Zhu Q., Zhu H. 2016. Tribological behavior of hydrogenated diamond-like carbon on polished alumina substrate with chromium interlayer for biomedical application, *Biotribology*, 7, 1–10.
119. Choudhury D., Morita T., Sawae Y., Lackner J.M., Towler M., Krupka I. 2016. A novel functional layered diamond like carbon coating for orthopedics applications, *Diamond and Related Materials*, 61, 56–69.
120. Choudhury D., Lackner J., Fleming R.A., Goss J., Chen J., Zou M. 2017. Diamond-like carbon coatings with zirconium-containing interlayers for orthopedic implants, *Journal of the Mechanical Behavior of Biomedical Materials*, 68, 51–61.
121. Han S.X., Ning Z.W., Chen K., Zheng J. 2017. Preparation and tribological properties of Fe-hydroxyapatite bioceramics, *Biosurface and Biotribology*, 3(2), 75–81.
122. Xu L., Zhang D., Chen K., Yang X., Wang Q., Qi J. 2017. Tribological behavior of diamondlike carbon film-deposited Ti6Al4V alloy swinging against ultrahigh molecular weight polyethylene in fetal bovine serum, *The Journal of Tribology*, 139(3), 031301.
123. Qin L., Feng X., Hafezi M., Zhang Y., Guo J., Dong G., Qin Y. 2018. Investigating the tribological and biological performance of covalently grafted chitosan coatings on Co–Cr–Mo alloy, *Tribology International*, 127, 302–312.
124. Daavari M., Atapour M., Mohedano M., Arrabal R., Matykina E., Taherizadeh A. 2021. Biotribology and biocorrosion of MWCNTs-reinforced PEO coating on AZ31B Mg alloy, *Surfaces and Interfaces*, 22, 100850.
125. Ortega-Saenz J.A., Alvarez-Vera M., Hernandez-Rodriguez M.A.L. 2013. Biotribological study of multilayer coated metal-on-metal hip prostheses in a hip joint simulator, *Wear*, 301(1–2), 234–242.
126. Zhang H., Zhang S., Luo J., Liu Y., Qian S., Liang F., Huang Y. 2013. Investigation of Protein Adsorption Mechanism and Biotribological Properties at Simulated Stem-Cement Interface, *The Journal of Tribology* 135(3), 032301.
127. Stevenson H., Parkes M., Austin L., Jaggard M., Akhbari P., Vaghela U., Williams H.R.T., Gupte C., Cann P. 2018. The development of a small-scale wear test for CoCrMo specimens with human synovial fluid, *Biotribology*, 14, 1–10.
128. Zhang J., Chen Z., Gao Y., Zhang X., Guo L., Jin Z. 2019. Computational wear prediction for impact of kinematics boundary conditions on wear of total knee replacement using two cross-shear models, *The Journal of Tribology*. 141(11), 111201.
129. Bergiers S., Hothi H., Richards R., Henckel J., Hart A. 2019. Quantifying the bearing surface wear of retrieved hip replacements, *Biosurface and Biotribology*, 5(1), 28–33.
130. Affatato S., Merola M., Ruggiero A. 2019. Tribological performances of total knee prostheses: Roughness measurements on medial and lateral compartments of retrieved femoral components, *Measurement*, 135, 341–347.
131. Affatato S., Ruzzi S., Milosevic M., Ruggiero A. 2020. Wear characterization and contact surfaces analysis of menisci and femoral retrieved components in bi-condylar knee prostheses, *Journal of the Mechanical Behavior of Biomedical Materials*, 110, 103959.
132. de Villiers D., Collins S. 2020. Wear of large diameter ceramic-on-ceramic hip bearings under standard and microseparation conditions, *Biotribology*, 21, 100117.
133. Kennedy F.E., Currier B.H., Van Citters D.W., Currier J.H., Collier J.P., Mayor M.B. 2003 Oxidation of ultra-high molecular weight polyethylene and its influence on contact fatigue and pitting of knee bearings, *Tribology Transactions*, 46(1), 111–118.
134. Williams P.A., Yamamoto K., Masaoka T., Oonishi H., Clarke I.C. 2007. Highly cross-linked polyethylenes in hip replacements: improved wear performance or paradox? *Tribology Transactions*, 50(2), 277–290.

135. Qing-Liang W., Ge S. 2007. Comparison of biotribology of swine compact bone against UHMWPE, *Journal of China University of Mining and Technology*, 17(1), 133–137.
136. Lie J.-L., Zhu Y.-Y., Wang Q.-L., Ge S. 2008. Biotribological behavior of ultra high molecular weight polyethylene composites containing bovine bone hydroxyapatite, *Journal of China University of Mining and Technology*, 18(4), 606–612.
137. Takeichi Y., Higashiyama T., Nakahigashi T., Tanaka Y., Tsujioka M., Uemura M. 2008. The effect of sandblasting of UHMWPE substrate on the wear resistance of hydrogen-containing carbon coating, *Tribology*, 3(2), 94–99.
138. Plumlee K., Schwartz C.J. 2009. Improved wear resistance of orthopaedic UHMWPE by reinforcement with zirconium particles, *Wear*, 267(5–8), 710–717.
139. Ge S., Wang S., Huang X. 2009. Increasing the wear resistance of UHMWPE acetabular cups by adding natural biocompatible particles, *Wear*, 267(5–8), 770–776.
140. Wang Q., Liu J., Ge S. 2009. Study on biotribological behavior of the combined joint of CoCrMo and UHMWPE/BHA composite in a hip joint simulator, *Journal of Bionic Engineering*, 6(4), 378–386.
141. Harun M.N., Wang F.C., Jin Z.M., Fisher J. 2009. Long-term contact-coupled wear prediction for metal-on-metal total hip joint replacement, *Proceedings of the Institution of Mechanical Engineers, Part J: Journal of Engineering Tribology*, 223(7), 993–1001.
142. Schwartz C.J., Bahadur S. 2009. Investigation of an Approach to Balance Wear Resistance and Mechanical Properties of Crosslinked UHMWPE. *Tribology Letters*, 34, 125–131.
143. Galetz M.C., Glatzel U. 2010. Molecular deformation mechanisms in UHMWPE during tribological loading in artificial joints. *Tribology Letters*, 38, 1–13.
144. Suñer S., Bladen C.L., Gowland N., Tipper J.L., Emami N. 2014. Investigation of wear and wear particles from a UHMWPE/multi-walled carbon nanotube nanocomposite for total joint replacements, *Wear*, 317(1–2), 163–169.
145. Chen G., Ni Z., Qian S., Zhao Y. 2016. Biotribological behaviour of Vitamin E-blended highly cross-linked UHMWPE in a hip joint simulator, *Industrial Lubrication and Tribology*, 68(5), 548–553.
146. Dantas T.A., Abreu C.S., Costa M.M., Miranda G., Silva F.S., Dourado N., Gomes J.R. 2017. Bioactive materials driven primary stability on titanium biocomposites, *Materials Science and Engineering: C*, 77, 1104–1110.
147. Nečas D., Sawae Y., Fujisawa T., Nakashima K., Morita T., Yamaguchi T., Vrbka M., Křupka I., Hartl M. 2017. The influence of proteins and speed on friction and adsorption of metal/UHMWPE contact pair, *Biotribology*, 11, 51–59.
148. Sava M.M., Munteanu B., Renault E., Berthier Y., Trunfio-Sfarghiu A.M. 2018. Tribological analysis of UHMWPE tibial implants in unicompartmental knee replacements: from retrieved to in vitro studies, *Biotribology*, 13, 1–15.
149. Liu D., Wang Q., Zhang D., Wang J., Zhang X. 2019. Torsional friction behavior of contact interface between PEEK and CoCrMo in Calf Serum, *Journal of Tribology*, 141(1), 011602.
150. Mattei L., Di Puccio F., Ciulli E., Pauschitz A. 2020. Experimental investigation on wear map evolution of ceramic-on-UHMWPE hip prosthesis, *Tribology International*, 143, 106068.

2 Lubrication of Hip and Knee Joint Replacements
The Contribution of Experiments and Numerical Modeling

D. Nečas
Brno University of Technology, Brno, Czechia

M. Marian
Friedrich-Alexander-University Erlangen-Nuremberg, Erlangen, Germany

Y. Sawae
Kyushu University, Fukuoka, Japan

CONTENTS

2.1 Introduction: The Importance of Lubrication 33
2.2 Experimental Investigations 35
    2.2.1 Experimental Methods 35
    2.2.2 Hip Replacements 36
    2.2.3 Knee Replacements 43
2.3 Numerical Analyses 45
    2.3.1 Hard-on-Soft Hip Replacements 46
    2.3.2 Hard-on-Hard Hip Replacements 47
    2.3.3 Knee Replacements 51
2.4 Conclusions 52
References 53

2.1 INTRODUCTION: THE IMPORTANCE OF LUBRICATION

Total hip and knee arthroplasties (THAs, TKAs) have become routine techniques for patients suffering from joint diseases. Thanks to these surgeries, millions of patients worldwide can return to normal life every year [1, 2]. As illustrated in Figure 2.1, THAs typically consist of a femoral stem and head moving in the acetabular cup

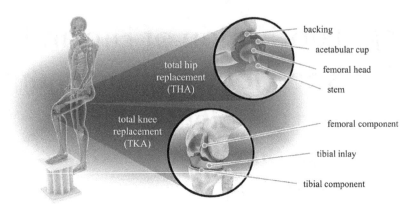

FIGURE 2.1 Total hip and knee arthroplasties in the human body and their structure.

embedded in the pelvis or sometimes a backing. In turn, TKAs mainly involve a femoral component rubbing against the bearing surface of the tibial plateau. In daily life, the artificial joints, which are lubricated by synovial fluid, experience complex and dynamic movements and loads. While hard head-on-soft cup (hard-on-soft), as well as hard head-on-hard cup (hard-on-hard) pairings, can be found for THAs, TKAs always comprise a hard femur-on-soft tibia couple. The implants can differ in their geometric features, partly also patient-specific. Generally, biocompatible materials are used. For the hard components, this includes ceramics (alumina or zirconia; only for THAs) and metals (stainless steel, cobalt-chromium, or titanium alloy), and for the soft components, polymers, primarily ultrahigh molecular weight or highly crosslinked polyethylene (UHMWPE, HXLPE). Despite the unprecedented development in terms of implant design, materials, or surgical techniques and equipment, the limited service life of the replacements represents a persisting challenge. Based on the extensive retrospective analyses, it is assumed that artificial hips and knees may survive for approximately 15 to 25 years [3, 4]. However, it needs to be assumed that this is still not enough, especially in the case of young active patients. Moreover, it is expected that a rapid increase of especially knee surgeries will occur in the next three decades [5]. Since implant failure is associated with a subsequent need for revision surgery, it is desired to further improve the implants to survive longer. When searching for the factors leading to implant failure, aseptic loosening due to osteolysis plays an important role [6]. It should be noted that osteolysis is affected by the interaction of tissues with wear particles released during joint articulation to a certain extent. Although recent investigations showed a promising improvement, deeper knowledge on tribological performance is a key toward "unlimited" survival. In that case, wear rate analysis seems to be fundamental; however, it needs to be assumed that wear is just a consequence of lubrication mechanisms and associated friction processes. The particular importance of lubrication has been highlighted in recent years [7, 8]. Artificial joints may not replicate the behavior of natural synovial joints. Synovial cartilage is an amazing biphasic structure enabling joint operation under an extremely low level of friction. Various lubrication mechanisms were revealed for joint cartilage in addition to typical lubrication regimes [9]. In contrast to cartilage, it is suggested

Lubrication of Hip and Knee Joint Replacements

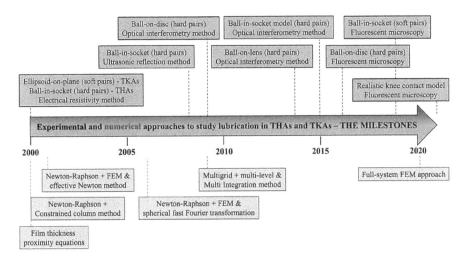

FIGURE 2.2 Experimental and numerical milestones toward understanding the lubrication mechanisms of THAs and TKAs.

that the replacements usually operate in a boundary or mixed regime [10, 11]. To conclude, lubrication indisputably influences the performance of hip and knee implants. While the behavior of natural synovial cartilage may be an inspiration for further development, it is essential to understand the lubrication behavior of artificial joints completely. It has been promoted by renowned experts in the field of (bio-) tribology that experimental measurements should be supported by numerical modeling and vice versa. Ideally, experimental and numerical data should coincide, enabling clear findings. As indicated in the chart of some important milestones in Figure 2.2, considerable efforts have been made and published in this regard over the past decades. The present chapter provides a detailed overview of experimental and numerical approaches toward revealing implant lubrication behavior, while the main findings and suggestions for future research are summarized at the end of the chapter.

2.2 EXPERIMENTAL INVESTIGATIONS

2.2.1 Experimental Methods

Regarding experimental investigations, many measurement methods and approaches have been introduced since the 1950s. Focusing on lubrication analysis, attention is paid to film thickness inside the contact, lubricant flow, lubricant composition, temperature distribution, or fluid pressure. In general, electrical, optical, or acoustic methods may be adopted [12]. For the investigation of lubrication mechanisms in artificial joints, the following have been applied over the last two decades:

- electrical resistance techniques,
- optical interferometry,
- fluorescent microscopy, and
- acoustic methods

Each specific method has some limitations which require the application of simplified laboratory models. Regarding electrical methods, ceramic and polyethylene representing conventional implant materials exhibit very low electrical resistance and capacitance, which means that only metal-on-metal implants may be studied. Further, electrical techniques exhibit lower accuracy than optical methods and provide only quantitative information about the film thickness inside the contact without the visual information, i.e., distribution of film over the contact zone or behavior of lubricant constituents may not be observed. In contrast, optical methods provide the visual content; however, one of the contact bodies needs to be transparent; thus real implant material combinations cannot be studied. Independently of the applied method, simplification in laboratory model for the examination of lubrication mechanisms in joint implants may come from (i) geometry, (ii) material, (iii) contact mechanics, (iv) lubricant, or (v) test conditions.

2.2.2 Hip Replacements

Pilot experimental investigations of hard-on-hard hip implants using the electrical resistivity method were introduced at the beginning of the millennium. Dowson et al. [13] applied a real geometrical ball-in-socket arrangement, focusing on the determination of surface separation during the walking cycle. For metal-on-metal pair, the presence of proteins in the lubricant was found to be essential for efficient lubrication while the thicker film was detected for more concentrated serum. The data suggested that the contact operated in the mixed lubrication regime while cyclic separation was attributed to elastohydrodynamic action. Surprisingly, a relatively weak bond of proteins to the metal substrate was detected, contrasting with some later observations of the adsorption phenomenon. The same methodological approach was subsequently employed for testing of a ceramic-on-ceramic bearing pair [14]. However, the contact surfaces had to be modified to ensure sufficient conductivity. Therefore, a thin titanium nitride layer was applied to the ceramic substrate, which affected the behavior to some extent. This approach led to considerable voltage fluctuations attributed to a combination of surface asperities contact and partial coating detachment. These fluctuations disabled to bring clear findings regarding the dependence of cycle phase and film formation. Thus, the authors further concentrated on metal pairs, investigating the effect of implant geometry and cycle dynamics [15, 16].

Regarding the nominal diameter of the femoral head, the authors found that small implants exhibited no separation, indicating operation in boundary lubrication regime, potentially leading to elevated wear rate. The partial surface separation was observed with increased diameter, while the largest head showed sufficient protection by the thick lubricating film [15]. The subsequent investigation extended the knowledge focusing on the effect of diametric clearance [16]. Experimental data revealed that a lower clearance led to greater film thickness. The authors have also shown that physiological conditions caused more severe lubrication conditions. Therefore, it may be concluded from investigations with the electrical resistivity method that the implants should generally be larger with smaller diametric clearance, while real physiological operating conditions should be applied in laboratory

Lubrication of Hip and Knee Joint Replacements

investigations. The hypothesis about the positive influence of small clearance was later confirmed utilizing the acoustic method based on ultrasonic reflection [17] and optical interferometry [18]. However, ultrasonic measurements showed that too small clearance might have a rather negative impact leading to thinner lubricating film [17]. Furthermore, recent clinical observations revealed an increased failure risk of large metal-on-metal implants having a small clearance. Despite the implant design was supported by extensive simulator testing, the prediction failed to reveal potential causes leading to extensive wear [19]. Finally, while a smaller clearance ensures better surface compliance, leading to a larger contact area and more favorable pressure distribution and running-in wear, the effect on steady-state wear is insignificant [20]. To sum up, the geometry of the implants needs to be balanced to provide optimal lubrication performance.

Assuming some limitations of the electrical and acoustic methods, later investigations dealt with optical measurement methods based on the direct in situ observation of the contact area. The first paper in 2009 from Mavraki and Cann [21] adopted the optical interferometry method while measuring lubricant film thickness in the contact lubricated by simple protein solution mimicking synovial fluid (SF) and bovine serum (BS) as a reference lubricant. The experiments were realized in a simplified well-established ball-on-disk configuration, where the contact of a steel ball and a transparent glass disk was considered. The measurements were performed under pure rolling conditions (no-slip) while film thickness was studied as a rolling speed function. At the end of the experiments, the authors observed a very thin adsorbed layer of proteins on the contact surfaces which was supported by the formation of the hydrodynamic film during the rotation and increasing with elevated speed for BS. Focusing on the model SF, the film was rather constant over the speed range. The subsequent paper adopted the same approach, revealing the influence of kinematic conditions, contact pressure, and temperature [22]. The tests were also performed under pure sliding with the metal ball rotating against a stationary glass disk (see Figure 2.3). In contrast to pure rolling, severe sliding led to a rapid decrease

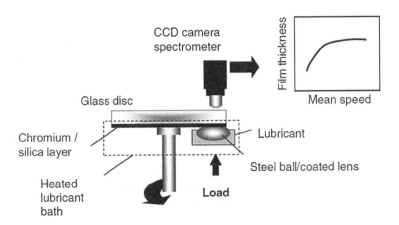

FIGURE 2.3 Ball-on-disk device combined with optical interferometry for measuring thin films [22] (reprinted with permission).

of film thickness, indicating limited adsorption ability as the proteins have been wiped off. The important role of contact pressure is one of the main outcomes of the study. For this purpose, the metal ball was substituted by a metal-coated convex glass lens. It was assumed that lower pressure enhanced lubrication properties, especially at lower speeds. This fact needs to be considered when interpreting results of concentrated non-conformal contacts (such as ball-on-disk) because the real hip is highly conformal while the surfaces fit together with high geometrical precision. Therefore, this study may be considered as one of the first explorations pointing at the importance of surface conformity. Regarding temperature effects, no considerable changes in film thickness were observed for ambient and body temperature. In the following studies, Myant et al. [23] replaced the steel ball with the original CoCrMo femoral head. More emphasis was put on the role of albumin and γ-globulin, dominant constituents of SF. Static experiments based on simple loading without motion were done to clarify the adsorption behavior. It was shown that γ-globulin exhibited a better ability to form an adsorbed layer. On the contrary, the adsorption layer of albumin was very thin and independent of protein concentration. Subsequent time tests with simple protein solutions performed at constant load and relatively low speed showed qualitatively similar behavior. During the test, protein agglomerations of high viscosity, periodically increasing instantaneous film thickness were found to be formed at the contact inlet. These gel-like inlet phases were described in detail in the following study, where a clear correlation between the length of the phase in a longitudinal direction and film thickness was reported [24]. The authors later confirmed previous assumptions that biological protein-containing liquids do not exhibit Newtonian behavior. Specifically, an apparent shear-thinning effect was observed, giving an implication for numerical simulations. Concerning the shear-thinning behavior, it was later revealed that this effect is even more pronounced when the solution contains hyaluronic acid (HA), which is mainly responsible for non-Newtonian fluid nature [25]. All the previous studies employing ball-on-disk optical devices considered metal components. The comparison of metal and ceramic femoral head behavior under BS lubrication was presented later. Vrbka et al. [26] performed time tests at three speeds under pure rolling, two speeds at positive sliding (the disk rotates faster than the ball), and one speed at negative sliding (the ball rotates faster than the disk). Under rolling conditions, a time-increasing tendency with the positive effect of elevated speed was observed for the metal head. The movement of the proteins through the contact is shown in Figure 2.4. Ceramic also showed an increasing trend; however, the rise was not as steep. Once the slip was introduced, the behavior completely changed. Under positive sliding, the film rapidly jumped after the experiment started. After reaching the maximum, it dropped and became very thin for the rest of the test. This tendency was observed independently of head material. Under negative sliding, a negligible film was detected throughout the experiment for both heads. The importance of the applied conditions was further proven by a study that focused on the effect of type of motion on the thickness of the calf serum (CS) film. Myant et al. [27] tested three types of motions, finding that transition from simple unidirectional to reversal motion better mimicking joint function led to a rapid decrease of the lubricant film. Apparently, the methodology based on the use of simple ball-on-disk configuration combined with unidirectional motion suffers from some limitations.

Lubrication of Hip and Knee Joint Replacements

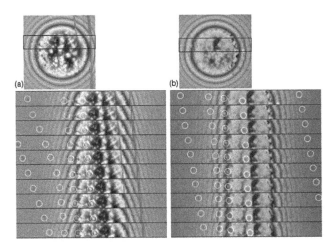

FIGURE 2.4 A sequence of contact images showing the passage of the proteins through the contact for metal (a) and ceramic (b) femoral head [26] (reprinted with permission).

However, it needs to be emphasized that these simplified models have always helped to understand the fundamentals, enabling us to go deeper in investigations. The gained knowledge was summarized in a paper defining protein aggregation lubrication regime [28]. In this reference, multiple theoretical aspects of SF lubrication were summarized, while some similarities and differences against classical elastohydrodynamic lubrication (EHL) theory are highlighted.

Following some implications from previous research mostly related to the issue of surface conformity, i.e., contact pressure, the experimental methodology was subsequently modified by fixing a concave glass lens at the bottom of the glass disk [29]. Only pure negative sliding (the ball rotates against a fixed lens) could be applied. In contrast to previous observations where negative sliding led to nearly zero lubricant film, conformal arrangement led to an immediate jump of film thickness to its maximum right after the start of the test. The film then continuously decreased and stabilized within a relatively short time at a level higher than surface roughness, ensuring sufficient separation of surfaces. Since the role of conformity was shown to be fundamental, the next step was to achieve full surface compliance corresponding to real implant coupling. For this purpose, a simple simulator based on a pendulum principle was developed by Vrbka et al. [30]. The uniqueness of this simulator was in the real contact arrangement, where the femoral head swings in a model of the acetabular cup made of optical glass. The latter was fixed in the base frame while the head was attached to the swinging pendulum arm. The developed methodology was subsequently used to investigate various parameters of implants and lubricants on film formation. The first published study from Nečas et al. [18] focused on the effect of implant material, nominal diameter, and clearance on BS lubricating film. The simulator was also equipped with electromagnetic motors, enabling continuous swinging flexion-extension (FE) motion (see Figure 2.5). An initial set of experiments based on repeated loading and unloading without the presence of swinging motion

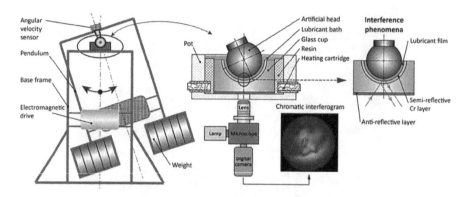

FIGURE 2.5 Pendulum hip joint simulator for film thickness investigation considering real contact conformity [18] (reprinted with permission).

was conducted to reveal adsorption behavior in more detail. Another experiment focused on the role of material using a metal femoral head led to a continuous increase of the adsorbed layer with each following loading cycle. However, ceramic exhibited very unstable behavior followed by repeated adsorption and desorption, indicating the weaker bonds between the proteins and the contact surface. Subsequent swinging tests revealed the important role of implant geometry. Concerning the effect of nominal diameter, the smaller implant generally supported the formation of the thicker lubricating film. Nevertheless, the size of the clearance was found to be essential. For both tested diameters, lower clearance led to considerable improvement of film formation, while larger clearance caused the film to be very thin and practically constant. The second part of the study dealt with the role of model lubricant [31]. BS was used as a reference, and two model fluids containing albumin, γ-globulin, HA, and phospholipids (PLs) in a concentration mimicking healthy and pathological SF were applied. Despite the protein content in the model, SFs were nearly double compared to BS, the adsorbed film was lower for model fluids for both metal and ceramic heads. The effect of SF constituents was found to be fundamental under swinging. The importance of HA was specifically highlighted, finding that increased content of HA led to substantially thicker lubricating film compared to BS and low-content HA model fluid. The study later points to the importance of the interaction of the constituents since the behavior of simple solutions showed remarkably different results compared to complex films. While HA was found to play an important role in a fluid mixture, simple HA failed to form any measurable film shortly after the experiments started. The study implied that the use of CS or BS of unknown composition is not the best choice when investigating implant lubrication conditions. The detailed information about the composition and content of the fluid should always be known, helping to explain the obtained results. The methodology consisting of a combination of the pendulum and optical interferometry was later successfully employed in a study describing the potential of surface texturing [32]. The authors compared various shapes of micro-dimples made on the femoral head, finding that the fully-developed film thickness was up to 3.5 times higher compared to the non-textured implant. This study is very promising when searching for new ways of development toward extended implant lifespan.

A number of the above investigations focused on the behavior of SF constituents, frequently investigating simple solutions or mixtures. However, the applied approaches did neither allow for a clear understanding of constituent interactions nor an assessment of the behavior of specific molecules in a mixture. This drawback comes from the nature of the applied measurement method. The references employed the optical interferometry technique for the measurement of thin films. Despite the high accuracy of the method, it should be noted that this approach determined the film thickness quantitatively from the general point of view. Therefore, there is no chance to identify individual ingredients in the film. To get deeper knowledge on film formation mechanism in hip joints, aiming at the role of specific constituents, optical interferometry was supplemented by fluorescent microscopy, enabling to concentrate at specific fluorescently stained constituents in the lubricant.

The first study was introduced in 2016 by Nečas et al. [33]. The authors made a little step back in terms of the experimental configuration since the method previously has not been applied to investigate implant lubrication. Therefore, the experiments were realized in a simple ball-on-disk arrangement while the contact of metal femoral head and glass disk was observed using both the above methods. A mixture of albumin and γ-globulin was applied as the test lubricant. Initially, the contact was observed using optical interferometry to evaluate the overall film thickness development. Subsequently, the experiments were repeated twice with fluorescently stained albumin being combined with non-stained γ-globulin and vice versa. This approach enabled concentration on each specific constituent while the contact was lubricated by the mixture. As a result, qualitative information about the intensity (i.e., dimensionless film thickness) of each specific protein was obtained (Figure 2.6). By scaling the data against interferometry results, mutual interaction and the role of specific constituents could be assessed. The experiments were realized under pure rolling and both positive and negative sliding, finding that overall trends well-corresponded to previous observations [26]. In terms of the proteins, it was found that γ-globulin forms mostly a thin adhered layer while further film enhancement was attributed to albumin.

Similar behavior was also observed for alumina and zirconia toughened ceramic femoral heads [34]. A great benefit of fluorescent microscopy is the ability to investigate non-reflective compliant materials. Therefore, there is the option of studying polymers mimicking the behavior of polyethylene implant components. The combination of methodologies based on the use of interferometry and fluorescent microscopy resulted in a two-part publication dealing with lubrication mechanisms in hard-on-soft [35] and hard-on-hard [36] hip implants. The acetabular cup was made from transparent polymethyl methacrylate (PMMA) to investigate a hard-on-soft contact. The latter has mechanical, physical, and surface properties comparable to polyethylene. Two different types of tests were performed while both the adsorption and the dynamic film were observed. Thirteen different lubricants were applied, being of various complexity, and always based on one of the constituents (albumin, γ-globulin, HA) to be fluorescently stained and combined with other non-stained components. Thus, the lubrication mechanism could be revealed, highlighting the

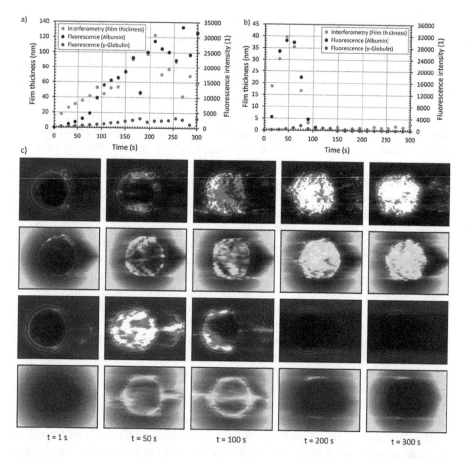

FIGURE 2.6 Film thickness development for the metal femoral head in a ball-on-disk configuration using optical interferometry and fluorescent microscopy for lower (a) and higher (b) speed under positive sliding conditions. (c) Fluorescent images of the contact zone corresponding to film thickness development (a) [33] (reprinted with permission).

interaction of γ-globulin with HA and phospholipids when forming a thin adsorbed boundary layer, enabling further layering of albumin. For the hard pairing, the same lubricants were used while the data of both studies were compared, see for example Figure 2.7. It was found that HA generally supports a thicker lubricating film when mixed with other constituents; however, this effect is considerably influenced by the protein content. The study further highlighted the importance of contact nature when examining lubrication processes within artificial hips. Differences between soft and hard pairs were observed, especially under swinging motion. While the film had a decreasing tendency for hard pairs, the PMMA cup application led to film enhancement. This finding supports previous suggestions related to the sensitivity of the SF film on contact pressure. On the contrary, despite thicker films, soft pairs exhibited higher friction accompanied by faster damping of swinging motion when the driving

Lubrication of Hip and Knee Joint Replacements

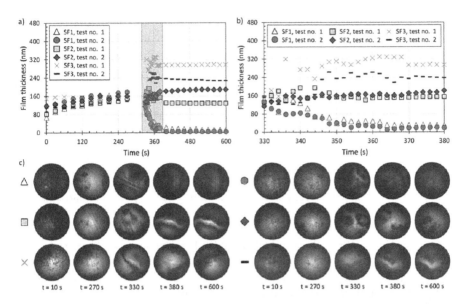

FIGURE 2.7 Repeatability test of film thickness development in a ball-on-cup configuration for hard-on-soft bearing pair (a). Detail of the gray zone (b). Respective optical interferograms [36] (reprinted with permission).

motors of the pendulum were cut-off. This implies the role of internal friction within the lubricating film.

2.2.3 KNEE REPLACEMENTS

Many papers dealt with the lubrication mechanisms within THAs. The situation is quite different for TKAs where only a limited number of experimental studies may be found. The point is that a knee implant has a very complicated geometry. Further, hard-on-hard pairs are not used in TKAs. The majority of implants consist of a metal femoral component articulating with a polyethylene tibial insert securely fixed in the tibial part. As in the case of hips, the first investigation dealing with the lubrication performance of artificial knee was carried out employing an electrical resistivity method. The initial paper published in the 1980s showed the potential contribution of the elastomeric artificial cartilage layer on the tibial components to enhance lubrication performance. The experiments were realized in the knee joint simulator with two knee prosthesis models with a different tibial component. The first setup combined the metal femoral component and a platinum-coated UHMWPE tibial component, while another model used a flat conductive silicone rubber as artificial cartilage instead of the concaved PE tibia. Substantially improved elastohydrodynamic lubricant film formation was observed for silicone rubber specimens compared with UHMWPE [37]. However, the following study showed that the rubber exhibited unacceptably high friction, while much better results were achieved for a polyvinyl alcohol (PVA) hydrogel layer mimicking cartilage [38]. The papers were later followed by Ohtsuki et al. [39]. The authors tested the contact of a metal ball in contact with a silicone rubber flat layer, focusing on the effect of contact geometry. The main conclusion of this study was that a transverse geometry generally supports the formation of a stable lubricating layer compared to a longitudinal one. A further study concentrated mostly on wear and friction analysis of TKA; however, the authors also partially dealt with lubrication [40]. Data obtained based on the experiments with various model lubricants corresponded well to previous observations for a hard-on-soft hip implant, showing that the adsorbed layer may contribute to wear protection of rubbing surfaces despite elevated friction. The first study introducing a suitable methodological approach for TKA lubrication investigation was recently introduced. Nečas et al. [41] developed a knee joint simulator allowing for in situ observation of the contact together with the application of transient dynamics mimicking ISO standards for knee testing. Specifically, the simulator enables control of the cycle frequency, axial load, FE motion, and anterior/posterior translation. The experimental approach was based on previous experience with hip implants [35]. Therefore, the contact of the metal femoral component sliding against a real-shaped model of the tibial insert made from PMMA was observed using fluorescent microscopy. In the pilot study, the authors focused on simulator debugging and observation of contact shape and migration over the simplified walking cycle under lubrication by a mixture of albumin and γ-globulin. Subsequently, the authors further enhanced the observation, focusing on the interaction of SF constituents considering more complex model fluids containing proteins, HA, and phospholipids [42]. The results showed the considerable influence of adsorbed proteins on the visual appearance of the contact zone. Further, a very positive stabilizing effect of HA and phospholipids on the lubricating layer was observed. This study also discussed the potential limitations of the methodological approach, focusing on the issue of measurement repeatability, contact mechanics, surface roughness, surface wettability, mechanical, physical, and chemical properties. The investigation resulted in the last paper published in early 2021 [43]. In that case, real kinematic conditions and transient loading were applied while investigating both lateral and medial compartments under a real frequency of 1 Hz. Lubrication strategy complied with the previous paper on hips [35], since it was found very effective in revealing the mutual interactions of SF constituents. Besides, a feasibility study with mineral oil as the test lubricant was performed, enabling comparison of experimental data and numerical modeling. The developed numerical model is described in the subsequent section. The influence of interrupted loading was examined as well. The results showed a good correlation between experimental and numerical approaches. Regarding the lubrication performance, the medial compartment exhibited worse conditions in general. Further, it was found that interrupted walking leads to thinning of the lubricant layer, which may be crucial regarding the consequent wear rate. Therefore, rest periods in walking are suggested, enabling the film to be recovered, preventing the surfaces against mutual contact. Based on the data for various model fluids, an illustrative theoretical model of a lubricating layer within TKA was proposed. The designed methodology for the investigation of knee implant lubrication is shown in Figure 2.8.

Lubrication of Hip and Knee Joint Replacements

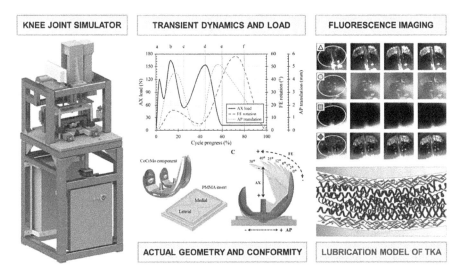

FIGURE 2.8 Experimental methodology for the investigation of knee implant lubrication [43] (reprinted with permission).

2.3 NUMERICAL ANALYSES

Theoretical considerations and numerical analyses have accompanied the experimental investigations on lubrication mechanisms in joint replacements from the very beginning. In line with early findings on natural joints, it was evident that the lubrication mechanisms are also driven by the interplay of SF hydrodynamics and rheology as well as the elastic deformation of the bearing surfaces; all these aspects need to be appropriately considered. Attempts solely focusing on pure hydrodynamic lubrication, e.g., from [44–47], were therefore quickly supplanted by those based upon the EHL theory. Pioneering work was notably done by the groups around Jin and Dowson, who first attempted to predict fluid film parameters for hard-on-soft and hard-on-hard hip implants [48] as well as knee replacements [49] utilizing simplified proximity equations [50] derived for isoviscous EHL contacts with linear elastic materials [51] as well as layered elastohydrodynamic contacts [52], respectively. In the following, also due to the progress and novel insights in the field of EHL simulations for concentrated contacts, the numerical modeling approaches have been continuously developed and expanded to cover more and more implant configurations and relevant phenomena. In order to solve for the fluid film pressure and lubricant gap distribution, the governing equations of most numerical studies generally included:

- The **Reynolds differential equation** [53] written either in polar or cartesian coordinates to describe the hydrodynamic pressure build-up between the mating surfaces.
- **Elasticity equations** to account for the elastic deformation of the contacting bodies.
- The **lubricant film equation** to describe the macro- and/or micro-geometry of the rubbing surfaces

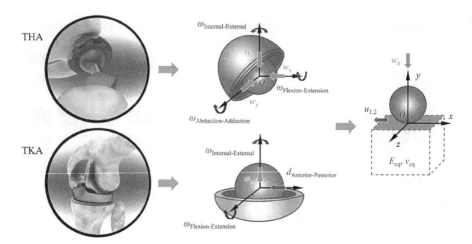

FIGURE 2.9 From contacts in THAs and TKAs to a model ball-in-socket configuration and their abstraction to a ball-on-plane geometry.

- The **load balance equation** to ensure an equilibrium of forces between generated hydrodynamic pressure and applied load.
- **Rheological lubricant models**, i.e., mathematical descriptions of the viscosity behavior of the SF.

Various methods have been developed to solve and couple the system of equations, which, besides numerical aspects, especially regarding the Reynolds and elasticity equation, can be distinguished by the considered material pairing and the geometric model conception. As illustrated in Figure 2.9, the contacts in hip and knee replacements can be interpreted as a conformal ball-in-socket pairing or abstracted to a contact between a rigid ball and a plane with equivalent elastic properties (ball-on-plane pairing) as classically done in "hard" elastohydrodynamics. While a majority of works assumed incompressibility and Newtonian behavior, few studies also considered shear-thinning effects. This was then represented, for example, by Cross [54] or Carreau [55] models with two Newtonian plateaus.

Regarding hip replacements, Mattei et al. [56] already provided a comprehensive overview of numerical modeling. Thus, only the most relevant and more recent work for the elastohydrodynamic lubrication in hard-on-soft and hard-on-hard hip implants will be presented in the following before the contributions on the simulation of lubrication in knee replacements are discussed.

2.3.1 Hard-on-Soft Hip Replacements

Initially, Jalali-Vahid et al. [57] analyzed the EHL film formation for hard-on-soft implants based upon the Newton-Raphson (N-R) method. Thereby, the Reynolds equation was adapted in spherical coordinates for a ball-in-socket setup and discretized by finite and backward difference schemes, while the constrained column model was utilized for calculating the elastic deformation. It could be shown that an alternative calculation with the simplified ball-on-plane concept led to an overestimation of the lubricant film for the studied configuration [58]. Moreover, despite the positive impact of a larger femoral head radius, a smaller radial clearance as well as higher thickness and lower elastic modulus of the acetabular cup on increasing the fluid film thickness, it was expected that the lubricant thickness is more in the range of typical roughness, i.e., mixed lubrication is present [59]. A transient extension of the numerical approach considering dynamic stresses revealed a combination of entrainment and squeeze effects being largely responsible for generating and maintaining a stable fluid film [60]. Yet, calculated values were very close to those from a quasi-static estimation using averaged speed and load [61].

Wang and Jin [62] adapted the methodology from [60] to solve the Reynolds equation by the N-R approach with finite-difference (FD) discretization, while the elastic deformation of the femoral head and UHMWPE acetabular cup (ball-in-socket) was determined by the spherical fast Fourier transformation (SFFT) method. To this end, the displacement coefficients were determined beforehand by the finite element method (FEM), resulting in significantly reduced computational costs. Thus, it could be shown that the cup inclination angle and the internal-external (IE) rotation had a subordinate role for the fluid film and pressure formation and that these were rather dominated by the FE motion [63].

2.3.2 Hard-on-Hard Hip Replacements

Apart from the aforementioned studies, a majority of numerical work was done for hard-on-hard implants. As such, Jagatia and Jin [64] applied the N-R solution of the equation system consisting of a finite and backward difference discretized Reynolds equation as well as the effective Newton method [65] accounting for elastic deformation through displacement coefficients that were initially determined by a FEM simulation, potentially even including the effects of a polymer backing and allowing a transferability to hip resurfacing prostheses [66]. Thus, it was shown that the equivalent ball-on-plane geometry assumption delivers similar results to a calculation with the ball-in-socket configuration if the deformed contact radius is smaller than the cup wall thickness [67]. Jalali-Vahid et al. [68] also came to a similar conclusion based upon their N-R scheme introduced earlier. With this approach and the ball-on-plane simplification, transient analyses were also performed by Williams et al. [69] with a focus on dynamic load and speed. These and the studies of Jalali-Vahid et al. [70] on the start-up conditions indicated significant differences in the film thicknesses compared to a quasi-static perspective.

As for hard-on-soft pairings, the utilization of the SFFT method provided significant advances in numerical efficiency for hard-on-hard implants under dynamic loading and motion conditions as well. Wang and Jin [71] also showed the crucial role of squeeze effects in transient simulations, especially at reversal points of the motion where the entrainment speed momentarily turns zero while the hydrodynamic pressure was rather driven by the load than by the velocities. Similar to hard-on-soft implants, the acetabular cup inclination angle was shown to play a minor role in fluid film and pressure formation. However, Liu et al. [72] revealed that certain geometrical parameters, as well as the bearing construction, influence the lubrication conditions.

Thereby, more conformal bearings, i.e., a lower clearance and a larger femoral head radius, as well as a sandwich cup with polyethylene backing instead of a monolithic cup were reported to promote film formation due to larger contact areas and squeeze effects carrying the load. Also, macroscopic geometry changes due to wear during running-in improved conformity and thus lubrication [73]. These findings basically matched well with numerical results on hip resurfacing prostheses [74]. Wang and Jin [75], as well as Wang et al. [76], showed for quasi-static conditions that a non-sphericity caused by manufacturing deviations or deliberately designed also has a tremendous impact on the contact condition in dependency of orientation and magnitude, even having potential for improving fluid film formation. Gao et al. [77] extended the numerical model toward mixed lubrication by reducing the Reynolds equation when the fluid film collapsed in accordance with Hu and Zhu [78]. Thus, it could be shown that, in addition to the macro-geometry, the micro-geometry may also have a decisive influence on the lubricant film formation [79]. Therefore, deliberately inserted micro-textures could potentially have beneficial effects on the reduction of the solid asperity contact ratio, particularly under boundary or mixed lubrication, while they had an adverse effect in the full film regime.

The introduction of the multigrid (MG) instead of the N-R method allowed a further considerable improvement in numerical stability and accuracy [80]. Thus, the effects of transient 3D physiological loading and motion on the fluid film formation could be studied, for which Gao et al. [81] predicted a substantial variation of the film thickness distribution with time and location under different operating conditions. Thereby, significant differences in the derived values were reported compared to unidirectional loads and movements, see Figure 2.10.

Also driven by the progress in the field of classical hard EHL point contacts, the multi-level and multi-integration (MLMI) technique [82] subsequently received considerable attention for calculating the deformations in hard-on-hard hip replacements considering a ball-in-socket [80] or a ball-on-plane geometry [83] with particular advantages for time-transient calculations. As such, Gao et al. [84] demonstrated a

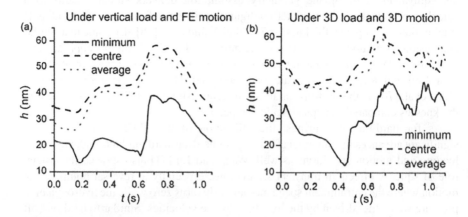

FIGURE 2.10 Variation of the minimum, center, and average film thickness during a convergent walking cycle under vertical load and flexion-extension motion (a) as well as 3D load and motion (b) [81] (reprinted with permission).

Lubrication of Hip and Knee Joint Replacements

significant influence of the fluid film formation in dependency of different walking patterns with entrainment and squeeze effects being largely responsible. The latter permitted a separating lubricant film to be maintained even during shorter intermittent breaks. Also, Meng et al. [85] studied the influence of non-spherical bearing surfaces under transient conditions. Thus, an alpharabola femoral head and cup were found to enlarge the fluid film compared to conventional spherical bearings due to considerable squeeze film action. It was also shown that a larger head radius and a lower clearance, as well as ceramic-on-ceramic or ceramic-on-metal instead of metal-on-metal implants, can have a positive effect on the contact conditions [86].

Based upon their investigations under steady-state conditions with viscosity properties obtained by Yao et al. [87], Wang et al. [88] found only neglectable differences regarding fluid film and pressure between a Newtonian und the non-Newtonian fluid model. Thus, most numerical studies on hip replacements considered a Newtonian behavior of the SF, and shear-thinning effects were neglected. For viscosity, low values were simply assumed, which were valid for higher shear rates and are similar to water. However, by expanding their transient MG/MLMI-based EHL simulation approach with a shear-thinning Cross model while assuming an averaged shear rate in the gap height direction, Gao et al. [89] pointed out the significant effect of non-Newtonian behavior on the contact conditions, see Figure 2.11. The higher viscosity at low shear rates substantially increased the calculated film thickness for physiological load cycles, stressing the importance of appropriate rheological models. Also, the crucial role of powerful squeeze effects to maintain greater film thickness for the shear-dependent viscosity was highlighted. Thus, fluid film lubrication was reported during the swing phase, while mixed or boundary lubrication were likely to appear during the stance phase. Again, a smaller clearance was found to be positive for lubricating film formation.

The steady progress in numerical modeling allowed the investigation of more and more effects and phenomena and eventually led to wear prediction expansion. Although lubrication analysis and wear simulation were done separately for a very long time, a combined consideration has clear advantages with respect to relevance and accuracy due to mutual relations [56]. For this purpose, EHL simulation models were extended with regard to the analysis of mixed lubrication conditions [90]. Thus, various predictions of wear behavior could subsequently be elaborated on the basis

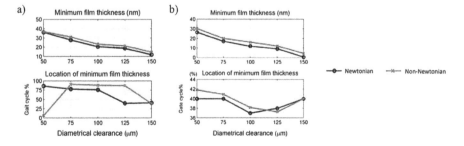

FIGURE 2.11 Magnitudes and locations of the minimum film thickness against hip joint clearance for a simulator (a) and physiological walking pattern (b) [89] (reprinted with permission).

of the timely and locally resolved lubrication conditions [91, 92]. As pointed out by Liu et al. [93], the motion inputs have considerable influence on the predicted lubrication and consequently also the wear behavior. Therefore, Ruggiero et al. [94] introduced a sophisticated numerical framework that efficiently couples the determination of motion characteristics from a musculoskeletal biomechanical multibody simulation with a lubricant film calculation. Mixed lubrication was considered by a load-sharing concept, the Reynolds equation was discretized by FD and solved by iterative Newton method cycles, while the local elastic deformation was calculated by a simplified Hertzian approximation [95] or the constrained column model [96], respectively.

Since this chapter focuses more on joint replacement lubrication and neither on wear modeling nor biomechanical musculoskeletal simulation, those aspects shall not be elaborated further. Instead, the interested reader is referred to a review paper from Mattei et al. [56] or other chapters of this book. Anyways, their outcome and accuracy are sensitive to how well the lubrication conditions present in the implants are predicted. The corresponding EHL simulation models were widely verified and cross-checked by mesh convergence studies or comparisons with numerical models for dry conditions [86, 97]. In addition, indirect validation was partly carried out by comparisons with data on frictional torque [90] or observed wear phenomena in physical hip simulators [98]. However, these approaches cannot adequately address all factors, and certain error sources inevitably remain. Merely, a direct comparison between simulations and experimental investigations under most similar conditions, as described in the previous section of this chapter, can bring more clarity in this respect. This was recently enabled by Lu et al. [99] by validating results from their numerical model based upon MG and MLMI against fluid film measurements from a pendulum hip joint simulator with an optical imaging system and a CoCr-on-glass bearing pair. While simulation and experiments showed excellent agreement in studies with a low-viscosity mineral oil without macromolecular agglomeration and whose rheological behavior was well known, this was not directly the case for the BS used as substitute SF, due to discrepancies between the fluid behavior and the rheological model adapted from literature [24] (Figure 2.12). Only by introducing a new

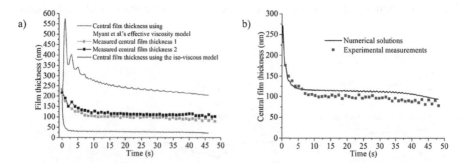

FIGURE 2.12 Comparison between the experimentally measured and numerically calculated central film thicknesses at the equilibrium position of the pendulum for the isoviscous and initial effective viscosity model (a) as well as the new entrainment velocity-effective viscosity relation (b) [99] (reprinted with permission).

entrainment velocity-effective viscosity relation based on a modified Cross model, a satisfactory agreement was found. This once again underlined the importance of an adequate description of the fluid and also shear-thinning effects.

2.3.3 KNEE REPLACEMENTS

There are significantly fewer numerical studies on knee implants compared to the works discussed here. As applies to the experimental work, this can be attributed to the more complex geometries and the fact that hard-on-soft pairings are usually used in TKAs. Basically, the few numerical models for knee replacements were strongly driven by the findings and advances in the modeling of hip implants. Substantial simplifications still limited initial studies in terms of geometry, kinematics, and load [100–102]. It was not until Su et al. [103] performed complete time-dependent EHL simulations under physiological loading and motion of a gait cycle using a MG/FD approach to solve the Reynolds equation while the elastic deformation was incorporated by the constrained column model. Thereby, a ball-on-plane geometry with a finite thickness of the tibial plateau and Newtonian fluid behavior was assumed. Hence, they were able to show that squeeze effects play a crucial role in maintaining the fluid film during the stance phase, while the entrainment velocity was largely responsible for forming the film formation in the swing phase. Certain geometric design parameters could also support reducing the pressures and increasing the lubricant film height. In particular, high joint conformity and a larger tibial inlay thickness with a lower Young's modulus proved to be advantageous. Nevertheless, the calculated lubricant film heights were of the order of typical roughness, which would occasionally suggest mixed lubrication conditions [104].

Later, Gao et al. [105] utilized their numerical model based upon the MG and SFFT method to account for the lubrication in TKAs considering a ball-in-socket geometry and shear-thinning by a Cross model. However, the main focus of this work was put on wear modeling and the influence of surface texturing. In this respect, it could be shown for the examined cases that the lateral condyle could benefit from textures, while this is not the case for the medial compartment. It was also shown that the hydrodynamic pressures decreased, and the lubricant film height tended to increase with the wear-related changes in macro-geometry, i.e., an increase in conformity. The evolutions over the gait cycle basically showed a similar character as already reported by Su et al. [103], but the underlying mechanisms were not the main focus here.

Recently, Marian et al. [106] adapted the full-system approach from Habchi et al. [107] to numerically model soft EHL contacts in TKAs. In contrast to most of the previously applied and described approaches, the Reynolds equation was not weakly/iteratively but strongly/fully coupled with the elastic deformation of the ball-on-plane pairing. This was facilitated by solving both with FEM [108]. Mixed lubrication conditions could be included via a load-sharing concept. Furthermore, by using a generalized Reynolds equation, the assumption of constant shear stresses, density, and viscosity in the lubricant gap height direction could be resolved for the first time. Thus, thermal and shear-thinning effects by a Carreau or Cross model could be taken into account, whereas the integral and velocity term, as well as the energy equation,

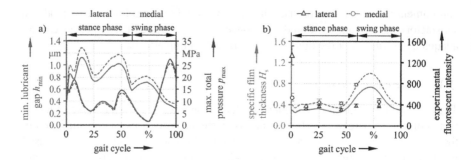

FIGURE 2.13 Minimum lubricant gap and maximum pressure over one gait cycle (a), mean film height and comparison with experimental data at various time steps (b) [106] (reprinted with permission).

were coupled iteratively. Initially, the numerical model was directly validated against optical fluorescent measurements on a knee simulator under lubrication of a low-viscosity mineral oil [42], where good agreement was found (Figure 2.13). Thereby, the medial compartment was more heavily stressed, experienced higher pressures, and smaller minimum film heights as well as higher probability for solid asperity contact compared to the lateral condyle. The overall lubricant gap was smaller in the stance phase, where load and geometry played a dominant role, whereas the swing phase was determined by geometry and kinematics. Generally, the fluid film formation was largely affected by reversal points of motion, whereby the collapse of the lubrication film could be prevented by transient squeeze effects. Thus, it could be estimated that the stance phase and the zero entrainment speed points promote wear and are crucial for the TKA service life, especially in the medial condyle. Further investigations were carried out to study the influence of the modeling strategy. It was found that the complexity of numerical modeling had a large effect on calculation results and accuracy, especially for the fluid film height. Thereby, transient squeeze effects and shear-thinning fluid characteristics are crucial. It was also shown that a radius of the femoral component that varies with the FE motion and the consideration of a finite thickness of the tibial plateau needs to be considered. Finally, it was revealed that the individual rheological SF parameters have a large impact on fluid film formation. Particularly noteworthy is that the whole numerical modeling approach was based on the utilization of solvers from commercially available multiphysics software. Thus, it is expected that the research focus can be shifted from numerical aspects even more toward physical modeling in the future.

2.4 CONCLUSIONS

An outstanding improvement in knowledge about lubrication of hip and knee joint replacements has been achieved over the last two decades. Experimental investigations as well as numerical modeling brought us many new findings and suggestions for further research, toward the extension of implant longevity, preventing the need for revising surgeries. Therefore, the impact is not only social in terms of patient´s convenience, but also in economic site assuming that the costs associated with revisions are often two or three times higher compared to primary surgeries. Focusing on the contribution of experiments, various approaches based on electrical resistivity, acoustic, optical interferometry, or fluorescent microscopy methods were introduced. These revealed the importance of surface conformity and radial clearance, the effects of load, speed, temperature, or the type of applied motion on fluid film formation. Thanks to optical methods, the role of specific SF constituents was further elaborated and lubrication mechanisms within both THA and TKA were revealed. From a numerical perspective, various approaches have been developed to solve and couple the Reynolds equation for the hydrodynamics and the elastic deformation. This has started with Newton-Raphson and constrained column methods, the latter being successively supplanted by a SFFT and later by a multi-level multi-integration method, and the former by multigrid methods. Therefore, simulation models based on FDs with specially developed solution algorithms can mostly be found, whereby a fully coupled FEM approach based on commercial multiphysics software has also been applied recently. While assuming a simplified, equivalent ball-on-plane geometry is appropriate for hard-on-hard hip replacements as well as TKAs, a more accurate ball-in-socket configuration needs to be taken into account for hard-on-soft THAs. The numerical work was also able to show the importance of material and geometry properties, i.e., surface conformity and radial clearance or the importance of squeeze effects under dynamic load and motion. In addition, recent works in particular highlighted the relevance of the rheological properties of the SF.

Overall, it must be noted that all the employed experimental methods, due to limited access into real joints, and numerical modeling, due to simplifications, model conceptions, and mathematical descriptions, always comply with certain assumptions. Thus, these can only provide certain insights into lubrication mechanisms of real joint implants. It is, therefore, especially remarkable that experiment and simulation have recently come closer and closer and we have now reached a level where both can be directly compared and validated. This validity represents the basic requirement for all implications to improved implant designs derived on the basis of the developed theories.

However, there are still many phenomena and effects to be explored. In the future, researchers should further improve the experimental approaches as well as the numerical models to approach even more realistic joint conditions. The phenomenon of adsorption [109–111] is still yet to be investigated in more detail. Further, we should follow new trends in materials and manufacturing abilities while focusing on coatings [112], surface treatment [113], or micro-texturing [32, 112, 114]. Finally, we should follow the composition and behavior of real human SFs when suggesting model lubricants to get clinically relevant data. To conclude, there are still enormous abilities for future research toward extended or unlimited service life of hip and knee joint replacements.

REFERENCES

1. Kurtz, S., K. Ong, E. Lau, F. Mowat, and M. Halpern. 2007. "Projections of Primary and Revision Hip and Knee Arthroplasty in the United States from 2005 to 2030". *The Journal of Bone & Joint Surgery*, 89 (4): 780–785. doi:10.2106/JBJS.F.00222.

2. Price, A.J., A. Alvand, A. Troelsen, J.N. Katz, G. Hooper, A. Gray, A. Carr, and D. Beard. 2018. "Knee Replacement". *The Lancet* 392 (10158): 1672–1682. doi:10.1016/S0140-6736(18)32344-4.
3. Evans, J.T., J.P. Evans, R.W. Walker, A.W. Blom, M.R. Whitehouse, and A. Sayers. 2019. "How Long Does a Hip Replacement Last? A Systematic Review and Meta-Analysis of Case Series and National Registry Reports with More than 15 Years of Follow-Up". *The Lancet* 393 (10172): 647–654. doi:10.1016/S0140-6736(18)31665-9.
4. Cook, R., P. Davidson, and R. Martin. "More Than 80% of Total Knee Replacements Can Last for 25 Years". *BMJ*. doi:10.1136/bmj.l5680.
5. Inacio, M.C.S., E.W. Paxton, S.E. Graves, R.S. Namba, and S. Nemes. 2017. "Projected Increase in Total Knee Arthroplasty in the United States – An Alternative Projection Model". *Osteoarthritis and Cartilage* 25 (11): 1797–1803. doi:10.1016/j.joca.2017.07.022.
6. Gallo, J., S.B. Goodman, Y.T. Konttinen, M.A. Wimmer, and M. Holinka. 2013. "Osteolysis around Total Knee Arthroplasty: A Review of Pathogenetic Mechanisms". *Acta Biomaterialia* 9 (9): 8046–8058. doi:10.1016/j.actbio.2013.05.005.
7. Jin, Z.M., M. Stone, E. Ingham, and J. Fisher. 2006. "(V) Biotribology". *Current Orthopaedics* 20 (1): 32–40. doi:10.1016/j.cuor.2005.09.005.
8. Serro, A.P., K. Degiampietro, R. Colaço, and B. Saramago. 2010. "Adsorption of Albumin and Sodium Hyaluronate on Uhmwpe: A Qcm-D and Afm Study". *Colloids and Surfaces B: Biointerfaces* 78 (1): 1–7. doi:10.1016/j.colsurfb.2010.01.022.
9. Ruggiero, A. 2020. "Milestones in Natural Lubrication of Synovial Joints". *Frontiers in Mechanical Engineering* 6 (July). doi:10.3389/fmech.2020.00052.
10. Scholes, S.C., A. Unsworth, and A.A.J. Goldsmith. 2000. "A Frictional Study of Total Hip Joint Replacements". *Physics in Medicine and Biology* 45 (12): 3721–3735. doi:10.1088/0031-9155/45/12/315.
11. Dowson, D., and Z.-M. Jin. 2006. "Metal-On-Metal Hip Joint Tribology". *Proceedings of the Institution of Mechanical Engineers, Part H: Journal of Engineering in Medicine* 220 (2): 107–118. doi:10.1243/095441105X69114.
12. Albahrani, S.M.B., D. Philippon, P. Vergne, and J.M. Bluet. 2015. "A Review of In Situ Methodologies for Studying Elastohydrodynamic Lubrication". *Proceedings of the Institution of Mechanical Engineers, Part J: Journal of Engineering Tribology* 230 (1): 86–110. doi:10.1177/1350650115590428.
13. Dowson, D., C.M. McNie, and A.A.J. Goldsmith. 2000. "Direct Experimental Evidence Of Lubrication In A Metal-On-Metal Total Hip Replacement Tested In A Joint Simulator". *Proceedings of the Institution of Mechanical Engineers, Part C: Journal of Mechanical Engineering Science* 214 (1): 75–86. doi:10.1243/0954406001522822.
14. Smith, S.L., D. Dowson, A.A.J. Goldsmith, R. Valizadeh, and J.S. Colligon. 2001. "Direct Evidence of Lubrication in Ceramic-On-Ceramic Total Hip Replacements". *Proceedings of the Institution of Mechanical Engineers, Part C: Journal Of Mechanical Engineering Science* 215 (3): 265–268. doi:10.1243/0954406011520706.
15. Smith, S.L., D. Dowson, and A.A.J. Goldsmith. 2001. "The Effect of Femoral Head Diameter Upon Lubrication and Wear of Metal-On-Metal Total Hip Replacements". *Proceedings of the Institution of Mechanical Engineers, Part H: Journal of Engineering in Medicine* 215 (2): 161–170. doi:10.1243/0954411011533724.
16. Smith, S.L., D. Dowson, and A.A.J. Goldsmith. 2006. "The Effect of Diametral Clearance, Motion and Loading Cycles Upon Lubrication of Metal-On-Metal Total Hip Replacements". *Proceedings of the Institution of Mechanical Engineers, Part C: Journal of Mechanical Engineering Science* 215 (1): 1–5. doi:10.1243/0954406011520454.

17. Brockett, C.L., P. Harper, S. Williams, G.H. Isaac, R.S. Dwyer-Joyce, Z. Jin, and J. Fisher. 2008. "The Influence of Clearance on Friction, Lubrication and Squeaking in Large Diameter Metal-On-Metal Hip Replacements". *Journal of Materials Science: Materials in Medicine* 19 (4): 1575–1579. doi:10.1007/s10856-007-3298-9.
18. Nečas, D., M. Vrbka, F. Urban, J. Gallo, I. Křupka, and M. Hartl. 2017. "In Situ Observation of Lubricant Film Formation in THR Considering Real Conformity: The Effect of Diameter, Clearance and Material". *Journal of the Mechanical Behavior of Biomedical Materials* 69: 66–74. doi:10.1016/j.jmbbm.2016.12.018.
19. Medley, J.B. 2016. "Can Physical Joint Simulators Be Used to Anticipate Clinical Wear Problems of New Joint Replacement Implants Prior to Market Release?". *Proceedings of the Institution of Mechanical Engineers, Part H: Journal of Engineering in Medicine* 230 (5): 347–358. doi:10.1177/0954411916643902.
20. Fisher, J. 2011. "Bioengineering Reasons for the Failure of Metal-On-Metal Hip Prostheses". *The Journal of Bone and Joint Surgery*. British Volume 93-B (8): 1001–1004. doi:10.1302/0301-620X.93B8.26936.
21. Mavraki, A. and P.M. Cann. 2009. "Friction and Lubricant Film Thickness Measurements on Simulated Synovial Fluids". *Proceedings of the Institution of Mechanical Engineers, Part J: Journal of Engineering Tribology* 223 (3): 325–335. doi:10.1243/13506501JET580.
22. Mavraki, A., and P.M. Cann. 2011. "Lubricating Film Thickness Measurements with Bovine Serum". *Tribology International* 44 (5): 550–556. doi:10.1016/j.triboint.2010.07.008.
23. Myant, C., R. Underwood, J. Fan, and P.M. Cann. 2012. "Lubrication of Metal-On-Metal Hip Joints: The Effect of Protein Content and Load on Film Formation and Wear". *Journal of the Mechanical Behavior of Biomedical Materials* 6: 30–40. doi:10.1016/j.jmbbm.2011.09.008.
24. Myant, C., and P. Cann. 2013. "In Contact Observation of Model Synovial Fluid Lubricating Mechanisms". *Tribology International* 63: 97–104. doi:10.1016/j.triboint.2012.04.029.
25. Shinmori, H., M. Kubota, T. Morita, T. Yamaguchi, and Y. Sawae. 2020. "Effects of Synovial Fluid Constituents on Friction between UHMWPE and CoCrMo". *Tribology Online* 15 (4): 283–292. doi:10.2474/trol.15.283.
26. Vrbka, M., T. Návrat, I. Křupka, M. Hartl, P. Šperka, and J. Gallo. 2013. "Study of Film Formation in Bovine Serum Lubricated Contacts under Rolling/Sliding Conditions". *Proceedings of the Institution of Mechanical Engineers, Part J: Journal of Engineering Tribology* 227 (5): 459–475. doi:10.1177/1350650112471000.
27. Myant, C.W., and P. Cann. 2014. "The Effect of Transient Conditions on Synovial Fluid Protein Aggregation Lubrication". *Journal of the Mechanical Behavior of Biomedical Materials* 34: 349–357. doi:10.1016/j.jmbbm.2014.02.005.
28. Myant, C., and P. Cann. 2014. "On the Matter of Synovial Fluid Lubrication: Implications for Metal-On-Metal Hip Tribology". *Journal of the Mechanical Behavior of Biomedical Materials* 34: 338–348. doi:10.1016/j.jmbbm.2013.12.016.
29. Vrbka, M., I. Křupka, M. Hartl, T. Návrat, J. Gallo, and A. Galandáková. 2014. "In Situ Measurements of Thin Films In Bovine Serum Lubricated Contacts Using Optical Interferometry". *Proceedings of the Institution of Mechanical Engineers, Part H: Journal of Engineering in Medicine* 228 (2): 149–158. doi:10.1177/0954411913517498.
30. Vrbka, M., D. Nečas, M. Hartl, I. Křupka, F. Urban, and J. Gallo. 2015. "Visualization of Lubricating Films between Artificial Head and Cup With Respect to Real Geometry". *Biotribology* 1–2: 61–65. doi:10.1016/j.biotri.2015.05.002.

31. Nečas, D., M. Vrbka, D. Rebenda, J. Gallo, A. Galandáková, L. Wolfová, I. Křupka, and M. Hartl. 2018. "In Situ Observation of Lubricant Film Formation in THR Considering Real Conformity: The Effect of Model Synovial Fluid Composition". *Tribology International* 117: 206–216. doi:10.1016/j.triboint.2017.09.001.
32. Choudhury, D., D. Rebenda, S. Sasaki, P. Hekrle, M. Vrbka, and M. Zou. 2018. "Enhanced Lubricant Film Formation through Micro-Dimpled Hard-On-Hard Artificial Hip Joint: An In-Situ Observation of Dimple Shape Effects". *Journal of the Mechanical Behavior of Biomedical Materials* 81: 120–129. doi:10.1016/j.jmbbm.2018.02.014.
33. Nečas, D., M. Vrbka, F. Urban, I. Křupka, and M. Hartl. 2016. "The Effect of Lubricant Constituents on Lubrication Mechanisms in Hip Joint Replacements". *Journal of the Mechanical Behavior of Biomedical Materials* 55: 295–307. doi:10.1016/j.jmbbm.2015.11.006.
34. Nečas, D., M. Vrbka, I. Křupka, M. Hartl, and A. Galandáková. 2016."Lubrication within Hip Replacements – Implication for Ceramic-On-Hard Bearing Couples". *Journal of the Mechanical Behavior of Biomedical Materials* 61: 371–383. http://dx.doi.org/10.1016/j.jmbbm.2016.04.003.
35. Nečas, D., M. Vrbka, A. Galandáková, I. Křupka, and M. Hartl. 2019. "On The Observation of Lubrication Mechanisms within Hip Joint Replacements. Part I: Hard-On-Soft Bearing Pairs". *Journal of the Mechanical Behavior of Biomedical Materials* 89: 237–248. doi:10.1016/j.jmbbm.2018.09.022.
36. Nečas, D., M. Vrbka, J. Gallo, I. Křupka, and M. Hartl. 2019. "On the Observation of Lubrication Mechanisms within Hip Joint Replacements. Part II: Hard-On-Hard Bearing Pairs". *Journal of the Mechanical Behavior of Biomedical Materials* 89: 249–259. doi:10.1016/j.jmbbm.2018.09.026.
37. Murakami, T., and N. Ohtsuki. 1987. "Paper Xii(Iii) Lubricating Film Formation In Knee Prostheses Under Walking Conditions". In *Fluid Film Lubrication – Osborne Reynolds Centenary, Proceedings of the 13Th Leeds–Lyon Symposium on Tribology, Held In Bodington Hall, The University Of Leeds*, 387–392. Tribology Series. Elsevier. doi:10.1016/S0167-8922(08)70968-4.
38. Sawae, Y., T. Murakami, H. Higaki, and S. Moriyama. 1996. "Lubrication Property of Total Knee Prostheses with PVA Hydrogel Layer as Artificial Cartilage". *JSME International Journal. Ser. C, Dynamics, Control, Robotics, Design And Manufacturing* 39 (2): 356–364. doi:10.1299/jsmec1993.39.356.
39. Ohtsuki, N., T. Murakami, S. Moriyama, and H. Higaki. 1997. "Influence of Geometry of Conjunction on Elastohydrodynamic Film Formation in Knee Prostheses with Compliant Layer". In *Elastohydrodynamics – '96 Fundamentals And Applications In Lubrication And Traction, Proceedings of the 23Rd Leeds-Lyon Symposium on Tribology Held in the Institute of Tribology, Department of Mechanical Engineering*, 349–359. Tribology Series. Elsevier. doi:10.1016/S0167-8922(08)70464-4.
40. Flannery, M., E. Jones, and C. Birkinshaw. 2008. "Analysis of Wear And Friction of Total Knee Replacements Part Ii: Friction and Lubrication as a Function of Wear". *Wear* 265 (7–8): 1009–1016. doi:10.1016/j.wear.2008.02.023.
41. Nečas, D., K. Sadecká, M. Vrbka, J. Gallo, A. Galandáková, I. Křupka, and M. Hartl. 2019. "Observation of Lubrication Mechanisms in Knee Replacement: A Pilot Study". *Biotribology* 17: 1–7. doi:10.1016/j.biotri.2019.02.001.
42. Nečas, D., K. Sadecká, M. Vrbka, A. Galandáková, M.A. Wimmer, J. Gallo, and M. Hartl. 2021. "The Effect of Albumin and Γ-Globulin on Synovial Fluid Lubrication: Implication for Knee Joint Replacements". *Journal of the Mechanical Behavior of Biomedical Materials* 113. doi:10.1016/j.jmbbm.2020.104117.

43. Nečas, D., M. Vrbka, M. Marian, B. Rothammer, S. Tremmel, S. Wartzack, A. Galandáková, J. Gallo, M.A. Wimmer, I. Křupka, and M. Hartl, 2021. "Towards the Understanding of Lubrication Mechanisms in Total Knee Replacements – Part I: Experimental Investigations". *Tribology International* 156: 1–13. doi:10.1016/j.triboint.2021.106874.
44. Goenka, P.K., and J.F. Booker. 1980. "Spherical Bearings: Static and Dynamic Analysis via the Finite Element Method." *Journal of Lubrication Technology* 102 (3): 308–318. doi:10.1115/1.3251522.
45. Jin, Z.M., and D. Dowson. 1999. "A Full Numerical Analysis of Hydrodynamic Lubrication in Artificial Hip Joint Replacements Constructed from Hard Materials." *Proceedings of the Institution of Mechanical Engineers, Part C: Journal of Mechanical Engineering Science* 213 (4): 355–370. doi:10.1243/0954406991522310.
46. Meyer, D.M., and J.A. Tichy. 2003. "3-D Model of a Total Hip Replacement in Vivo Providing Hydrodynamic Pressure and Film Thickness for Walking and Bicycling." *Journal of Biomechanical Engineering* 125 (6): 777–784. doi:10.1115/1.1631585.
47. Pascau, A., B. Guardia, J.A. Puertolas, and E. Gómez-Barrena. 2009. "Knee Model of Hydrodynamic Lubrication during the Gait Cycle and the Influence of Prosthetic Joint Conformity." *Journal of Orthopaedic Science: Official Journal of the Japanese Orthopaedic Association* 14 (1): 68–75. doi:10.1007/s00776-008-1287-6.
48. Jin, Z.M., D. Dowson, and J. Fisher. 1997. "Analysis of Fluid Film Lubrication in Artificial Hip Joint Replacements with Surfaces of High Elastic Modulus". *Proceedings of the Institution of Mechanical Engineers, Part H: Journal of Engineering in Medicine* 211 (3): 247–256. doi:10.1243/0954411971534359.
49. Jin, Z.M., D. Dowson, J. Fisher, N. Ohtsuki, T. Murakami, H. Higaki, and S. Moriyama. 1998. "Prediction of Transient Lubricating Film Thickness in Knee Prostheses with Compliant Layers." *Proceedings of the Institution of Mechanical Engineers. Part H, Journal of Engineering in Medicine* 212 (3): 157–164. doi:10.1243/0954411981533935.
50. Marian, M., M. Bartz, S. Wartzack, and A. Rosenkranz. 2020a. "Non-Dimensional Groups, Film Thickness Equations and Correction Factors for Elastohydrodynamic Lubrication: A Review." *Lubricants* 8 (10): 95. doi:10.3390/lubricants8100095.
51. Hamrock, B.J., and D. Dowson. 1978. "Elastohydrodynamic Lubrication of Elliptical Contacts for Materials of Low Elastic Modulus I—Fully Flooded Conjunction." *Journal of Lubrication Technology* 100 (2): 236–245. doi:10.1115/1.3453152.
52. Jin, Z.M., D. Dowson, and J. Fisher. 1993. "Fluid Film Lubrication in Natural Hip Joints." In *Thin Films in Tribology, Proceedings of the 19th Leeds-Lyon Symposium on Tribology Held at the Institute of Tribology, University of Leeds* 25: 545–555. Tribology Series: Elsevier.
53. Reynolds, O. 1886. "On the Theory of Lubrication and Its Application to Mr. Beauchamp Tower's Experiments, Including an Experimental Determination of the Viscosity of Olive Oil." *Philosophical Transactions of the Royal Society of London* 177: 157–234.
54. Cross, M.M. 1965. "Rheology of Non-Newtonian Fluids: A New Flow Equation for Pseudoplastic Systems." *Journal of Colloid Science* 20 (5): 417–437. doi:10.1016/0095-8522(65)90022-X.
55. Carreau, P.J. 1972. "Rheological Equations from Molecular Network Theories." *Transactions of the Society of Rheology* 16 (1): 99–127. doi:10.1122/1.549276.
56. Mattei, L., F. Di Puccio, B. Piccigallo, and E. Ciulli. 2011. "Lubrication and Wear Modelling of Artificial Hip Joints: A Review." *Tribology International* 44 (5): 532–549. doi:10.1016/j.triboint.2010.06.010.

57. Jalali-Vahid, D., M. Jagatia, Z.M. Jin, and D. Dowson. 2000. "Elastohydrodynamic Lubrication Analysis of UHMWPE Hip Joint Replacements." In *Thinning Films and Tribological Interfaces, Proceedings of the 26th Leeds-Lyon Symposium on Tribology.* Vol. 38, 329–339. Tribology Series: Elsevier.
58. Jalali-Vahid, D., M. Jagatia, Z.M. Jin, and D. Dowson. 2001. "Prediction of Lubricating Film Thickness in a Ball-In-Socket Model with a Soft Lining Representing Human Natural And Artificial Hip Joints". *Proceedings of the Institution of Mechanical Engineers, Part J: Journal of Engineering Tribology* 215(4):363–372. doi:10.1243/1350650011543600.
59. Jalali-Vahid, D., M. Jagatia, Z.M. Jin, and D. Dowson. 2001. "Prediction of Lubricating Film Thickness in Uhmwpe Hip Joint Replacements". *Journal of Biomechanics* 34 (2): 261–266. doi:10.1016/S0021-9290(00)00181-0.
60. Jalali-Vahid, D., and Z.M. Jin. 2001. "Transient Elastohydrodynamic Lubrication Analysis of Ultra-High Molecular Weight Polyethylene Hip Joint Replacements." *Proceedings of the Institution of Mechanical Engineers, Part C: Journal of Mechanical Engineering Science* 216 (4): 409–420. doi:10.1243/0954406021525205.
61. Jalali-Vahid, D., Z.M. Jin, and D. Dowson. 2003a. "Elastohydrodynamic Lubrication Analysis of Hip Implants with Ultra High Molecular Weight Polyethylene Cups under Transient Conditions." *Proceedings of the Institution of Mechanical Engineers, Part C: Journal of Mechanical Engineering Science* 217 (7): 767–777. doi:10.1243/095440603767764417.
62. Wang, F.C., and Z.M. Jin. 2004. "Prediction of Elastic Deformation of Acetabular Cups and Femoral Heads for Lubrication Analysis of Artificial Hip Joints." *Proceedings of the IMechE* 218 (3): 201–209. doi:10.1243/1350650041323331.
63. Wang, F.C., and Z.M. Jin. 2005. "Elastohydrodynamic Lubrication Modeling of Artificial Hip Joints under Steady-State Conditions". *Journal of Tribology* 127 (4): 729–739. doi:10.1115/1.1924460.
64. Jagatia, M., and Z.M. Jin. 2001. "Elastohydrodynamic Lubrication Analysis of Metal-on-Metal Hip Prostheses under Steady State Entraining Motion." *Proceedings of the Institution of Mechanical Engineers. Part H, Journal of Engineering in Medicine* 215 (6): 531–541. doi:10.1243/0954411011536136.
65. Wang, D. 1994. "Elastohydrodynamic Lubrication of Point Contacts for Layers of 'Soft' Solids and for 'Monolithic' 'Hard' Materials in the Transient Bouncing Ball Problem." PhD Thesis, University of Leeds, UK. https://books.google.de/books?id=MM05vwEACAAJ.
66. Udofia, I.J., and Z.M. Jin. 2003. "Elastohydrodynamic Lubrication Analysis of Metal-on-Metal Hip-Resurfacing Prostheses." *Journal of Biomechanics* 36 (4): 537–544. doi:10.1016/S0021-9290(02)00422-0.
67. Wang, W.-Z., F.-C. Wang, Z.-M. Jin, D. Dowson, and Y.-Z. Hu. 2009. "Numerical Lubrication Simulation of Metal-on-Metal Artificial Hip Joint Replacements: Ball-in-Socket Model and Ball-on-Plane Model." *Proceedings of the IMechE* 223 (7): 1073–1082. doi:10.1243/13506501JET581.
68. Jalali-Vahid, D., Z.M. Jin, and D. Dowson. 2003. "Isoviscous Elastohydrodynamic Lubrication of Circular Point Contacts with Particular Reference to Metal-on-Metal Hip Implants." *Proceedings of the IMechE* 217(5):397–402. doi:10.1243/135065003322445313.
69. Williams, S., D. Jalali-Vahid, C. Brockett, Z. Jin, M.H. Stone, E. Ingham, and J. Fisher. 2006. "Effect of Swing Phase Load on Metal-on-Metal Hip Lubrication, Friction and Wear." *Journal of Biomechanics*, 2274–2281. doi:10.1016/j.jbiomech.2005.07.011.
70. Jalali-Vahid, D, Z.M. Jin, and D. Dowson. 2006. "Effect of Start-up Conditions on Elastohydrodynamic Lubrication of Metal-on-Metal Hip Implants." *Proceedings of the IMechE* 220 (3): 143–150. doi:10.1243/13506501JET150.

71. Wang, F., and Z. Jin. 2008. "Transient Elastohydrodynamic Lubrication of Hip Joint Implants." *Journal of Tribology Transaction of ASME* 130 (1). doi:10.1115/1.2806200.
72. Liu, F., Z. Jin, P. Roberts, and P. Grigoris. 2007. "Effect of Bearing Geometry and Structure Support on Transient Elastohydrodynamic Lubrication of Metal-on-Metal Hip Implants." *Journal of Biomechanics*, 1340–1349. doi:10.1016/j.jbiomech.2006.05.015.
73. Liu, F., Z.M. Jin, F. Hirt, C. Rieker, P. Roberts, and P. Grigoris. 2005. "Effect of Wear of Bearing Surfaces on Elastohydrodynamic Lubrication of Metal-on-Metal Hip Implants." *Proceedings of the Institution of Mechanical Engineers. Part H, Journal of engineering in medicine* 219 (5): 319–328. doi:10.1243/095441105X34356.
74. Liu, F., Z. Jin, P. Roberts, and P. Grigoris. 2006. "Importance of Head Diameter, Clearance, and Cup Wall Thickness in Elastohydrodynamic Lubrication Analysis of Metal-on-Metal Hip Resurfacing Prostheses." *Proceedings of the Institution of Mechanical Engineers. Part H, Journal of Engineering in Medicine* 220 (6): 695–704. doi:10.1243/09544119JEIM172.
75. Wang, F.C., and Z.M. Jin. 2007. "Effect of Non-Spherical Bearing Geometry on Transient Elastohydrodynamic Lubrication in Metal-on-Metal Hip Joint Implants." *Proceedings of the IMechE* 221 (3): 379–389. doi:10.1243/13506501JET249.
76. Wang, F.C., S.X. Zhao, A.F. Quiñonez, H. Xu, X.S. Mei, and Z.M. Jin. 2009. "Nonsphericity of Bearing Geometry and Lubrication in Hip Joint Implants." *Journal of Tribology Transactions of ASME* 131 (3). doi:10.1115/1.3118782.
77. Gao, L., P. Yang, I. Dymond, J. Fisher, and Z. Jin. 2010. "Effect of Surface Texturing on the Elastohydrodynamic Lubrication Analysis of Metal-on-Metal Hip Implants." *Tribology International* 43 (10): 1851–1860. doi:10.1016/j.triboint.2010.02.006.
78. Hu, Y.-Z., and D. Zhu. 2000. "A Full Numerical Solution to the Mixed Lubrication in Point Contacts." *Journal of Tribology* 122 (1): 1. doi:10.1115/1.555322.
79. Gao, L.M., Q.E. Meng, F. Liu, J. Fisher, and Z.M. Jin. 2010. "The Effect of Aspherical Geometry and Surface Texturing on the Elastohydrodynamic Lubrication of Metal-on-Metal Hip Prostheses under Physiological Loading and Motions." *Proceedings of the Institution of Mechanical Engineers, Part C: Journal of Mechanical Engineering Science* 224 (12): 2627–2636. doi:10.1243/09544062JMES2193.
80. Gao, L.M., Q.E. Meng, F.C. Wang, P.R. Yang, and Z.M. Jin. 2007. "Comparison of Numerical Methods for Elastohydrodynamic Lubrication Analysis of Metal-on-Metal Hip Implants: Multi-Grid Verses Newton-Raphson." *Proceedings of the IMechE* 221 (2): 133–140. doi:10.1243/13506501JET228.
81. Gao, L., F. Wang, P. Yang, and Z. Jin. 2009. "Effect of 3D Physiological Loading and Motion on Elastohydrodynamic Lubrication of Metal-on-Metal Total Hip Replacements." *Medical Engineering & Physics* 31 (6): 720–729. doi:10.1016/j.medengphy.2009.02.002.
82. Venner, C.H., and A.A. Lubrecht. 2000. *Multilevel Methods in Lubrication*. 1. Auflage. Amsterdam: Elsevier.
83. Mattei, L., B. Piccigallo, K. Stadler, E. Ciulli, and F. Di Puccio. 2009. "EHL Modeling of Hip Implants Based on a Ball-on-Plane Configuration." *Ancona, Italy: AIMETA*, 161–173.
84. Gao, L., J. Fisher, and Z. Jin. 2011. "Effect of Walking Patterns on the Elastohydrodynamic Lubrication of Metal-on-Metal Total Hip Replacements." *Proceedings of the IMechE* 225 (6): 515–525. doi:10.1177/1350650110396802.
85. Meng, Q.E., F. Liu, J. Fisher, and Z.M. Jin. 2011. "Transient Elastohydrodynamic Lubrication Analysis of a Novel Metal-on-Metal Hip Prosthesis with a Non-Spherical Femoral Bearing Surface." *Proceedings of the Institution of Mechanical Engineers. Part H, Journal of Engineering in Medicine* 225 (1): 25–37. doi:10.1243/09544119JEIM795.

86. Meng, Q., F. Liu, J. Fisher, and Z. Jin. 2013. "Contact Mechanics and Lubrication Analyses of Ceramic-on-Metal Total Hip Replacements." *Tribology International* 63: 51–60. doi:10.1016/j.triboint.2012.02.012.
87. Yao, J.Q., M.P. Laurent, T.S. Johnson, C.R. Blanchard, and R.D. Crowninshield. 2003. "The Influences of Lubricant and Material on Polymer/CoCr Sliding Friction." *Wear* 255 (1–6): 780–784. doi:10.1016/S0043-1648(03)00180-7.
88. Wang, W.-Z., Z.M. Jin, D. Dowson, and Y.Z. Hu. 2008. "A Study of the Effect of Model Geometry and Lubricant Rheology upon the Elastohydrodynamic Lubrication Performance of Metal-on-Metal Hip Joints." *Proceedings of the IMechE* 222 (3): 493–501. doi:10.1243/13506501JET363.
89. Gao, L., D. Dowson, and R.W. Hewson. 2016. "A Numerical Study of Non-Newtonian Transient Elastohydrodynamic Lubrication of Metal-on-Metal Hip Prostheses." *Tribology International* 93: 486–494. doi:10.1016/j.triboint.2015.03.003.
90. Wang, F.C., C. Brockett, S. Williams, I. Udofia, J. Fisher, and Z.M. Jin. 2008. "Lubrication and Friction Prediction in Metal-on-Metal Hip Implants." *Physics in Medicine and Biology*, 53 (5): 1277–1293. doi:10.1088/0031-9155/53/5/008.
91. Gao, L., D. Dowson, and R.W. Hewson. 2017. "Predictive Wear Modeling of the Articulating Metal-on-Metal Hip Replacements." *Journal of Biomedical Materials Research. Part B, Applied Biomaterials* 105 (3): 497–506. doi:10.1002/jbm.b.33568.
92. Gao, L., Z. Hua, and R. Hewson. 2018. "Can a "Pre-Worn" Bearing Surface Geometry Reduce the Wear of Metal-on-Metal Hip Replacements? – a Numerical Wear Simulation Study." *Wear* 406–407: 13–21. doi:10.1016/j.wear.2018.03.010.
93. Liu, F., J. Fisher, and Z. Jin. 2013. "Effect of Motion Inputs on the Wear Prediction of Artificial Hip Joints." *Tribology International* 63: 105–114. doi:10.1016/j.triboint.2012.05.029.
94. Ruggiero, A., A. Sicilia, and S. Affatato. 2020. "In Silico Total Hip Replacement Wear Testing in the Framework of ISO 14242-3 Accounting for Mixed Elasto-Hydrodynamic Lubrication Effects." *Wear* 460–461: 203420. doi:10.1016/j.wear.2020.203420.
95. Ruggiero, A., and A. Sicilia. 2020. "Lubrication Modeling and Wear Calculation in Artificial Hip Joint During the Gait." *Tribology International* 142: 105993. doi:10.1016/j.triboint.2019.105993.
96. Ruggiero, A., and A. Sicilia. 2020. "A Mixed Elasto-Hydrodynamic Lubrication Model for Wear Calculation in Artificial Hip Joints." *Lubricants* 8 (7): 72. doi:10.3390/lubricants8070072.
97. Meng, Q. 2010. "Elastohyrodynamic Lubrication in Metal-on-Metal Artificial Hip Joints with Aspherical Bearing Surfaces and Complex Structures." PhD thesis, University of Leeds.
98. Dowson, D., C. Hardaker, M. Flett, and G.H. Isaac. 2004. "A Hip Joint Simulator Study of the Performance of Metal-on-Metal Joints: Part II: Design." *The Journal of Arthroplasty* 19 (8 Suppl 3): 124–130. doi:10.1016/j.arth.2004.09.016.
99. Lu, X., D. Nečas, Q. Meng, D. Rebenda, M. Vrbka, M. Hartl, and Z. Jin. 2020. "Towards the Direct Validation of Computational Lubrication Modelling of Hip Replacements." *Tribology International* 146: 106240. doi:10.1016/j.triboint.2020.106240.
100. Tandon, P.N., and S. Jaggi. 1979. "A Model for the Lubrication Mechanism in Knee Joint Replacements." *Wear* 52 (2): 275–284. doi:10.1016/0043-1648(79)90068-1.
101. Kennedy, F.E., D.W. van Citters, K. Wongseedakaew, and M. Mongkolwongrojn. 2007. "Lubrication and Wear of Artificial Knee Joint Materials in a Rolling/Sliding Tribotester." *Journal of Tribology* 129 (2): 326. doi:10.1115/1.2464130.

102. Mongkolwongrojn, M., K. Wongseedakaew, and F.E. Kennedy. 2010. "Transient Elastohydrodynamic Lubrication in Artificial Knee Joint with Non-Newtonian Fluids." *Tribology International* 43 (5–6): 1017–1026. doi:10.1016/j.triboint.2009.12.041.
103. Su, Y., Z. Fu, P. Yang, and C. Wang. 2010. "A Full Numerical Analysis of Elastohydrodynamically Lubrication in Knee Prosthesis under Walking Condition." *Journal of Mechanics in Medicine and Biology* 10 (4): 621–641. doi:10.1142/S0219519410003605.
104. Su, Y., P. Yang, Z. Fu, Z. Jin, and C. Wang. 2011. "Time-Dependent Elastohydrodynamic Lubrication Analysis of Total Knee Replacement under Walking Conditions." *Computer Methods in Biomechanics and Biomedical Engineering* 14 (6): 539–548. doi:10.1080/10255842.2010.485569.
105. Gao, L., Z. Hua, R. Hewson, M.S. Andersen, and Z. Jin. 2018. "Elastohydrodynamic Lubrication and Wear Modelling of the Knee Joint Replacements with Surface Topography." *Biosurface and Biotribology* 4 (1): 18–23. doi:10.1049/bsbt.2017.0003.
106. Marian, M., C. Orgeldinger, B. Rothammer, D. Nečas, M. Vrbka, I. Křupka, M. Hartl, M.A. Wimmer, S. Tremmel, and S. Wartzack. 2020b. "Towards the Understanding of Lubrication Mechanisms in Total Knee Replacements – Part II: Numerical Modeling." *Tribology International*, 106809. doi:10.1016/j.triboint.2020.106809.
107. Habchi, W., I. Demirci, D. Eyheramendy, G. Morales-Espejel, and P. Vergne. 2007. "A Finite Element Approach of Thin Film Lubrication in Circular EHD Contacts." *Tribology International* 40 (10–12): 1466–1473. doi:10.1016/j.triboint.2007.01.017.
108. Habchi, W. 2018. *Finite Element Modeling of Elastohydrodynamic Lubrication Problems*. Newark: John Wiley & Sons Incorporated. https://ebookcentral.proquest.com/lib/gbv/detail.action?docID=5322515.
109. Parkes, Maria, Connor Myant, Philippa M. Cann, and Janet S.S. Wong. 2014. "The Effect of Buffer Solution Choice on Protein Adsorption and Lubrication". *Tribology International* 72: 108–117. doi:10.1016/j.triboint.2013.12.005.
110. Parkes, Maria, Connor Myant, Philippa M. Cann, and Janet S.S. Wong. 2015. "Synovial Fluid Lubrication: The Effect of Protein Interactions on Adsorbed and Lubricating Films". *Biotribology* 1–2: 51–60. doi:10.1016/j.biotri.2015.05.001.
111. Nečas, D., Y. Sawae, T. Fujisawa, K. Nakashima, T. Morita, T. Yamaguchi, M. Vrbka, I. Křupka, and M. Hartl. 2017. "The Influence of Proteins and Speed on Friction and Adsorption of Metal/Uhmwpe Contact Pair". *Biotribology* 11: 51–59. doi:10.1016/j.biotri.2017.03.003.
112. Choudhury, D., F. Urban, M. Vrbka, M. Hartl, and I. Krupka. 2015. "A Novel Tribological Study on Dlc-Coated Micro-Dimpled Orthopedics Implant Interface". *Journal of the Mechanical Behavior of Biomedical Materials* 45: 121–131. doi:10.1016/j.jmbbm.2014.11.028.
113. Dong, Y., P. Svoboda, M. Vrbka, D. Kostal, F. Urban, J. Cizek, P. Roupcova, H. Dong, I. Krupka, and M. Hartl. 2016. "Towards Near-Permanent Cocrmo Prosthesis Surface by Combining Micro-Texturing and Low Temperature Plasma Carburising". *Journal of the Mechanical Behavior of Biomedical Materials* 55: 215–227. doi:10.1016/j.jmbbm.2015.10.023.
114. Nečas, D., H. Usami, T. Niimi, Y. Sawae, I. Křupka, and M. Hartl. 2020. "Running-In Friction of Hip Joint Replacements Can Be Significantly Reduced: The Effect of Surface-Textured Acetabular Cup". *Friction* 8: 1137–1152. doi:10.1007/s40544-019-0351-x.

3 Computational Modeling of Biotribology on Artificial Knee Joints

Liming Shu
The University of Tokyo, Tokyo, Japan

Xijin Hua
University of Cambridge, Cambridge, United Kingdom

Naohiko Sugita
The University of Tokyo, Tokyo, Japan

CONTENTS

3.1 Introduction 63
3.2 Artificial Knee Joint 64
3.3 Biotribology of Artificial Knee Joint 66
    3.3.1 Lubrication Mechanism of Artificial Knee Joint 66
    3.3.2 Wear Mechanism of Artificial Knee Joint 68
3.4 Computational Modeling of Wear in Artificial Knee 69
    3.4.1 In Vitro Knee Wear Simulator 69
    3.4.2 Numerical Wear Simulator 70
    3.4.3 Elastohydrodynamic Lubrication and Wear Modeling of Artificial Knee Joint 74
        3.4.3.1 Mixed Lubrication Modeling 74
        3.4.3.2 Wear Modeling 75
    3.4.4 Effect of Daily Activities 76
    3.4.5 Patient-Specific Wear Simulator 76
3.5 Outlook 80
Appendix: Fortran User Subroutine (Umeshmotion) for 2D Wear Testing 81
References 86

3.1 INTRODUCTION

As the most important joint of the human body, the knee joint has an extremely complex anatomical structure and mechanical environment. Because the knee joint is the main joint of the lower extremities, it is susceptible to diseases such as trauma and osteoarthritis, which leads to the highest occurrence of knee disease among all bone and joint diseases. In people over 60 years of age, more than 80% of patients have radiographic signs of osteoarthritis of the knee joint, and 50% of them are painful.

DOI: 10.1201/9781003139270-3

Knee replacement surgery is the most effective method for treating this disease, which was first performed in 1968 [1]. Hitherto, 4,700,621 primary total knee replacements (TKRs) were performed in the US in 2010, which has greatly improved the quality of life [2]. TKR is a very successful method for curing these knee diseases. The prosthesis survival rate has been reported to be approximately 90% in 10 years and 80% in 20 years [3, 4]. However, it has been noted that 11%–19% of primary TKR patients are unsatisfied with the surgical outcome, while approximately 6% require revision surgery due to operative complications [5–7]. The fact that an implant "survived" does not mean user satisfaction. The patient may still be in pain or suffer from the lack of function of the knee prosthesis.

Polyethylene wear remains a major limitation of the service life of TKR in patients, especially in younger patients. It has been reported that the revision rate of TKR for patients under 60 years was five times higher than that for patients over 70 years of age. More than 20% of these revisions were caused by wear of the tibial insert [8, 9]. In vitro knee wear simulators have been developed and widely used in the preclinical evaluation of implant designs to understand the polyethylene wear mechanisms of bearing materials [10–13]. However, they only focused on a single basic daily activity (walking), which does not meet the requirements of an increasing number of younger patients. Further, although in vitro testing is invaluable for preclinical evaluation, it is relatively time-consuming and costly. An in vitro knee wear simulator operating at one Hz requires approximately two months to complete a 5 million cycle test [14]. Hence, computational methods for preclinical wear testing of TKR under various dynamic loading conditions have been studied owing to the lower cost and calculation time of such methods [13, 15, 16]. In this section, a state-of-the-art introduction of computational biotribology on artificial knee joints is presented.

3.2 ARTIFICIAL KNEE JOINT

More than 150 types of prostheses have been designed and evaluated since the 1950s to mimic the biomechanics of a normal knee joint [17]. Knee prostheses can be divided into three types based on whether the femorotibial joint is constrained or not, which is known as constrained (hinged) TKR, unconstrained (cruciate-retaining design, posterior stabilized design) TKR, and semi-constrained (medial pivot design) TKR. Additionally, the unconstrained and semi-constrained TKR could also be divided into fixed and mobile bearings based on whether polyethylene can rotate on the tibial tray component. Figure 3.1 presents a typical mobile-bearing cruciate-retaining TKR design that is composed of a femoral component (FC), tibial insert (TI), tibial tray (TT), and patella button (PB). Generally, during TKR, the lower end of the thigh bone is removed and replaced with the FC, and the upper end of the lower leg bone is removed and replaced with the TT component. The TI was placed between the FC and TT in the TKR system. The posterior surface of the patella was cemented to the patella using bone cement. The TI and PB components interact with the FC and restore the functionality of the cartilage and the menisci in a normal knee joint.

The materials used to fabricate the FC and TT components are generally cobalt chromium molybdenum alloy (CoCrMo). The TI and PB components are usually made up of ultra-high-molecular-weight polyethylene (UHMWPE), which has high abrasion resistance. Both CoCrMo and UHMWPE were biocompatible, with a low

Computational Modeling of Biotribology

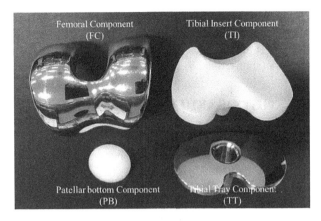

FIGURE 3.1 Components of a normal knee prosthesis.

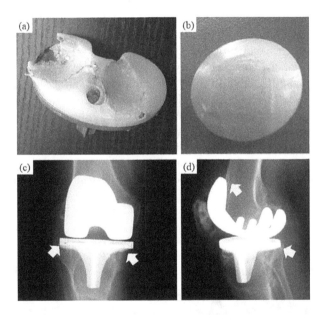

FIGURE 3.2 Wear (a, b) and loosening (c, d) of the artificial knee joint.

coefficient of contact friction. Since the late 1990s, highly cross-linked UHMWPE was introduced into the TI and PB design to reduce wear and debris-induced osteolysis following joint arthroplasty. High-cross-linked UHMWPE was developed by exposing UHMWPE to gamma radiation to break up intramolecular bonds and produce free radicals that promote cross-linking across multiple polymer chains, thereby increasing the overall density and improving the wear characteristics. It is worth noting that different wear mechanisms were found between different conventional and highly cross-linked UHMWPE, which will be explained in the next section.

Figure 3.2 illustrates the wear and loosening of TKR, which is one of the main reasons for TKR failure. Friction caused by joint surfaces rubbing against each other wears away the surface of the implant, causing bone loss and loosening of the implants. The factors influencing wear mechanism and amount of wear generation include joint kinematics, implant design, material properties, micromotion between the TI and backing metal tray, and alignment of the TKR components.

3.3 BIOTRIBOLOGY OF ARTIFICIAL KNEE JOINT

3.3.1 Lubrication Mechanism of Artificial Knee Joint

A normal knee joint is surrounded by a membrane and the synovium, which produces a small amount of thick fluid known as synovial fluid. The synovial fluid helps to nourish the cartilage and maintain the slipperiness of the knee. The efficiency of lubrication has a remarkable influence on the lifetime of the TKR. Thus, the role of synovial fluid in the lubrication of TKR or the lubrication mechanism has attracted great interest in recent years. In engineering, lubrication can be divided into three regimes: boundary, mixed, and hydrodynamic lubrication. According to previous studies on lubrication of TKR, the lubrication between the FC and TI mainly occurs in the mixed lubrication region. In 2021, Nečas et al. [18] and Marian et al. [19] presented a comprehensive investigation of the lubrication mechanisms in TKR from novel experimental and numerical analyses. They used mercury lamp-induced fluorescence to observe the lubricant film formation and confirmed mixed lubrication between the TI and FC components. Notably, the film formation is sensitive to the geometry of the TKR design and loading. Nečas et al. [18] found that film formation was partially disrupted on the medial side of the TKR because of the high contact pressure between the FC and TI components.

Figure 3.3 presents the lubrication model, which considers the behavior of the individual constituents in the model synovial fluid. The main components of synovial

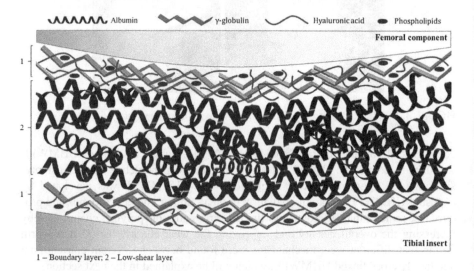

FIGURE 3.3 Lubrication model of TKA [18].

Computational Modeling of Biotribology

fluid are albumin, γ-globulin, hyaluronic acid, and phospholipids. The adsorption characteristics of the different proteins in the synovial fluid led to a layered arrangement of proteins and subsequently form a special boundary lubrication film. γ-globulin exhibits stronger adsorption on hydrophobic surfaces. UHMWPE is known as a highly hydrophobic material, and CoCrMo is neither hydrophobic nor hydrophilic. Thus, a stable, thin, and uniform γ-globulin film is formed on the contact surfaces of the femoral and TI components. The albumin film is formed between two γ-globulin layers owing to its good ability to attach to the boundary layer. Further, the α-helix of albumin creates strong mutual bonds, enhancing the lubricating film.

Marian et al. [19] developed a fully coupled transient 3D model for a soft elastohydrodynamically lubricated contact based on the generalized Reynolds equation and the finite element method, as shown in Figure 3.4. A good agreement was found between the numerical model and the experimental investigation by Nečas et al. [18].

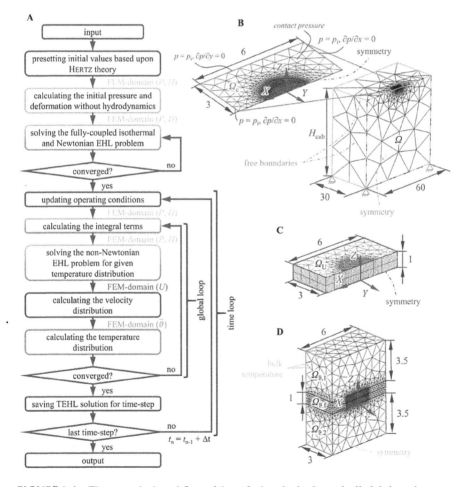

FIGURE 3.4 The numerical workflow of the soft elastohydrodynamically lubricated contact based upon the generalized Reynolds equation and finite element method [19].

They presented the medial side of the TKR prone to solid asperity contact instead of mixed lubrication owing to the high contact pressure. Additionally, the individual rheological synovial fluid parameters would also significantly affect the lubrication condition of the TKR.

3.3.2 Wear Mechanism of Artificial Knee Joint

Despite numerous attempts to develop a detailed theoretical basis for wear models, wear prediction remains largely a part of empirical science. In 1957, Archard and Hirst found that the wear depth at each location is dependent on its sliding distance and contact pressure (CP), which is known as the classical Archard's wear law [20]:

$$H_{wear} = kpS, \tag{3.1}$$

where H_{wear} is the wear depth, k is a constant wear factor, p is the CP, and S is the sliding distance between the contact pairs. The mass loss (m_{wear}) owing to wear can be calculated by integrating the wear depth as follows:

$$m_{wear} = k\rho \int SpdA. \tag{3.2}$$

where ρ is the density, and dA is the difference in the contact area. The constant wear coefficient (k) was acquired using a one-direction roll-on-plane experiment.

Many extended Archard's wear laws have been established for the wear estimation of TKR. Innocenti et al. [21] highlighted that the friction coefficient (μ) has a significant effect on the wear of the contact pair. To include the friction parameter in Archard's wear law, the extended model is expressed as follows:

$$m_{wear} = k\rho\left(1+3\mu^2\right)^{0.5} \int SpdA, \tag{3.3}$$

Wang et al. [22] and Kang et al. [23] demonstrated that the cross-shear (CS) ratio and CP significantly affect the wear coefficient during pin-on-plate wear testing on highly cross-linked UHMWPE. The CS ratio is defined as the fraction of the total friction work that is perpendicular to the principal molecular orientation (PMO) of the polyethylene chains:

$$CS = \frac{\Sigma_{inc} W_\perp}{\Sigma_{inc}\left(W_\perp + W_\parallel\right)}, \tag{3.4}$$

where inc is the increment of the whole wear simulation, and $W_\perp$ and $W_\parallel$ are the frictional work parallel and perpendicular to the PMO direction, respectively.

For the adapted Archard's wear law with consideration of the CS ratio [24], the mass loss can be expressed as:

$$m_{wear} = \rho \int SC\left(\text{fun}(CS)\right)dA. \tag{3.5}$$

Computational Modeling of Biotribology

where $C(\text{fun}(CS))$ is the non-dimensional wear coefficient that depends on the CS ratio. However, Abdelgaied et al. [25] highlighted that the constant wear coefficient is also dependent on the CP and material properties of the bearing material. Thus, a renewed adapted Archard's wear law is expressed as:

$$m_{wear} = \rho \int SC\left(\text{fun}\left(CS, \frac{CP}{E}\right)\right) dA, \tag{3.6}$$

where $C(\text{fun}(CS, CP/E))$ is the non-dimensional wear coefficient that depends on the CS ratio and CP on the contact surfaces, and E is the elastic modulus of the bearing material.

3.4 COMPUTATIONAL MODELING OF WEAR IN ARTIFICIAL KNEE

3.4.1 In Vitro Knee Wear Simulator

Retrieval analysis of implant components plays an important role in determining the efficacy of new designs and provides an invaluable resource for laboratory investigations. Table 3.1 illustrates the measured wear rates of different TKR designs in the in vivo wear measurements. The mobile-bearing TKR generally exhibited a lower wear rate than that of the fixed-bearing TKR. This difference may be explained by the rotational freedom between the TI and TT components.

Several types of in vitro wear simulators have been used to investigate the anti-wear performance of artificial knee joints in the design phase. The Stanmore knee simulator is one of the most widely used knee simulators in wear testing. The simulator can be divided into two types according to the different controlled approaches: displacement- and force-controlled knee simulators. The testing was performed on the synovial fluid of bovine to mimic the biotribological condition of TKR in humans. In the force-controlled knee simulator, four non-linear springs are arranged parallelly around the TT component, simplifying the ligament constraints in a knee joint. Based on the actual knee joint laxity, the translation and rotation resistances were set to 9.3 N/mm and 0.36 N·m/°, respectively. Most of the wear testing followed the ISO standard (14243) and American Society for Testing and Materials (ASTM) standard (732) to unify the experimental conditions. The flexion–extension (F–E) rotation,

TABLE 3.1
Measurement of Wear Rate in TKR

TKR	Bearing	Wear rate (mm/year)	Reference
PFC Synatomic (DePuy)	Fixed	0.35	[26]
Interax (Stryker)	Fixed	0.23	[27]
Unicompartmental (Biomet)	Mobile	0.02	[28]
Anatomic Graduated Component (Biomet)	Fixed	0.10	[29]
Low Contact Stress (DePuy)	Mobile	0.053	[30]

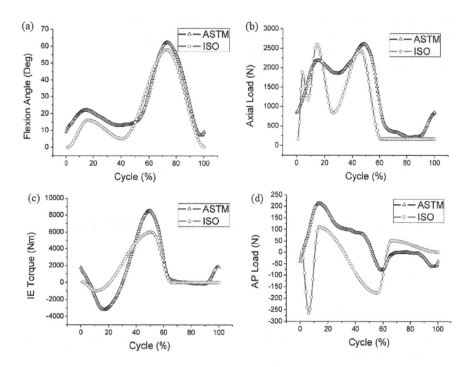

FIGURE 3.5 The boundary condition from ISO 1423-1: 2009 and ASTM F3141: 2017 [31].

axial force, anterior–posterior (A–P) force, and internal–external (I–E) torque were set as the inputs of wear testing to mimic the joint loading of TKR patients, as shown in Figure 3.5. A significant difference in both the magnitude and trend can be found between the ISO standard (14243) and the ASTM standard (732). Some researchers have stated that the ASTM standard (732) presented a condition similar to that of human gait [31].

3.4.2 Numerical Wear Simulator

The numerical wear simulator has attracted great interest in the last two decades owing to the high cost and time-consuming nature of in vitro wear testing. The majority of computational wear studies of artificial knee joints have focused on the TI and PB components. According to Archard's wear law, it is necessary to calculate the sliding distance (kinematics) and CP between the contact pairs. Numerical wear simulations can be divided into multi-body dynamics (MD) simulations and finite element (FE) simulations. Table 3.2 presents a simple comparison between the MD and FE methods. It is difficult to acquire accurate CP using the MD method owing to the rigid body assumption. Thus, with the modern advancement in computer technology, most state-of-the-art wear simulators have been developed based on the FE method. Figure 3.6 illustrates a typical force-controlled FE wear model that was created based on the Stanmore knee simulator. It can be found that the wear simulator is

TABLE 3.2
Difference between Multi-body Dynamics (MD) Simulation and Finite Element (FE) Simulation

Parameter	Finite Element Method	MD
Assumption	Body – deformable	Rigid body
Shape	Shape changes	No shape change
Output variables (Common)	Stress, Strain, Strain rate	Acceleration, Velocity, Loads on moving bodies
Efficiency	Slow	Fast

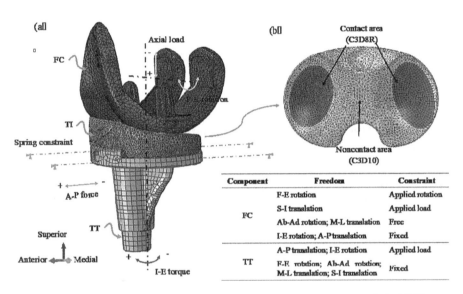

FIGURE 3.6 FE model with force-control loading conditions for wear prediction [32].

still created based on the simplified knee models (Stanmore knee simulator) that do not consider the muscle force and interaction between the femur and patella.

Figure 3.7 presents the computational workflow of the wear simulation. The CP, slide distance, CS ratio, wear depth calculation, and geometry updating were incorporated into a single function. The constant wear factor or non-dimensional wear coefficient should first be determined from the pin-on-disk experiment to calculate the wear depth.

Table 3.3 summarized the typical constant wear factor from the latest research. A significant difference could be found among previous studies. In comparison with the in vitro experimental results (Figure 3.8a), a much higher predicted accuracy was found on the results based on the adapted Archard wear model from Abdelgaied et al., [25] (Figure 3.8b) than that based on the classical Archard-based wear model from Innocenti et al. [21] (Figure 3.8c). In other words, it is necessary to consider the effect of CP and CS on wear factor in computational wear modeling.

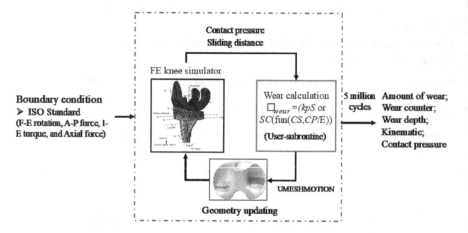

FIGURE 3.7 The computational workflow in wear simulation [32].

TABLE 3.3
Constant Wear Factor in TKR Wear Simulation

Polyethylene Type	Constant Wear Factor	Reference
Non-cross-linked	$1.03 \pm 0.22\text{e-}7$ mm^3/Nm	[33]
Non-cross-linked	$10^{-8.895} \times (8.517 \times 10^{-5} + 9.365 \times CS)^{0.148}$	[24]
Moderately cross-linked	$10^{-8.964} \times (3.4823 \times 10^{-6} + 2.057 \times CS)^{0.191}$	[24]
Highly cross-linked	$1.837\text{e-}8$ mm^3/Nm	[21]
Highly cross-linked	$10^{-9} \times [1.47 \times (1 - \exp(-116.21 \times CS)) \times (0.84 + 450.23 \times (CP/E)^{1.49})]$	[25]

The surface geometry should be updated based on the wear loss calculated. The direction of wear on each node was normal to the contact surface, and the magnitude was the predicted wear depth at the end of each increment. Each loading cycle was divided into small increments, and the wear was calculated for each increment and summed over the entire cycle. Two types of alternative surface adaptation strategies are used in geometrical updating: node translation and adaptive meshing (Figure 3.9). The node translation approach adjusts the surface node directly from the calculated wear depth, whereas adaptive meshing allows the user to specify a region of elements in which Abaqus can automatically adjust the interior nodes to maintain the element quality. Thus, adaptive meshing has better prediction accuracy for CP and stress than node translation. This is because the latter can increase the stress concentration and convergence problem owing to poor element quality. A sample code for the 2D wear simulation based on the classical Archard's wear law is added in this chapter's Appendix.

With the calculated wear depth in a single loading cycle, the total wear was calculated by multiplying the linear wear depths of the nodes with the number of cycles in an update interval, after which the surface topography was adjusted accordingly. Five

Computational Modeling of Biotribology

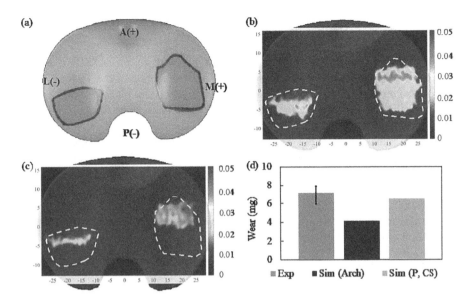

FIGURE 3.8 Comparison of the predicted wear contour by (a) Archard-based wear contour, (b) the adapted Archard-based wear contour, and (c) experimental results. (d) Comparison of the amount of wear mass in the experiment (Exp), classical Archard-based model (Sim (Arch)), and adapted Archard-based wear model (Sim (P, CS)) [32].

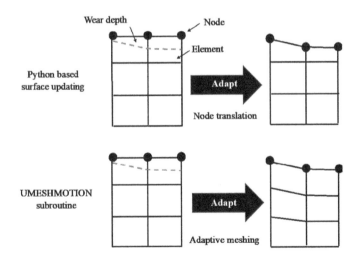

FIGURE 3.9 Comparison of two alternative surface adaptation strategies in wear simulation.

million cycles (mc) were conducted for each test, as per ISO 14243–1:2009 standards. However, it would still take an exceedingly long calculation time as the surface updates every loading cycle. Thus, a large update interval (0.1 to 0.2 mc) was used for a total of 5 mc based on a convergence study on the effect of the update interval on the wear rate.

3.4.3 ELASTOHYDRODYNAMIC LUBRICATION AND WEAR MODELING OF ARTIFICIAL KNEE JOINT

Mixed lubrication in the knee joint is believed to be an important factor in the wear of TKR. The integration of lubrication into the wear modeling of the TKR is therefore important to accurately predict implant wear. However, the challenge of addressing lubrication in wear modeling lies in the complicated wear mechanism when lubrication is involved, particularly for multiple contacts and complicated geometry in the knee joint. By assuming the contacts between the femoral condyles and TI as ball-in-socket geometry with uniform curvature radii, Gao et al. [34] recently developed an advanced lubrication-wear model for lubricated knee joints in which the lubrication parameters were coupled in the wear factor through an adapted Archard wear formula [35].

The advanced lubrication-wear modeling was composed of two parts: mixed lubrication modeling and wear modeling.

3.4.3.1 Mixed Lubrication Modeling

For mixed lubrication modeling, a full film regime was first considered, in which the thin film lubrication was governed by the Reynolds equation formulated in spherical coordinates (θ, φ) [36]:

$$\frac{\partial}{\partial \varphi}\left(\frac{h^3}{\eta}\frac{\partial p}{\partial \varphi}\right) + \sin\theta \frac{\partial}{\partial \theta}\left(\frac{h^3}{\eta}\sin\theta \frac{\partial p}{\partial \theta}\right) = -6R^2 \sin^2\theta \left(\omega \frac{\partial h}{\partial \varphi} + 2\frac{\partial h}{\partial t}\right) \quad (3.7)$$

where p is the fluid pressure, h is the fluid film thickness, η is the viscosity of the joint synovial fluid, R is the uniform curvature radius of the TI, and w is the flexion-extension angular rotation speed. The film thickness (h) including both the rigid geometric gap and elastic deformation (δ) between the two bearing surfaces, was calculated as:

$$h(\varphi, \theta) = c - e_x \sin\theta\cos\varphi - e_y \sin\theta\sin\varphi - e_z\cos\theta + \delta(p) \quad (3.8)$$

where c is the radial clearance and e_x, e_y, and e_z are the eccentricity components. The elastic deformation (δ) of the tibial surface was determined to be proportional to the local pressure.

When the calculated film thickness (h) was smaller than the thickness of $h_B = 20$ nm, which was assumed to be the thickness of the molecular layer of synovial fluid absorbed on the surface [37], the lubrication regime was switched to the boundary lubrication mode. In this case, the film thickness was assumed to be equal to the thickness h_B, i.e. $h(p) = h_B$, and the elastic deformation and pressure were calculated using Eq. 9 and Eq. 10, respectively [34]:

$$h_0 = c - e_x \sin\theta\cos\varphi - e_y \sin\theta\sin\varphi - e_z\cos\theta + \delta(\varphi, \theta) \quad (3.9)$$

$$\delta(\varnothing, \theta) = \iint_{\varnothing\theta} K(\varnothing - \varnothing', \theta - \theta', \theta_m) p(\varnothing', \theta') d\theta d\varnothing \quad (3.10)$$

Computational Modeling of Biotribology

An equivalent spherical discrete convolution (ESDC) technique [38] and multi-level multi-integration (MLMI) [39] were used to calculate the surface elastic deformation. K represents the influence coefficient of the elastic surfaces, and θ_m is the fixed mean latitude.

3.4.3.2 Wear Modeling

An advanced wear model, which coupled the mixed lubricated condition of TKR, was developed and adopted to predict the bearing surface wear evolution in the implant. The wear model was based on an adapted Archard wear formula [35], in which the wear factor was proposed as a power function of the "λ ratio," which is defined as the ratio of film thickness to the average surface roughness (R_a). The linear wear rate of the implant was calculated as [34]:

$$\text{wear rate} = \begin{cases} k_\omega p v \left(\dfrac{1}{\lambda}\right)^a, & \text{if } \lambda < 3 \\ 0, & \text{if } \lambda \geq 3 \end{cases} \tag{3.11}$$

$$\lambda = h / R_a \tag{3.12}$$

where k_w is the constant wear parameter, and the power term (a) determines how sensitive the transition to wear occurs with a decreasing film thickness.

The relative sliding speed of the articular surfaces was calculated using the following equation:

$$v = \sqrt{v_\theta^2 + v_\varphi^2} \tag{3.13}$$

$$\begin{cases} v_\theta = -R\omega_x \sin\varphi \\ v_\varphi = -R\omega_x \cos\varphi \cos\theta \end{cases} \tag{3.14}$$

Once the wear rate and the sliding speed were calculated, the linear wear at an arbitrary point (i, j) on the bearing surface at the k_{th} time step in one gait cycle could be derived using the following equation:

$$W_L^{i,j}(k) = k_w p_{i,j} v_{i,j} \nabla t \left(\dfrac{R_a}{h_{i,j}}\right)^a \tag{3.15}$$

The wear depth in one cycle at point (i, j) was summer as:

$$W_{L\_cyc}^{i,j} = \sum_{k=1}^{n} W_L^{i,j}(k) \tag{3.16}$$

Within N gait cycles, if the change in the surface profile due to wear was not large enough to alter the lubrication, the wear depth per N cycles at the point (i, j) was calculated as:

$$W_{L\_tot}^{i,j} \simeq N \cdot W_{L\_cyc}^{i,j} \tag{3.17}$$

And the volume wear was calculated as a product of the linear wear and the area of the mesh cell with that point as vertex:

$$W_{vol} = \sum_{i=1}^{m}\sum_{i=1}^{m}\left(W_{L-tot}^{i,j} \times A_{i,j}\right) \qquad (3.18)$$

The area of each mesh cell on the assumed spherical surface was approximated as the area of the trapezoid because the curvature was small enough compared to the cup radius:

$$A_{i,j} \approx \left(\frac{\pi R}{m}\right)^2 \cdot \sin\theta_{i,j} \qquad (3.19)$$

It is assumed that the surface profile of the implant does not alter the lubrication state within N gait cycles. However, after a certain number of cycles when the worn surface geometry was large enough to affect the pressure and film thickness, the surface profile needed to be updated for the lubrication simulation, and new pressures and film thicknesses were obtained and used to calculate the following cycles.

3.4.4 Effect of Daily Activities

Walking profiles, which is the most prevalent motor task [40], have been widely applied in wear testing of TKR implants. However, it is known that the type of daily activity has a significant effect on the wear rate of polyethylene bearings. Higher local contact stress and kinematics were found during squatting, rising from a chair, and going up and down stairs [41], which can affect prosthesis durability by activating different polyethylene wear and failure mechanisms. During the development of in silico polyethylene wear simulation of TKR, different wear behaviors of various activities should be considered, other than walking [42–45]. Table 3.4 summarizes the wear factor under different daily activities from the simulation and experiment. A significant difference in the wear factor may be caused by different geometrical designs and material properties of TIs. According to the computational results from Shu et al. [32], the wear risk of daily activities can be ranked in the order of squatting, walking upstairs, level walking, walking-ISO, walking downstairs, standing and sitting, and cycling.

3.4.5 Patient-Specific Wear Simulator

Patient-specific, also called subject-specific, means customizing the object to the precise anatomy, physiology, mechanics, and kinematics of a single person. The knee joint was subjected to substantial external loading during different daily activities. These loadings, along with the kinematics and anatomy of the knee joint, vary from person to person, which impacts the wear behavior of the knee joint replacements. Therefore, patient-specific wear modeling has been developed to improve the

TABLE 3.4
Comparison of Wear Factor of Knee Prosthesis due for Activity

Activity	Computational Wear Factor from Shu et al. [32] (mg/mc)	Computational Wear Factor from Abdelgaied et al. [25] (mg/mc)	Experimental Wear Factor from Abdelgaied et al. [25] (mg/mc)	Experimental Wear Factor from Reinders et al. [44] (mg/mc)
Walking-ISO	1.32	4.09	5.28	5.59
Level walking	1.57	–	–	17.90
Squatting	2.57	3.37	3.18	–
Standing and sitting	0.63	–	–	2.64
Walking upstairs	1.71	5.10	6.46	8.08
Walking downstairs	1.20	–	–	6.40

accuracy of the model and accelerate implant design. As opposed to the conventional wear simulation, where the load and motions in ISO 14243 were adopted as input, the patient-specific wear modeling normally used patient-specific forces, patient-specific joint motions, or both as inputs.

There are three elements for patient-specific wear modeling: patient-specific knee loading, patient-specific knee kinematics, and patient-specific implant. Based on these three elements, patient-specific wear modeling can be divided into three categories:

(1) *Patient-specific in vivo kinematic data.* Early attempts at patient-specific wear modeling used patient-specific in vivo kinematics as inputs, combining a dynamic contact model and a computational wear model [46]. First, in vivo fluoroscopic kinematics data (anterior-posterior translation, internal-external rotation, and flexion) were collected from a total knee arthroplasty patient. Subsequently, a dynamic contact model was developed and used to perform two simulations: a forward dynamics simulation that predicted the contact forces and remaining kinematics (axial translation, varus-valgus rotation, and medial-medial lateral translation) and a subsequent inverse dynamics simulation that predicted accurate CPs and slip velocities. Finally, the calculated CPs and slip velocities were input into a computational wear model to predict the implant wear. The implant wear in this model was given by the total damage depth, which is the sum of the material removal due to mild wear and surface deformation due to compressive creep. The main limitation of this method was that there was no advancement to the kinematics due to the change in implant geometry resulting from the wear. Because the load distribution on the articular surface of the implant and the kinematics of the knee joint determine the implant wear, which in turn can alter the load distribution and kinematics, the

interaction among the knee joint load, kinematics, and implant wear are vitally important, and a novel patient-specific wear model that takes into account the interaction should be developed.

(2) *Multiscale modeling couples a musculoskeletal multi-body dynamics (MBD) model, an FE TKR model, and a wear model.* By applying the musculoskeletal MBD model, a patient-specific computational weal modeling framework that couples a patient-specific lower-limb musculoskeletal MBD model and an FE TKR wear model was developed [40]. The patient-specific musculoskeletal MBD model integrates the patient's body anatomy, body inertia, mass distribution, and gait pattern and applies the principles of rigid body dynamics and statics to the body to predict the joint reaction forces and torques, muscle forces, and motion of the knee joint, based on the motion capture data and ground reaction forces measured from the gait lab. In the modeling framework, a patient-specific musculoskeletal MBD model with an instrumented knee implant was developed, which was used to calculate the medial, lateral, and total tibia-femoral (TF) and patellofemoral (PF) contact forces, ligament forces, and knee joint motions during gait. These outputs were then inputted into a detailed FE model for the same knee implant as the boundary conditions. The CP and the sliding distance of the implants were then calculated from the FE model and given as input to a wear model developed by Abdelgaied et al. [25] to calculate the wear and creep in the implant. The geometry of the implant was also updated and then imported to the musculoskeletal MBD model to calculate the new joint load and movements. This process was repeated until the required cycle was completed. The entire process of the patient-specific computational Weibull modeling framework is shown in Figure 3.10. Because

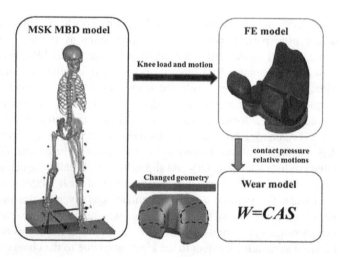

FIGURE 3.10 A patient-specific wear modeling framework combined a patient-specific musculoskeletal multi-body dynamics model, a detailed FE total knee replacement model, and a wear model [48].

Computational Modeling of Biotribology

the variation of the implant geometry has been reported to affect the load and motion of the knee joint in the musculoskeletal MBD model [47], the novelty of this modeling framework is that the updated worn geometry of the implants calculated by the wear model is exported to the musculoskeletal MBD model for new load and motion prediction.

(3) *Patient-specific TKR*. In contrast to the above three wear models, this type of modeling used the conventional wear formulation described in Section 3.4.2, but with a patient-specific TKR, to reduce implant wear [49, 50], optimizing implant design [51], and designing a unicompartmental TKR [52]. In these models, the patient-specific implant model was developed using an existing 3D model of the knee joint with actual anatomical geometries that were created based on the computed tomography (CT) and magnetic resonance imaging (MRI) of the patient. Specifically, the FC of the implant was created using the anatomic articulating surface geometry of the femoral bone on the sagittal and coronal planes, where three patient-specific "J" curves for the trochlear groove and the medial and lateral condyles were developed. The tibial component was designed according to the outline of the patient's tibia. A typical design workflow for a patient-specific knee implant is shown in Figure 3.11. [13] When the femoral and tibial components of the TKR were created, an FE model for the TKR was developed, and a conventional wear model described

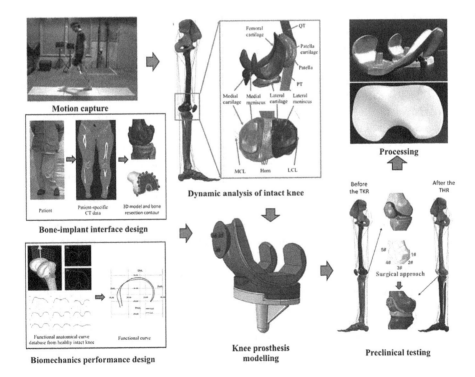

FIGURE 3.11 The design of patient-specific TKR [13].

in Section 3.4.2, for example, the knee kinematics measured from the Stanmore knee simulator, and the CPs and sliding distance predicted from the FE model were input to Archard's wear law to calculate the implant wear.

3.5 OUTLOOK

In-depth knowledge of the biotribology of an artificial knee joint could significantly enhance the service life of a total knee replacement and thus improve the quality of life of the patients. Wear testing from either experimental or computational aspects has provided an efficient approach for the preclinical analysis of artificial knee joints. It fosters advances in biomechanics analysis, better decision-making in surgery, and acceleration of the design of implant updates. However, the practical and widespread use of the presented method will still be limited until the following challenges are overcome.

(1) Lubrication plays an important role in joint replacement wear. Studies on lubrication and wear of both hip and knee joints have highlighted the importance and necessity of including wear and lubrication in the numerical simulation of joint replacements [11, 18]. However, owing to the complex geometry and the lubrication mechanism of TKR, the lubrication theory and calculations applied to the TKR are severely lacking. The primary study on the lubrication and wear of TKR conducted by Gao et al. [34] is limited, as they assume the contact between the femoral and tibial components as a ball-in-socket articulation. However, real TKR articulating surfaces are typically aspherical, and the roughness of the surface and the eastohydrodynamic lubrication (EHL) fluid film thickness is at the same level. Therefore, future work on developing a more realistic numerical lubrication and wear model should consider the real TKR surface geometry and surface roughness.

(2) Most of the wear simulators of the knee are created based on the classical Stanmore knee simulator. It does not consider the muscle force and interaction between the femur and patella. A higher fidelity knee simulator, considering the patellofemoral joint, muscle loading, and patient-specific differences, should be considered in future studies. For instance, higher prediction accuracy was achieved by combining the FE method with musculoskeletal modeling [53].

(3) The knee joint is subjected to substantial external loading during routine activities. However, current studies on TKR wear have mainly focused on normal gait. With the development of kinematics and kinetics studies of the human body, comprehensive wear modeling that considers different routine activities, such as running, upstairs, and downstairs, should be developed in the future. In particular, a multiscale modeling approach that couples a patient-specific musculoskeletal model and wear modeling should be conducted in the future.

(4) Current numerical simulations of the TKR were mainly focused on normal conditions. Future studies should consider simulating the biotribology of the TKR under adverse conditions, such as an off-the-shelf TKR, to gain a full understanding of the wear mechanism of the TKR in practice.

(5) Although wear modeling for TKR has been widely developed, few studies have been conducted in clinical practice. Future studies should also be conducted in clinical practice to exploit computational modeling. By comparing the results from the numerical simulation with the clinical observations, a complete understanding of the wear mechanism in TKR could be obtained. Further, wear modeling could be widely applied to special designs, such as unicompartmental knee arthroplasty, and by investigating the effect of various surgical techniques and implant component positions on TKR performance, it could be used to guide TKR surgery.

APPENDIX: FORTRAN USER SUBROUTINE (UMESHMOTION) FOR 2D WEAR TESTING

(Note: The loading condition is based on the study from McColl et al., [54])

```
C      USER INPUT FOR ADAPTIVE MESH CONSTRAINT
C      debris interfact is controlled by a function of stress, thickness
C      and so on.
C
       SUBROUTINE UMESHMOTION(UREF,ULOCAL,NODE,NNDOF,
     & LNODETYPE,ALOCAL,NDIM,TIME,DTIME,PNEWDT,
     & KSTEP,KINC,KMESHSWEEP,JMATYP,JGVBLOCK)
C
       INCLUDE 'ABA_PARAM.INC'
C
       DIMENSION ULOCAL(NDIM),JELEMLIST(100000)
       DIMENSION ALOCAL(NDIM,100000),TIME(2)
       DIMENSION JMATYP(100000),JGVBLOCK(100000)
C
       INTEGER flag1,cnt1
C
       INTEGER master
C
       REAL CPRESS,CSHEAR,CSLIP,COPEN,XCOORD,YCOORD,INCSLIP
C
       REAL CPRESS_R,CPRESS_L,INCSLIP_R,INCSLIP_L,grad_pr,grad_sl
C
       DIMENSION ARRAY(15)
C
       INTEGER LOCNUM,NELEMMAX
       CHARACTER PARTNAME
C
       REAL W_dist
C
       REAL X_error, Y_error
       common/wear/
```

```
     & ilastnode,
     & ilastnode2,
     & isclock,
     & imclock,
     & isnodes(2000),
     & imnodes(2000),
     & oldslip(2000),
     & tempslip(2000),
     & spress(2000),
     & sxcrd(2000),
     & sycrd(2000),
     & sincslip(2000),
     & islavereg(100000),
     & imasterreg(100000),
     & wearm(2000),
     & wears(2000)
C
C
      flag1=0
      cnt1=1
C
      master=0
C
C
      CPRESS_L=0
      CPRESS_R=0
      INCSLIP_L=0
      INCSLIP_R=0
      X_L=1.001*XCOORD
      X_R=0.999*XCOORD
C
h_crit=0.001
C
      NELEMMAX = 1000
      NELEMS = NELEMMAX
C
OPEN(unit=216,file='/home/shu/sh/debugref.txt',
     $     status='unknown')
OPEN(unit=217,file='/home/shu/sh/2Dva_185.txt',
     $     status='unknown')
ilastnode=NODE
      CALL
GETNODETOELEMCONN(NODE,NELEMS,JELEMLIST,JELEMTYPE,
     $     JRCD,JGVBLOCK)
      LOCNUM = 0
      JRCD = 0
```

```
      JTYP=0
      PARTNAME = ' '
C
      CALL GETPARTINFO(NODE,0,PARTNAME,LOCNUM,JRCD)
C
      CALL GETVRMAVGATNODE(NODE,JTYP,'CSTRESS',ARRAY,JRCD,
& JELEMLIST,NELEMS,JMATYP,JGVBLOCK)
      CPRESS = ARRAY(1)
      CSHEAR = ARRAY(2)
C
      CALL GETVRMAVGATNODE(NODE,JTYP,'CDISP',ARRAY,JRCD,
& JELEMLIST,NELEMS,JMATYP,JGVBLOCK)
      CSLIP = ARRAY(2)
      COPEN = ARRAY(1)
      CALL GETVRN(NODE,'COORD',ARRAY,JRCD,JGVBLOCK,LTRN)
      XCOORD=ARRAY(1)
      YCOORD=ARRAY(2)
      flag1=0
C
C
      IF((CPRESS==0).AND.(COPEN==-0.100000E+37))THEN
C
         master=1
IF(imasterreg(NODE)==0)THEN
imclock=imclock+1
imnodes(imclock)=NODE
imasterreg(NODE)=imclock
         END IF
C
      ELSE
C
IF(islavereg(NODE)==0)THEN
isclock=isclock+1
isnodes(isclock)=NODE
islavereg(NODE)=isclock
         END IF
C
spress(islavereg(NODE))=CPRESS
sxcrd(islavereg(NODE))=XCOORD
sycrd(islavereg(NODE))=YCOORD
C
tempslip(islavereg(NODE))=CSLIP
           INCSLIP=CSLIP-oldslip(islavereg(NODE))
         END IF
C    for debug
C
```

```
X_error_R=1
X_error_L=1
L_flag=0
R_flag=0
C
IF(master==1)THEN
        DO cnt1=1,isclock
C
IF(sxcrd(cnt1).GT.XCOORD)THEN
              IF(ABS(XCOORD-sxcrd(cnt1))<X_error_R)THEN
                CPRESS_R=spress(cnt1)
                INCSLIP_R=tempslip(cnt1)-oldslip(cnt1)
                X_R=sxcrd(cnt1)
X_error_R=ABS(XCOORD-sxcrd(cnt1))
R_flag=1
              END IF
            ELSE
              IF(ABS(XCOORD-sxcrd(cnt1))<X_error_L)THEN
                CPRESS_L=spress(cnt1)
                INCSLIP_L=tempslip(cnt1)-oldslip(cnt1)
                X_L=sxcrd(cnt1)
X_error_L=ABS(XCOORD-sxcrd(cnt1))
L_flag=1
              END IF
            END IF
          END DO
C
        IF(R_flag==0)THEN
          CPRESS=CPRESS_L
          INCSLIP=INCSLIP_L
        END IF
        IF(L_flag==0)THEN
          CPRESS=CPRESS_R
          INCSLIP=INCSLIP_R
        END IF
C
        IF(L_flag==0.AND.R_flag==0)THEN
          CPRESS=0
          INCSLIP=0
        END IF
        IF(L_flag==1.AND.R_flag==1)THEN
grad_pr=(CPRESS_R-CPRESS_L)/(X_R-X_L)
          CPRESS=CPRESS_L+grad_pr*(XCOORD-X_L)
grad_sl=(INCSLIP_R-INCSLIP_L)/(X_R-X_L)
          INCSLIP=INCSLIP_L+grad_sl*(XCOORD-X_L)
        END IF
     END IF
```

```
C
      IF(master==1)THEN
            UREF=1.925E-8
         END IF
      W_dist=(CPRESS)*ABS(INCSLIP)*UREF
C
         IF(KSTEP==1)THEN
      W_dist=0
         ELSE
      W_dist=W_dist*1000
      IF(master==0)THEN
            wears(islavereg(NODE))=wears(islavereg(NODE))+W_dist
         ELSE
      wearm(imasterreg(NODE))=wearm(imasterreg(NODE))+W_dist
         END IF

      WRITE(216,1000)KINC,PARTNAME,LOCNUM,wears(islavereg(NODE)),
     $              wearm(imasterreg(NODE)),sxcrd(islavereg(NODE))
      WRITE(217,2000)KINC,PARTNAME,LOCNUM,wears(islavereg(NODE)),
     $              CPRESS, INCSLIP, sxcrd(islavereg(NODE))
         end if
C
C
            ULOCAL(2)=ULOCAL(2)-W_dist
C        IF(W_dist.GT.h_crit)THEN
C        PNEWDT_0=PNEWDT
C          PNEWDT_1=0.99*h_crit/W_dist
C          IF(PNEWDT_1.LT.PNEWDT_0)THEN
C            PNEWDT=PNEWDT_1
C            WRITE (7,*) 'CHANGING TIME INCREMENT FROM ',PNEWDT_0
C            WRITE (7,*) 'TO ',PNEWDT
C            WRITE (7,*) 'BASED ON LOCNUM ',LOCNUM
C          END IF
C        END IF
C        write(19,*)'increment is inspected'
C
C
         IF(NODE==imnodes(imclock))THEN
            DO cnt1=1,isclock
               oldslip(cnt1)=tempslip(cnt1)
            END DO
         END IF
            ilastnode2=NODE
 1000 FORMAT(i6,10x,a10,10x,i4,10x,e13.6,10x,e13.6,10x,e13.6)
 2000 FORMAT(i6,10x,a10,10x,i4,10x,e13.6,10x,e13.6,10x,e13.6,10x,e13.6)
         RETURN
         END
```

REFERENCES

1. Jones GB. Arthroplasty of the knee by the Walldius prosthesis. *J Bone Joint Surg Br.* 1968;50: 505–510. Available: http://www.ncbi.nlm.nih.gov/pubmed/5726903.
2. Maradit Kremers H, Larson DR, Crowson CS, Kremers WK, Washington RE, Steiner CA, et al. Prevalence of Total Hip and Knee Replacement in the United States. *J Bone Joint Surg Am.* 2015;97: 1386–1397. doi:10.2106/JBJS.N.01141.
3. Berry DJ, Harmsen WS, Cabanela ME, Morrey BF. Twenty-five-year survivorship of two thousand consecutive primary Charnley total hip replacements: factors affecting survivorship of acetabular and femoral components. *J Bone Joint Surg Am.* 2002;84-A: 171–177. Available: http://www.ncbi.nlm.nih.gov/pubmed/11861721.
4. Bae DK, Song SJ, Park MJ, Eoh JH, Song JH, Park CH. Twenty-Year Survival Analysis in Total Knee Arthroplasty by a Single Surgeon. *J Arthroplasty.* 2012;27: 1297–1304.e1. doi:10.1016/j.arth.2011.10.027.
5. Bourne RB, Chesworth BM, Davis AM, Mahomed NN, Charron KDJ. Patient satisfaction after total knee arthroplasty: Who is satisfied and who is not? *Clin Orthop Relat Res.* 2010;468: 57–63. doi:10.1007/s11999-009-1119-9.
6. Pabinger C, Berghold A, Boehler N, Labek G. Revision rates after knee replacement: Cumulative results from worldwide clinical studies versus joint registers. *Osteoarthr Cartil.* 2013;21: 263–268. doi:10.1016/j.joca.2012.11.014.
7. Von Keudell A, Sodha S, Collins J, Minas T, Fitz W, Gomoll AH. Patient satisfaction after primary total and unicompartmental knee arthroplasty: An age-dependent analysis. *Knee.* 2014;21: 180–184. doi:10.1016/j.knee.2013.08.004.
8. National joint registry 15th annual report 2018. Natl Jt Regist England, Wales, *North Irel Isle Man.* 2018. doi:10.1038/nmat2505.
9. Ranawat AS, Mohanty SS, Goldsmith SE, Rasquinha VJ, Rodriguez JA, Ranawat CS. Experience with an all-polyethylene total knee arthroplasty in younger, active patients with follow-up from 2 to 11 years. *J Arthroplasty.* 2005;20: 7–11. doi:10.1016/j.arth.2005.04.027.
10. Kretzer JP, Reinders J, Sonntag R, Hagmann S, Streit M, Jeager S, et al. Wear in total knee arthroplasty – Just a question of polyethylene?: Metal ion release in total knee arthroplasty. *Int Orthop.* 2014;38: 335–340. doi:10.1007/s00264-013-2162-4.
11. O'Brien ST, Luo Y, Brandt JM. In-vitro and in-silico investigations on the influence of contact pressure on cross-linked polyethylene wear in total knee replacements. *Wear.* 2015;332–333: 687–693. doi:10.1016/j.wear.2015.02.048.
12. Miura H, Higaki H, Nakanishi Y, Mawatari T, Moro-Oka T, Murakami T, et al. Prediction of total knee arthroplasty polyethylene wear using the wear index. *J Arthroplasty.* 2002;17: 760–766. doi:10.1054/arth.2002.33546.
13. Shu L, Li S, Sugita N. Systematic review of computational modelling for biomechanics analysis of total knee replacement. *Biosurf Biotribol.* 2020;6: 3–11. doi:10.1049/bsbt.2019.0012.
14. Knight LA, Pal S, Coleman JC, Bronson F, Haider H, Levine DL, et al. Comparison of long-term numerical and experimental total knee replacement wear during simulated gait loading. *J Biomech.* 2007;40: 1550–1558. doi:10.1016/j.jbiomech.2006.07.027.
15. Willing R, Kim IY. Three dimensional shape optimization of total knee replacements for reduced wear. *Struct Multidiscip Optim.* 2009;38: 405–414. doi:10.1007/s00158-008-0281-0.
16. Kang K-T, Koh Y-G, Jung M, Nam J-H, Son J, Lee YH, et al. The effects of posterior cruciate ligament deficiency on posterolateral corner structures under gait- and squat-loading conditions. *Bone Jt Res.* 2017;6: 31–42. doi:10.1302/2046-3758.61.BJR-2016-0184.R1.

17. Carr BC, Goswami T. Knee implants – Review of models and biomechanics. *Mater Des.* 2009;30: 398–413. doi:10.1016/j.matdes.2008.03.032.
18. Nečas D, Vrbka M, Marian M, Rothammer B, Tremmel S, Wartzack S, et al. Towards the understanding of lubrication mechanisms in total knee replacements – Part I: Experimental investigations. *Tribol Int.* 2021;156: 106874. doi:10.1016/j.triboint.2021.106874.
19. Marian M, Orgeldinger C, Rothammer B, Nečas D, Vrbka M, Křupka I, et al. Towards the understanding of lubrication mechanisms in total knee replacements – Part II: Numerical modeling. *Tribol Int.* 2021;156. doi:10.1016/j.triboint.2020.106809.
20. Archard JF, Hirst W. The wear of metals under unlubricated conditions. *Proc R Soc A Math Phys Eng Sci.* 1956;236: 397–410. doi:10.1098/rspa.1956.0144.
21. Innocenti B, Labey L, Kamali A, Pascale W, Pianigiani S. Development and Validation of a Wear Model to Predict Polyethylene Wear in a Total Knee Arthroplasty: A Finite Element Analysis. *Lubricants.* 2014;2: 193–205. doi:10.3390/lubricants2040193.
22. Wang A. A unified theory of wear for ultra-high molecular weight polyethylene in multi-directional sliding. *Wear.* 2001;248: 38–47. doi:10.1016/S0043-1648(00)00522-6.
23. Kang L, Galvin AL, Brown TD, Jin Z, Fisher J. Quantification of the effect of cross-shear on the wear of conventional and highly cross-linked UHMWPE. *J Biomech.* 2008;41: 340–346. doi:10.1016/j.jbiomech.2007.09.005.
24. Abdelgaied A, Brockett CL, Liu F, Jennings LM, Jin Z, Fisher J. The effect of insert conformity and material on total knee replacement wear. *Proc Inst Mech Eng Part H J Eng Med.* 2014;228: 98–106. doi:10.1177/0954411913513251.
25. Abdelgaied A, Fisher J, Jennings LM. A comprehensive combined experimental and computational framework for pre-clinical wear simulation of total knee replacements. *J Mech Behav Biomed Mater.* 2018;78: 282–291. doi:10.1016/j.jmbbm.2017.11.022.
26. Benjamin J, Szivek J, Dersam G, Persselin S, Johnson R. Linear and volumetric wear of tibial inserts in posterior cruciate-retaining knee arthroplasties. *Clin Orthop Relat Res.* 2001; 131–138. doi:10.1097/00003086-200111000-00016.
27. Hoshino A, Fukuoka Y, Ishida A. Accurate in vivo measurement of polyethylene wear in total knee arthroplasty. *J Arthroplasty.* 2002;17: 490–496. doi:10.1054/arth.2002.32172.
28. Price AJ, Short A, Kellett C, Beard D, Gill H, Pandit H, et al. Ten-year in vivo wear measurement of a fully congruent mobile bearing unicompartmental knee arthroplasty. *J Bone Jt Surg – Ser B.* 2005;87: 1493–1497. doi:10.1302/0301-620X.87B11.16325.
29. Gill HS, Waite JC, Short A, Kellett CF, Price AJ, Murray DW. In vivo measurement of volumetric wear of a total knee replacement. *Knee.* 2006;13: 312–317. doi:10.1016/j.knee.2006.04.001.
30. Kop AM, Swarts E. Quantification of polyethylene degradation in mobile bearing knees: A retrieval analysis of the Anterior-Posterior-Glide (APG) and Rotating Platform (RP) Low ContactStress(LCS)knee.*ActaOrthop*.2007;78:364–370.doi:10.1080/17453670710013942.
31. Wang XH, Li H, Dong X, Zhao F, Cheng CK. Comparison of ISO 14243-1 to ASTM F3141 in terms of wearing of knee prostheses. *Clin Biomech.* 2019;63: 34–40. doi:10.1016/j.clinbiomech.2019.02.008.
32. Shu L, Hashimoto S, Sugita N. Enhanced In-Silico Polyethylene Wear Simulation of Total Knee Replacements During Daily Activities. *Ann Biomed Eng.* 2021;49: 322–333. doi:10.1007/s10439-020-02555-4.
33. O'Brien S, Luo Y, Wu C, Petrak M, Bohm E, Brandt JM. Computational development of a polyethylene wear model for the articular and backside surfaces in modular total knee replacements. *Tribol Int.* 2013;59: 284–291. doi:10.1016/j.triboint.2012.03.020.
34. Gao L, Hua Z, Hewson R, Andersen MS, Jin Z. Elastohydrodynamic lubrication and wear modelling of the knee joint replacements with surface topography. *Biosurf Biotribol.* 2018;4: 18–23. doi:10.1049/bsbt.2017.0003.

35. Sharif KJ, Evans HP, Snidle RW, Barnett D, Egorov IM. Effect of elastohydrodynamic film thickness on a wear model for worm gears. *Proc Inst Mech Eng Part J J Eng Tribol.* 2006;220: 295–306. doi:10.1243/13506501JET122.
36. Gao L, Wang F, Yang P, Jin Z. Effect of 3D physiological loading and motion on elastohydrodynamic lubrication of metal-on-metal total hip replacements. *Med Eng Phys.* 2009;31: 720–729. doi:10.1016/j.medengphy.2009.02.002.
37. Parkes M, Myant C, Cann PM, Wong JSS. The effect of buffer solution choice on protein adsorption and lubrication. *Tribol Int.* 2014;72: 108–117. doi:10.1016/j.triboint.2013.12.005.
38. Wang FC, Jin ZM. Prediction of elastic deformation of acetabular cups and femoral heads for lubrication analysis of artificial hip joints. *Proc Inst Mech Eng Part J Eng Tribol.* 2004;218: 201–208. doi:10.1243/1350650041323331.
39. Venner CH. Multigrid techniques: A fast and efficient method for the numerical simulation of elastohydrodynamically lubricated point contact problems. *Proc Inst Mech Eng Part J Eng Tribol.* 2000;214: 43–61. doi:10.1243/1350650001543007.
40. Morlock M, Schneider E, Bluhm A, Vollmer M, Bergmann G, Müller V, et al. Duration and frequency of every day activities in total hip patients. *J Biomech.* 2001;34: 873–881. Available: http://www.ncbi.nlm.nih.gov/pubmed/11410171.
41. Shu L, Yamamoto K, Kai S, Inagaki J, Sugita N. Symmetrical cruciate-retaining versus medial pivot prostheses: The effect of intercondylar sagittal conformity on knee kinematics and contact mechanics. *Comput Biol Med.* 2019;108: 101–110. doi:10.1016/j.compbiomed.2019.03.005.
42. Battaglia S, Belvedere C, Jaber SA, Affatato S, D'Angeli V, Leardini A. A new protocol from real joint motion data for wear simulation in total knee arthroplasty: Stair climbing. *Med Eng Phys.* 2014;36: 1605–1610. doi:10.1016/j.medengphy.2014.08.010.
43. Schwiesau J, Schilling C, Kaddick C, Utzschneider S, Jansson V, Fritz B, et al. Definition and evaluation of testing scenarios for knee wear simulation under conditions of highly demanding daily activities. *Med Eng Phys.* 2013;35: 591–600. doi:10.1016/j.medengphy.2012.07.003.
44. Reinders J, Sonntag R, Vot L, Gibney C, Nowack M, Kretzer JP. Wear testing of moderate activities of daily living using in vivo measured knee joint loading. *PLoS One.* 2015;10: 9–11. doi:10.1371/journal.pone.0123155.
45. Twiggs JG, Wakelin EA, Roe JP, Dickison DM, Fritsch BA, Miles BP, et al. Patient-Specific Simulated Dynamics After Total Knee Arthroplasty Correlate With Patient-Reported Outcomes. *J Arthroplasty.* 2018;33: 2843–2850. doi:10.1016/j.arth.2018.04.035.
46. Fregly BJ, Sawyer WG, Harman MK, Banks SA. Computational wear prediction of a total knee replacement from in vivo kinematics. *J Biomech.* 2005;38: 305–314. doi:10.1016/j.jbiomech.2004.02.013.
47. Chen Z, Zhang X, Ardestani MM, Wang L, Liu Y, Lian Q, et al. Prediction of in vivo joint mechanics of an artificial knee implant using rigid multi-body dynamics with elastic contacts. *Proc Inst Mech Eng Part H J Eng Med.* 2014;228: 564–575. doi:10.1177/0954411914537476.
48. Zhang J, Chen Z, Wang L, Li D, Jin Z. A patient-specific wear prediction framework for an artificial knee joint with coupled musculoskeletal multibody-dynamics and finite element analysis. *Tribol Int.* 2017;109: 382–389. doi:10.1016/j.triboint.2016.10.050.
49. Koh YG, Son J, Kwon OR, Kwon SK, Kang KT. Tibiofemoral conformity variation offers changed kinematics and wear performance of customized posterior-stabilized total knee arthroplasty. *Knee Surgery, Sport Traumatol Arthrosc.* 2019;27: 1213–1223. doi:10.1007/s00167-018-5045-9.

50. Koh YG, Park KM, Lee HY, Park JH, Kang KT. Prediction of wear performance in femoral and tibial conformity in patient-specific cruciate-retaining total knee arthroplasty. *J Orthop Surg Res*. 2020;15: 1–10. doi:10.1186/s13018-020-1548-4.
51. Koh Y-G, Jung K-H, Hong H-T, Kim K-M, Kang K-T. Optimal Design of Patient-Specific Total Knee Arthroplasty for Improvement in Wear Performance. *J Clin Med*. 2019;8: 2023. doi:10.3390/jcm8112023.
52. Koh YG, Park KM, Lee HY, Kang KT. Influence of tibiofemoral congruency design on the wear of patient-specific unicompartmental knee arthroplasty using finite element analysis. *Bone Jt Res*. 2019;8: 156–164. doi:10.1302/2046-3758.83.BJR-2018-0193.R1.
53. Shu L, Yamamoto K, Yao J, Saraswat P, Liu Y, Mitsuishi M, et al. A subject-specific finite element musculoskeletal framework for mechanics analysis of a total knee replacement. *J Biomech*. 2018;77: 146–154. doi:10.1016/j.jbiomech.2018.07.008.
54. McColl IR, Ding J, Leen SB. Finite element simulation and experimental validation of fretting wear. *Wear*. 2004;256: 1114–1127. doi:10.1016/j.wear.2003.07.001.

4 Development of a Multibody Biomechanical Model of the Human Upper Limb

Alessandro Ruggiero and Alessandro Sicilia
University of Salerno, Fisciano, Italy

CONTENTS

4.1 Introduction 91
4.2 Theoretical Approach 93
    4.2.1 Musculoskeletal System 93
    4.2.2 Kinematical Analysis 95
    4.2.3 Inverse Dynamics 100
    4.2.4 Hill Muscle Model 101
    4.2.5 Wrapping Muscles 104
    4.2.6 Static Optimization 106
4.3 Results and Discussion 110
4.4 Conclusions 118
List of Main Symbols 119
References 120

4.1 INTRODUCTION

In the framework of biomechanics, the dynamics of the human body play a key role, especially when the knowledge of the joint contact forces during certain kinematics is necessary. This can happen, for example, to analyze the joint loading, to define the lubrication regime of the natural and/or artificial synovial joints (hip, knee, ankle, etc.) and to estimate the friction and the wear of the contact surfaces [1–3], to predict articular diseases such as the osteoarthritis [4, 5], to design prostheses able to replace the natural joint [6, 7] or to investigate the prosthesis performance [8–10], etc. Regarding arthroplasty, the *in vitro* or *in vivo* approaches are adopted to study the biomechanical phenomena in the investigated joint. They are characterized by a wide deviation of the measurement results, since they are dependent on many parameters and vary from subject to subject [11–13], then so many experiments are required to define an average behavior of a certain physical system. For these reasons, the *in-silico* approaches are nowadays a challenge to overcome the described issues.

DOI: 10.1201/9781003139270-4

Concerning human motion simulations, several actual commercial software can solve inverse dynamics musculoskeletal problems. They are programmed by using "hidden" algorithms used to solve the motion problem, so, although they are usually computationally optimized, they are not fully controllable in terms of the involved parameters and solution techniques. A musculoskeletal system can be viewed as several bodies (bones) linked by joints allowing and constraining the relative motions between the bodies. The kinematical chain is moved by a complex actuation system, the muscles, modeled as deformable actuators connected to the bodies and controlled by neural excitation signals coming from the brain [14]. From a biomechanical point of view, many times is necessary to determine the joint contact forces in correspondence of a certainly known motion. One of the best ways to achieve the goal, avoiding direct measurements, is to solve the inverse dynamics problem by a multibody approach [15]: the subject's kinematic is acquired in a Motion Capture laboratory. The acquired data are processed to scale the subject musculoskeletal system and to obtain the degrees of freedom time evolution. The purpose is to find the driving actions on the musculoskeletal system following particular known kinematics and the resulting internal joint contact reactions. Then, the required input data to use the inverse dynamics approach are:

- the type, position, and kinematics of each joint in a suitable reference frame;
- the mass geometry and inertial properties of the body;
- the system topology (the bodies' connections through the joints);
- the degrees of freedom time evolution;
- the muscles topology and the attachment location;
- a muscle model with a suitable physiological activation criterion (muscular recruitment);
- the external forces time evolution.

Due to the redundancy of the muscles, the inverse dynamics problem has more unknown muscle forces than available equations. Therefore, static optimization is required to achieve the problem solution.

Many attempts to approach this issue are present in the scientific literature. Some authors propose biomechanical multibody models to investigate different phenomena. In [16], considering a simple upper extremity system subjected to gravity and to a concentrated force, the authors proposed the implementation of a muscle fatigue submodel, achieving a novel multibody algorithm. This approach allowed the authors to obtain interesting results regarding modification of the muscles activation and the number of recruited muscles after a loss of force production capacity. In [17] the authors described the main techniques adopted to solve the musculoskeletal system's inverse dynamics accounting for both muscular tissue dynamics and physiological criteria. They applied the model at the lower limb during the gait analysis of a geometrically reliable whole body. In [18] was shown the possible multibody analysis to approach a biomechanical craniofacial problem for both human and non-human applications.

In [19] an interesting overview of the multibody kinematic optimization was presented. The authors focused on the reliability of the kinematical analysis to be used

Multibody Biomechanics

with the upper limb modeling accounting for the motion of the soft tissue artifacts, the skin, which in general cause errors in the acquisition of the kinematics. In [20] the authors investigated the human spine developing an interesting multibody model obtained by the discretization of the intervertebral discs linked by a series of rotational joints. The obtained results allowed them to point out the utility of the model in the framework of the surgical field and the seating systems comfort. In this chapter, we propose an open multibody model able to solve the inverse dynamics of the human upper limb viewed as biomechanical system.

The model described here represents an extended version of a previous research paper by the same authors [21]. It is based on the constraints evaluation and the static optimization for the calculation of the muscular activations with a physiological criterion accounting for the actuation system realized by Hill muscles, both in a linear arrangement, through the fixed attachment points, and curved one, wrapped around surfaces fixed to the bodies. The model's trustworthiness is shown through a comparison with the inverse dynamics analysis results obtained from the software OpenSim focusing on an upper limb extremity subjected to simple kinematics.

4.2 THEORETICAL APPROACH

4.2.1 MUSCULOSKELETAL SYSTEM

The topology of a multibody model describes the set of n_B bodies and n_J joints with the information about joint links and the definition of the parent and child bodies. The parent body of a joint is the body in which the joint is defined in terms of reference frame, while the child bodies of a joint are the bodies subjected to the relative motion, linked through the joint to the parent body. In the proposed model the matrix T describes the topology with the ith row associated to the body i and the jth column associated to the joint j: for each column representing a joint, there is a 1 for the related parent body, a 2 for the related child bodies and a 0 otherwise, as expressed in (4.1). The ground was included as a parent body:

$$T = \begin{bmatrix} \cdots & \vdots & \cdots \\ \cdots & 0 & \cdots \\ \cdots & 1 & \cdots \\ \cdots & 2 & \cdots \\ \cdots & \vdots & \cdots \end{bmatrix} \begin{matrix} \vdots \\ no\,link \\ parent \\ child \\ \vdots \end{matrix} \quad (4.1)$$

The reference model in OpenSim is the "Arm26" [21], shown in Figure 4.1 together with the ground reference frame, the red muscles, the cyan wrapping surfaces, and the green bodies' mass centers. The model is constituted of 3 bodies and 2 joints. The bodies are identified in ground, humerus, and forearm (which is denoted with the complex of ulna, radius, and hand) while the joints are represented by the shoulder, which connects the humerus to the ground and the elbow, which links the forearm to the humerus.

The Lagrangian coordinates q_i describe each body i in the space (4.2) forming a 7 elements vector constituted by the mass center G_i, translation with respect to the

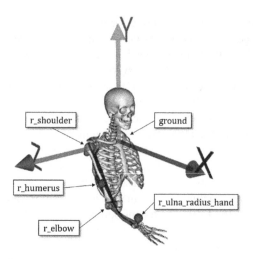

FIGURE 4.1 OpenSim arm26 model.

ground t_i and its orientation with respect to the ground reference frame, denoted by the unit quaternion $\boldsymbol{\theta}_i$:

$$q_i = \begin{bmatrix} t_i \\ \boldsymbol{\theta}_i \end{bmatrix} \qquad (4.2)$$

The unit quaternion $\boldsymbol{\theta}$, in (4.3), is a unit vector composed by the scalar real part θ_{Re} and the vector imaginary part $\boldsymbol{\theta}_{Im}$, which describes the orientation of a floating reference frame rotated with respect to a fixed one by the angle θ around the axis defined by the unit vector $\hat{v}$, in the fixed reference frame:

$$\begin{cases} \theta_{Re} = \cos\dfrac{\theta}{2} \\ \boldsymbol{\theta}_{Im} = \hat{v}\sin\dfrac{\theta}{2} \end{cases} \rightarrow \boldsymbol{\theta} = \begin{bmatrix} \theta_{Re} & \boldsymbol{\theta}_{Im}^T \end{bmatrix}^T \qquad (4.3)$$

The rotation matrix $\boldsymbol{R}$ obtained by the relative orientation is directly dependent on the quaternion $\boldsymbol{\theta}$ through the two matrices $\boldsymbol{E}$ and $\bar{\boldsymbol{E}}$, defined in (4.4):

$$\begin{cases} \boldsymbol{E}(\boldsymbol{\theta}) = \begin{bmatrix} -\boldsymbol{\theta}_{Im} & \theta_{Re}\boldsymbol{I} + \tilde{\boldsymbol{\theta}}_{Im} \end{bmatrix} \\ \bar{\boldsymbol{E}}(\boldsymbol{\theta}) = \begin{bmatrix} -\boldsymbol{\theta}_{Im} & \theta_{Re}\boldsymbol{I} - \tilde{\boldsymbol{\theta}}_{Im} \end{bmatrix} \end{cases} \rightarrow \boldsymbol{R}(\boldsymbol{\theta}) = \boldsymbol{E}(\boldsymbol{\theta})\bar{\boldsymbol{E}}(\boldsymbol{\theta})^T \qquad (4.4)$$

with $\boldsymbol{I}$ the 3×3 identity matrix and the tilde accent on a vector stands for its associated skew matrix (4.5):

$$\boldsymbol{u} = \begin{bmatrix} u_1 \\ u_2 \\ u_3 \end{bmatrix} \quad \tilde{\boldsymbol{u}} = \begin{bmatrix} 0 & -u_3 & u_2 \\ u_3 & 0 & -u_1 \\ -u_2 & u_1 & 0 \end{bmatrix} \qquad (4.5)$$

Multibody Biomechanics

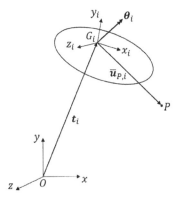

FIGURE 4.2 Locating a point fixed to a body.

The definition of the matrices E and $\bar{E}$ is enough to calculate the velocity angular vector in the fixed reference frame ω and in the floating one $\bar{\omega}$ together with their time derivatives (angular acceleration vectors) $\dot{\omega}$ and $\dot{\bar{\omega}}$, useful to find the time derivative of the rotation matrix $\dot{R}$, in (4.6):

$$\begin{cases} G = 2E \\ \bar{G} = 2\bar{E} \end{cases} \rightarrow \begin{cases} \omega = G\dot{\theta} = -\dot{G}\theta \\ \bar{\omega} = \bar{G}\dot{\theta} = -\dot{\bar{G}}\theta \end{cases} \begin{cases} \dot{\omega} = G\ddot{\theta} = -\ddot{G}\theta \\ \dot{\bar{\omega}} = \bar{G}\ddot{\theta} = -\ddot{\bar{G}}\theta \end{cases} \dot{R} = \tilde{\omega}R = R\tilde{\bar{\omega}} \quad (4.6)$$

With reference to Figure 4.2, the position r_P of any point P in the space fixed to the body i (joint, muscle attachment point, external force application point, etc.) can be found knowing its local position with respect to the body i, $\bar{u}_{P,i}$, and the body's Lagrangian coordinates q_i [22], through the (4.7):

$$r_P = t_i + R(\theta_i)\bar{u}_{P,i} \quad (4.7)$$

4.2.2 Kinematical Analysis

Due to the *a priori* time evolutions knowledge of the n_{dof} system's degrees of freedom, a kinematical analysis is possible considering the set of constraint equations during the time t, and resulting from the joint's kinematical behavior. With reference to an opportune set [23, 24] of the bodies' Lagrangian coordinates q, we have:

$$q = \begin{bmatrix} \vdots \\ q_i \\ \vdots \end{bmatrix} \quad (4.8)$$

A multibody system made of n_B bodies, which moves in a known way, is subjected to the constraint equations C made up by:

- n_{dof} rheonomic constraints which drive the degrees of freedom to move with the known trajectories (C_r);
- n_c scleronomic constraints due to the relative motions suppressed by the joints (C_s);
- $(n_B - 1)$ constraints which guarantee the unitary norm of the bodies quaternions (C_b).

Considering the mobility equation (4.9),

$$n_{dof} = 6(n_B - 1) - n_c \tag{4.9}$$

and concatenating the $7(n_B - 1)$ constraint equations, it is possible to reach the position analysis by solving the closed non-linear equations C, adopting the Newton iterative method (4.10):

$$C(q,t) = \begin{bmatrix} C_r(q,t) \\ C_s(q) \\ C_b(q) \end{bmatrix} = 0 \quad \rightarrow \quad q^{(k+1)} = q^{(k)} - C_q^{-1}\left(q^{(k)},t\right)C\left(q^{(k)},t\right) \tag{4.10}$$

The constraint Jacobian C_q in the equation (4.10) can be obtained differentiating with respect to the time the constraint equation set C, continuing with the velocity analysis and obtaining a linear system that provides the Lagrangian velocities $\dot{q}$ in the equation (4.11):

$$\dot{C}(q,\dot{q},t) = C_t + C_q\dot{q} = 0 \quad \rightarrow \quad C_q\dot{q} = -C_t \tag{4.11}$$

Going on to differentiating, another linear system is obtained in order to calculate the Lagrangian accelerations $\ddot{q}$, in the equation (4.12):

$$\ddot{C}(q,\dot{q},\ddot{q},t) = \dot{C}_t + \dot{C}_q\dot{q} + C_q\ddot{q} = 0 \quad \rightarrow \quad C_q\ddot{q} = -\left(\dot{C}_t + \dot{C}_q\dot{q}\right) \tag{4.12}$$

To build the vectors and the matrices involved in the kinematical analysis (C, C_q, C_t, $\dot{C}_q$, $\dot{C}_t$), it is necessary to describe the kinematical joint's behavior. In the proposed application, the shoulder and the elbow are considered as revolute joints J which allow only the relative rotation θ between the linked bodies i and j around the versor $\hat{v}$ fixed to the parent body i, as represented with reference to the elbow joint in the Figure 4.3.

The rheonomic constraint $C_{r,J}$ associated to the revolute joint J, is usually assumed considering that the scalar product between two vectors fixed to the bodies has to be equal to the cosine of the relative rotation θ [17, 24]. Due to the periodicity of trigonometric functions, the numerical solution of the position analysis does not conduct to a unique solution; hence, since all the joint rotations of the analysed upper limb model are executed in sagittal plane, the above constraint was modeled considering that the difference between the bodies' absolute angular coordinates φ (calculated from the equation (4.3)) projected on the rotation axis $\hat{v}$ has to be equal to the relative rotation θ, as written in the equation (4.13):

$$\begin{cases} \varphi_i = \theta_i\,\hat{v}_i \\ \varphi_j = \theta_j\,\hat{v}_j \end{cases} \quad \rightarrow \quad C_{r,J}(q,t) = \hat{v}^T R_i^T\left(\varphi_j - \varphi_i\right) - \theta(t) = 0 \tag{4.13}$$

Multibody Biomechanics

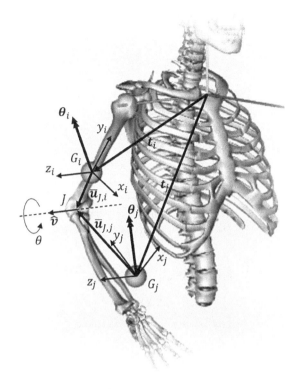

FIGURE 4.3 Elbow revolute joint.

The constraints $C_{s,J}$ is composed by a translational part and a rotational one [24], in the equation (4.14):

- the joint position calculated starting from the body i, $r_{J,i}$, has to be equal to the one seen by the body j, $r_{J,j}$;
- a vector fixed to body j, $\bar{s}_j$, parallel to the rotation axis $\hat{v}$, has to be orthogonal with respect to others two vectors fixed to the body i, $\bar{s}_{i1}$ and $\bar{s}_{i2}$, both orthogonal to the rotation axis $\hat{v}$ and to each other:

$$\begin{cases} r_{J,i} = t_i + R_i \bar{u}_{J,i} \\ r_{J,j} = t_j + R_j \bar{u}_{J,j} \\ s_j = R_j \bar{s}_j \\ s_{i1} = R_i \bar{s}_{i1} \\ s_{i2} = R_i \bar{s}_{i2} \end{cases} \rightarrow C_{s,J}(q) = \begin{bmatrix} r_{J,i} - r_{J,j} \\ s_{i1}^T s_j \\ s_{i2}^T s_j \end{bmatrix} = 0 \qquad (4.14)$$

The joint local positions $\bar{u}_{J,i}$ and $\bar{u}_{J,j}$ are provided by the geometry of the system; with reference to the Figure 4.4, the vectors $\bar{s}_j$, $\bar{s}_{i1}$ and $\bar{s}_{i2}$ are calculated considering the

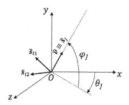

FIGURE 4.4 Revolute joint axis spherical transformation.

spherical rotation matrix $\boldsymbol{R}_v$ which rotates the reference frame of the body i or j leading the x axis to be parallel with respect to the rotation axis $\hat{v}$, achieving the (4.15):

$$\begin{cases} \hat{v} = \begin{bmatrix} \cos\varphi_J \cos\theta_J \\ \sin\varphi_J \\ \cos\varphi_J \sin\theta_J \end{bmatrix} \rightarrow \begin{cases} \theta_J = \arctan\left(\dfrac{\hat{v}_z}{\hat{v}_x}\right) \\ \varphi_J = \arctan\left(\dfrac{\hat{v}_y}{\sqrt{\hat{v}_x^2 + \hat{v}_z^2}}\right) \end{cases} \rightarrow \boldsymbol{R}_v = \begin{bmatrix} \bar{s}_j & \bar{s}_{i1} & \bar{s}_{i2} \end{bmatrix} \\ \boldsymbol{R}_y(\beta) = \begin{bmatrix} \cos\beta & 0 & \sin\beta \\ 0 & 1 & 0 \\ -\sin\beta & 0 & \cos\beta \end{bmatrix} \rightarrow \boldsymbol{R}_v = \boldsymbol{R}_y(-\theta_J)\boldsymbol{R}_z(\varphi_J) \\ \boldsymbol{R}_z(\gamma) = \begin{bmatrix} \cos\gamma & -\sin\gamma & 0 \\ \sin\gamma & \cos\gamma & 0 \\ 0 & 0 & 1 \end{bmatrix} \end{cases}$$

(4.15)

The time derivatives of the rheonomic constraint are reported in (4.16) (considering $\bar{G}\dot{\theta} = 0$):

$$\dot{C}_{r,J}(q,\dot{q},t) = -\hat{v}^T \bar{G}_i \dot{\theta}_i + \hat{v}^T R_i^T R_j \bar{G}_j \dot{\theta}_j - \dot{\theta}(t) = 0$$

$$\ddot{C}_{r,J}(q,\dot{q},\ddot{q},t) = -\hat{v}^T \bar{G}_i \ddot{\theta}_i + \hat{v}^T R_i^T R_j \bar{G}_j \ddot{\theta}_j + \hat{v}^T R_i^T \tilde{\omega}_i^T R_j \bar{G}_j \dot{\theta}_j + \hat{v}^T R_i^T \tilde{\omega}_j R_j \bar{G}_j \dot{\theta}_j - \ddot{\theta}(t) = 0$$

(4.16)

After collecting the terms, the (4.17) are obtained:

$$\dot{C}_{r,J} = \begin{bmatrix} 0 & -\hat{v}^T \bar{G}_i \end{bmatrix}\begin{bmatrix} \dot{i}_i \\ \dot{\theta}_i \end{bmatrix} + \begin{bmatrix} 0 & \hat{v}^T R_i^T R_j \bar{G}_j \end{bmatrix}\begin{bmatrix} \dot{i}_j \\ \dot{\theta}_j \end{bmatrix} - \dot{\theta}(t) = 0$$

$$\ddot{C}_{r,J} = \begin{bmatrix} 0 & -\hat{v}^T \bar{G}_i \end{bmatrix}\begin{bmatrix} \ddot{i}_i \\ \ddot{\theta}_i \end{bmatrix} + \begin{bmatrix} 0 & \hat{v}^T R_i^T R_j \bar{G}_j \end{bmatrix}\begin{bmatrix} \ddot{i}_j \\ \ddot{\theta}_j \end{bmatrix} + \begin{bmatrix} \dot{i}_i \\ \dot{\theta}_i \end{bmatrix} + \begin{bmatrix} 0 & \hat{v}^T R_i^T (\tilde{\omega}_i^T + \tilde{\omega}_j) R_j \bar{G}_j \end{bmatrix}\begin{bmatrix} \dot{i}_j \\ \dot{\theta}_j \end{bmatrix} - \ddot{\theta}(t) = 0$$

(4.17)

Multibody Biomechanics

The same scheme is adopted in order to find the time derivatives of the scleronomic constraints in the equations (4.18):

$$\dot{C}_{s,J}(q,\dot{q}) = \begin{bmatrix} \dot{t}_i - R_i \tilde{\bar{u}}_{J,i} \bar{G}_i \dot{\theta}_i - \dot{t}_j + R_j \tilde{\bar{u}}_{J,j} \bar{G}_j \dot{\theta}_j \\ -\bar{s}_j^T R_j^T R_i \tilde{\bar{s}}_{i1} \bar{G}_i \dot{\theta}_i - \bar{s}_{i1}^T R_i^T R_j \tilde{\bar{s}}_j \bar{G}_j \dot{\theta}_j \\ -\bar{s}_j^T R_j^T R_i \tilde{\bar{s}}_{i2} \bar{G}_i \dot{\theta}_i - \bar{s}_{i2}^T R_i^T R_j \tilde{\bar{s}}_j \bar{G}_j \dot{\theta}_j \end{bmatrix} = 0$$

$$\ddot{C}_{s,J}(q,\dot{q},\ddot{q}) = \begin{bmatrix} \ddot{t}_i - R_i \tilde{\bar{u}}_{J,i} \bar{G}_i \ddot{\theta}_i - R_i \tilde{\bar{\omega}}_i \tilde{\bar{u}}_{J,i} \bar{G}_i \dot{\theta}_i - \ddot{t}_j + R_j \tilde{\bar{u}}_{J,j} \bar{G}_j \ddot{\theta}_j \\ +R_j \tilde{\bar{\omega}}_j \tilde{\bar{u}}_{J,j} \bar{G}_j \dot{\theta}_j - \bar{s}_j^T R_j^T R_i \tilde{\bar{s}}_{i1} \bar{G}_i \ddot{\theta}_i - \bar{s}_j^T R_j^T (\tilde{\bar{\omega}}_j^T + \tilde{\bar{\omega}}_i) R_i \tilde{\bar{s}}_{i1} \bar{G}_i \dot{\theta}_i \\ -\bar{s}_{i1}^T R_i^T R_j \tilde{\bar{s}}_j \bar{G}_j \ddot{\theta}_j - \bar{s}_{i1}^T R_i^T (\tilde{\bar{\omega}}_i^T + \tilde{\bar{\omega}}_j) R_j \tilde{\bar{s}}_j \bar{G}_j \dot{\theta}_j - \bar{s}_j^T R_j^T R_i \tilde{\bar{s}}_{i2} \bar{G}_i \ddot{\theta}_i \\ -\bar{s}_j^T R_j^T (\tilde{\bar{\omega}}_j^T + \tilde{\bar{\omega}}_i) R_i \tilde{\bar{s}}_{i2} \bar{G}_i \dot{\theta}_i - \bar{s}_{i2}^T R_i^T R_j \tilde{\bar{s}}_j \bar{G}_j \ddot{\theta}_j - \bar{s}_{i2}^T R_i^T (\tilde{\bar{\omega}}_i^T + \tilde{\bar{\omega}}_j) R_j \tilde{\bar{s}}_j \bar{G}_j \dot{\theta}_j \end{bmatrix} = 0$$

(4.18)

Collecting the terms, the equations (4.19) are obtained:

$$\dot{C}_{s,J} = \begin{bmatrix} I & -R_i \tilde{\bar{u}}_{J,i} \bar{G}_i \\ 0 & -\bar{s}_j^T R_j^T R_i \tilde{\bar{s}}_{i1} \bar{G}_i \\ 0 & -\bar{s}_j^T R_j^T R_i \tilde{\bar{s}}_{i2} \bar{G}_i \end{bmatrix} \begin{bmatrix} \dot{t}_i \\ \dot{\theta}_i \end{bmatrix} + \begin{bmatrix} -I & R_j \tilde{\bar{u}}_{J,j} \bar{G}_j \\ 0 & -\bar{s}_{i1}^T R_i^T R_j \tilde{\bar{s}}_j \bar{G}_j \\ 0 & -\bar{s}_{i2}^T R_i^T R_j \tilde{\bar{s}}_j \bar{G}_j \end{bmatrix} \begin{bmatrix} \dot{t}_j \\ \dot{\theta}_j \end{bmatrix} = 0$$

$$\ddot{C}_{s,J} = \begin{bmatrix} I & -R_i \tilde{\bar{u}}_{J,i} \bar{G}_i \\ 0 & -\bar{s}_j^T R_j^T R_i \tilde{\bar{s}}_{i1} \bar{G}_i \\ 0 & -\bar{s}_j^T R_j^T R_i \tilde{\bar{s}}_{i2} \bar{G}_i \end{bmatrix} \begin{bmatrix} \ddot{t}_i \\ \ddot{\theta}_i \end{bmatrix} + \begin{bmatrix} -I & R_j \tilde{\bar{u}}_{J,j} \bar{G}_j \\ 0 & -\bar{s}_{i1}^T R_i^T R_j \tilde{\bar{s}}_j \bar{G}_j \\ 0 & -\bar{s}_{i2}^T R_i^T R_j \tilde{\bar{s}}_j \bar{G}_j \end{bmatrix} \begin{bmatrix} \ddot{t}_j \\ \ddot{\theta}_j \end{bmatrix}$$

$$+ \begin{bmatrix} 0 & -R_i \tilde{\bar{\omega}}_i \tilde{\bar{u}}_{J,i} \bar{G}_i \\ 0 & -\bar{s}_j^T R_j^T (\tilde{\bar{\omega}}_j^T + \tilde{\bar{\omega}}_i) R_i \tilde{\bar{s}}_{i1} \bar{G}_i \\ 0 & -\bar{s}_j^T R_j^T (\tilde{\bar{\omega}}_j^T + \tilde{\bar{\omega}}_i) R_i \tilde{\bar{s}}_{i2} \bar{G}_i \end{bmatrix} \begin{bmatrix} \dot{t}_i \\ \dot{\theta}_i \end{bmatrix} + \begin{bmatrix} 0 & R_j \tilde{\bar{\omega}}_j \tilde{\bar{u}}_{J,j} \bar{G}_j \\ 0 & -\bar{s}_{i1}^T R_i^T (\tilde{\bar{\omega}}_i^T + \tilde{\bar{\omega}}_j) R_j \tilde{\bar{s}}_j \bar{G}_j \\ 0 & -\bar{s}_{i2}^T R_i^T (\tilde{\bar{\omega}}_i^T + \tilde{\bar{\omega}}_j) R_j \tilde{\bar{s}}_j \bar{G}_j \end{bmatrix} \begin{bmatrix} \dot{t}_j \\ \dot{\theta}_j \end{bmatrix} = 0$$

(4.19)

Once the rheonomic and scleronomic constraints were evaluated, the ones related to the quaternions unitary norm are written, for each body, in the equation (4.20):

$$C_{b,i}(q) = \theta_i^T \theta_i - 1 = 0 \qquad (4.20)$$

The time derivatives of $C_{b,i}$ are calculated in (4.21):

$$\dot{C}_{b,i}(q,\dot{q}) = 2\theta_i^T \dot{\theta}_i = 0$$
$$\ddot{C}_{b,i}(q,\dot{q},\ddot{q}) = 2\theta_i^T \ddot{\theta}_i + 2\dot{\theta}_i^T \dot{\theta}_i = 0$$

(4.21)

Collecting the terms, the equations (4.22) were obtained:

$$\dot{C}_{b,i} = \begin{bmatrix} \mathbf{0} & 2\boldsymbol{\theta}_i^T \end{bmatrix} \begin{bmatrix} \dot{t}_i \\ \dot{\theta}_i \end{bmatrix} = 0$$

$$\ddot{C}_{b,i} = \begin{bmatrix} \mathbf{0} & 2\boldsymbol{\theta}_i^T \end{bmatrix} \begin{bmatrix} \ddot{t}_i \\ \ddot{\theta}_i \end{bmatrix} + \begin{bmatrix} \mathbf{0} & 2\dot{\boldsymbol{\theta}}_i^T \end{bmatrix} \begin{bmatrix} \dot{t}_i \\ \dot{\theta}_i \end{bmatrix} = 0$$
(4.22)

To extrapolate the submatrices to be associated with the related i and j bodies Lagrangian coordinates, each constraint k was written in the form of (4.23), so that the kinematical analysis can be solved:

$$\begin{cases} C_r(q,t) = a(q) - q_{dof}(t) \\ C_{r,t} = -\dot{q}_{dof} \\ C_{r,tt} = -\ddot{q}_{dof} \end{cases} \rightarrow \begin{cases} C_k(q,t) = 0 \\ \dot{C}_k(q,\dot{q},t) = C_{q,i}\dot{q}_i + C_{q,j}\dot{q}_j + C_{t,k} = 0 \\ \ddot{C}_k(q,\dot{q},\ddot{q},t) = C_{q,i}\ddot{q}_i + C_{q,j}\ddot{q}_j + \dot{C}_{q,i}\dot{q}_i + \dot{C}_{q,j}\dot{q}_j + \dot{C}_{t,k} = 0 \end{cases}$$
(4.23)

4.2.3 Inverse Dynamics

The solution of (4.10) over time provides all the needed for approaching the inverse dynamics. Considering the body i, with reference to the chosen generalized coordinates q_i, the motion equations include the mass matrix M_i, the centrifugal and Coriolis generalized force vector $Q_{v,i}$ and the external generalized force $Q_{e,i}$. As pointed out in the equation (4.24), the M_i and the $Q_{v,i}$ depend on the body mass m_i and inertia tensor evaluated in its local reference frame $\bar{I}_i$, while the $Q_{e,i}$ need the external force written in the ground reference frame F_e and its application point with respect to the body $\bar{u}_e$ [22]:

$$M_i = \begin{bmatrix} m_i I & 0 \\ 0 & \bar{G}_i^T \bar{I}_i \bar{G}_i \end{bmatrix} \quad Q_{v,i} = \begin{bmatrix} 0 \\ -2\dot{\bar{G}}_i^T \bar{I}_i \bar{\omega}_i \end{bmatrix} \quad Q_{e,i} = \begin{bmatrix} I & -R_i \tilde{\bar{u}}_e \bar{G}_i \end{bmatrix}^T F_e \quad (4.24)$$

Assembling the matrices and vectors in the ones related to the global multibody system, according to the Lagrangian coordinate vectors q, the motion equations (4.25) of the system, for a virtual displacement δq, is obtained. In (4.25) the work of the internal forces was considered through the constraint Jacobian C_q and the Lagrange multipliers λ:

$$\delta q^T \left(M\ddot{q} - Q_v - Q_e + C_q^T \lambda \right) = 0$$
(4.25)

Since the work of the internal forces was considered, the motion equations (4.25) are satisfied for any virtual displacement δq: in order to refer the bodies orientation

Multibody Biomechanics

to the local cartesian angular coordinates $\bar{\varphi}_i$, instead of the quaternion θ_i, a coordinate change was performed through the matrix J_q in the equation (4.26):

$$\delta q_i = \begin{bmatrix} \delta t_i \\ \delta \theta_i \end{bmatrix} = \begin{bmatrix} I & 0 \\ 0 & \frac{1}{4}G_i^T \end{bmatrix} \begin{bmatrix} \delta t_i \\ \delta \bar{\varphi}_i \end{bmatrix} = J_{q,i}\delta \bar{q}_i \quad \rightarrow \quad \delta \bar{q}^T J_q^T \left(M\ddot{q} - Q_v - Q_e + C_q^T \lambda \right) = 0 \tag{4.26}$$

The generalized force vector Q_c and the new constraint Jacobian $C_{\bar{q}}$ are defined in the equation (4.27), leading to the final form of the multibody motion equations:

$$\begin{cases} Q_c = J_q^T \left(M\ddot{q} - Q_v - Q_e \right) \\ C_{\bar{q}} = C_q J_q \end{cases} \rightarrow C_{\bar{q}}^T \lambda + Q_c = 0 \tag{4.27}$$

The coordinate transformation in the equation (4.26) allows to neglect the part of the Jacobian associated to the constraints needed to keep the quaternions' unitary norm: then the equation (4.27) becomes a closed linear system in which the unknowns are the Lagrange multipliers associated to the rheonomic constraints λ_r, representing the driving forces associated with each degree of freedom, and the ones related to the scleronomic constraints λ_s [24], as shown in the equation (4.28):

$$\begin{cases} C_{\bar{q}} = \begin{bmatrix} C_{\bar{q},r} \\ C_{\bar{q},s} \end{bmatrix} \\ \lambda = \begin{bmatrix} \lambda_r \\ \lambda_s \end{bmatrix} \end{cases} \rightarrow \begin{bmatrix} C_{\bar{q},r}^T & C_{\bar{q},s}^T \end{bmatrix} \begin{bmatrix} \lambda_r \\ \lambda_s \end{bmatrix} = -Q_c \tag{4.28}$$

The scleronomic multipliers λ_s are not equal to the joint reaction forces, because the actuation of the musculoskeletal system doesn't associate a single actuator to each degree of freedom. It is well known that there is a muscular redundancy and the muscular action is composed of a passive part, which has to be considered as a known internal force.

4.2.4 Hill Muscle Model

The Hill muscle model schematically represented in Figure 4.5, considers the muscle-tendon unit as a linear actuator between two attachment points A and B on the linked bodies. It is made by a series of the tendon SE with length l_t and the muscle, which is considered as a parallel between the contractile element CE and the passive element PE, with length l_m and inclined with respect to the action line, by the *pennation angle* α_p [25–27].

The total force F_m generated by the muscle-tendon series can be evaluated as the sum of the contractile element force F_{CE}, representing the active action of the contraction, and the passive contribute F_{PE}, provided by the muscular fibers' stiffness, calculated as a projection on the action direction, through the pennation angle α_p. F_{CE}

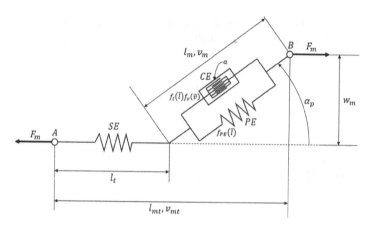

FIGURE 4.5 Hill muscle model.

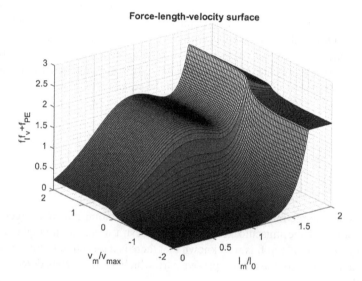

FIGURE 4.6 Hill model force-length-velocity relationships.

depends on the activation level a (a scalar number between 0 and 1) determined considering muscular recruitment criteria, add on the muscle fiber length l_m and deformation velocity v_m through the force-length-velocity relationships. F_{PE} depends only on the muscle fiber length l_m [27–29], as represented in (4.29) with reference to Figure 4.6. The force-length-velocity surface allows to point out the following:

- considering the force-length relation f_l, it is possible to observe that by increasing the muscle fiber length, the active force increases until it reaches a maximum isometric force F_0, in correspondence of the optimal fiber length l_0, then it decreases;
- the muscle generates a greater force than the maximum isometric one (in correspondence of zero deformation velocity) when it lengthens, with an

asymptotic behavior, and a lower force until it reaches the maximum contraction velocity v_{max}, beyond which it isn't able to produce actuation, following the force-velocity relation f_v;
- if the muscle length is greater than the optimal fiber length l_0, the passive element opposes a growing resistance until it reaches a maximum value following the relation f_{PE}:

$$\tilde{l} = \frac{l_m}{l_0} \quad \tilde{v} = \frac{v_m}{v_{max}}$$

$$f_l(\tilde{l}) = e^{\frac{(\tilde{l}-1)^2}{\gamma}} \quad f_v(\tilde{v}) = \begin{cases} 0 & \text{if } \tilde{v} < -1 \\ \dfrac{1+\tilde{v}}{1-\dfrac{\tilde{v}}{k_{CE,1}}} & \text{if } -1 \leq \tilde{v} < 0 \\ \dfrac{1+f_{max}\dfrac{\tilde{v}}{k_{CE,2}}}{1+\dfrac{\tilde{v}}{k_{CE,2}}} & \text{if } \tilde{v} \geq 0 \end{cases}$$

(4.29)

$$f_{PE}(\tilde{l}) = \begin{cases} 0 & \text{if } \tilde{l} < 1 \\ \dfrac{e^{k_{PE}\dfrac{\tilde{l}-1}{\varepsilon_0}}-1}{e^{k_{PE}}-1} & \text{if } 1 \leq \tilde{l} < 1+\varepsilon_1 \\ f_{PE,max} & \text{if } \tilde{l} \geq 1+\varepsilon_1 \end{cases}$$

$$\begin{cases} F_{CE} = af_l(\tilde{l})f_v(\tilde{v})F_0 \\ F_{PE} = f_{PE}(\tilde{l})F_0 \end{cases} \rightarrow F_m = (F_{CE}+F_{PE})\cos\alpha_p$$

Generally, it is widely assumed that the tendon dynamics is negligible, so that the tendon length l_t can be considered as a constant, and that the muscle width w_m keeps constant, even in correspondence of the muscle optimal fiber length l_0, when the muscle is inclined by the known optimal pennation angle α_0. Then, with reference to Figure 4.5, the equations (4.30) can be used to calculate the muscle length l_m, the muscle deformation velocity v_m and the pennation angle α_p, starting from the length l_{mt} and the deformation velocity v_{mt} of the muscle-tendon unit, which are known from the kinematical analysis [24].

$$\begin{cases} l_{mt} = l_t + l_m \cos\alpha_p \\ w_m = l_m \sin\alpha_p = l_0 \sin\alpha_0 \end{cases} \rightarrow \begin{cases} l_m = \sqrt{(l_0 \sin\alpha_0)^2 + (l_{mt}-l_t)^2} \\ \alpha_p = \arctan\left(\dfrac{l_0 \sin\alpha_0}{l_{mt}-l_t}\right) \\ v_m = \dot{l}_m = v_{mt}\cos\alpha_p \end{cases}$$

(4.30)

4.2.5 Wrapping Muscles

From a biomechanical point of view, some muscles are fixed to the bones by fixed points, while others can wrap around bony surfaces fixed to the bodies [30–32]. With the aim to locate the attachment points of the wrapped muscle, it is possible to model the curve followed by the wrapped muscle path by describing it as a geodesic on a wrapping bony surface [33, 34]. The surface spatial representation can be achieved accounting for two parameters u and v through the parametric equations $x(u,v)$, which satisfy the implicit surface equation $f(x) = 0$. The geodesic curve $c(s)$, along the curvilinear coordinate s, is evaluated as the constrained motion of a particle with mass m on the surface $x(u,v)$ in absence of external actions: then the equation of motion is assembled in (4.31), and it is solved in the forward dynamics verse. The particle is characterized by three degrees of freedom in the space, the translation q, while its mass m is arbitrary because its value affects only the Lagrange multiplier λ associated to the unique surface constraint C:

$$\begin{cases} q' = \dfrac{dq}{ds} \\ M = mI \\ C = f(q) \end{cases} \rightarrow \begin{cases} Mq'' + C_q^T \lambda = 0 \\ C(q) = 0 \end{cases} \quad (4.31)$$

By differentiating the constraint C with respect to the curvilinear coordinate s, the constraint Jacobian C_q and its derivative C_q' were obtained. The geodesic forward dynamics problem (4.32) is a closed non-linear differential algebraic equation which can be solved numerically, with the initial conditions r_0, the attachment point position, and $\hat{t}_0$, the tangent unit vector parallel to the surface calculated from the straight-line muscle line action projected on the surface tangent plane; the solution $q(s)$ is equal to the geodesic $c(s)$:

$$\begin{cases} C' = \nabla f(q) q' = C_q q' = 0 \\ C'' = \nabla f'(q) q' + \nabla f(q) q'' = C_q' q' + C_q q'' = 0 \end{cases}$$

$$\begin{cases} Mq'' + C_q^T \lambda = 0 \\ C_q q'' = -C_q' q' \end{cases} \rightarrow \begin{cases} \begin{bmatrix} M & C_q^T \\ C_q & 0 \end{bmatrix} \begin{bmatrix} q'' \\ \lambda \end{bmatrix} = \begin{bmatrix} 0 \\ -C_q' q' \end{bmatrix} \\ q(0) = r_0 \\ q'(0) = \hat{t}_0 \end{cases} \quad (4.32)$$

In the proposed model, with reference to Figure 4.7, in correspondence of each time instant, the model detects the contact between the straight-line muscles AB and

Multibody Biomechanics

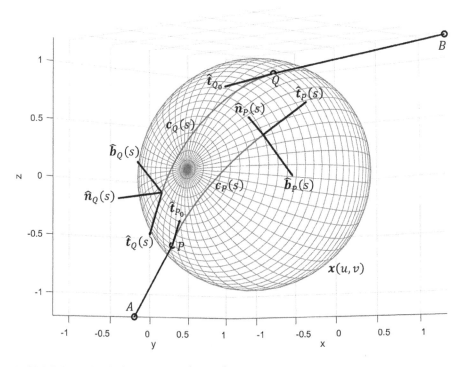

FIGURE 4.7 Geodesics on a wrapping surface.

the associated surfaces $x(u,v)$; then it calculates the geodesics starting from the two intersections P and Q on the surface, c_P and c_Q, varying the attachment points location until the original muscle AB is split into two straight-line muscle units AP and QB tangent to the surface while the related geodesics are collinear to each other in correspondence of the geodesics closest points P^* and Q^* [33].

The tangent, normal, and binormal unit vectors, $\hat{t}$, $\hat{n}$ and $\hat{b}$ are given in (4.33):

$$\hat{t} = c' = \begin{bmatrix} x_u & x_v \end{bmatrix} \begin{bmatrix} u' \\ v' \end{bmatrix}$$

$$\hat{n} = \frac{\nabla f}{|\nabla f|} \qquad (4.33)$$

$$\hat{b} = \hat{t} \times \hat{n}$$

The objective was to find the unknown geodesics initial positions, the attachment points location, described by the surface parameters (u_{0P}, v_{0P}) and (u_{0Q}, v_{0Q}) which set to zero the function f in (4.34). In this equation, the first two components impose the surface's tangency of the split muscles, while the last two components guarantee the geodesics' collinearity. The non-linear closed problem was solved by using the Newton iterative method with the numerical determination of the Jacobian J_f:

$$\varepsilon = \begin{bmatrix} u_{0P} \\ v_{0P} \\ u_{0Q} \\ v_{0Q} \end{bmatrix} \rightarrow \begin{cases} r_P = x(u_{0P}, v_{0P}) \\ r_Q = x(u_{0Q}, v_{0Q}) \end{cases} \rightarrow \begin{cases} \hat{t}_P = \dfrac{r_P - r_A}{|r_P - r_A|} \\ \hat{t}_Q = \dfrac{r_Q - r_B}{|r_Q - r_B|} \end{cases}$$

$$f(\varepsilon) = \begin{bmatrix} \hat{t}_P^T \hat{n}_P \\ \hat{t}_Q^T \hat{n}_Q \\ \hat{b}_{P^*}^T (r_{P^*} - r_{Q^*}) \\ \hat{b}_{P^*}^T \hat{t}_{Q^*} \end{bmatrix} = 0 \rightarrow \varepsilon^{(k+1)} = \varepsilon^{(k)} - J_f^{-1}(\varepsilon^{(k)}) f(\varepsilon^{(k)}) \quad (4.34)$$

The convergence of the Newton cycle allows the determination of the two geodesics c_P and c_Q joined in correspondence of the collinearity point. The resulting definitive muscle path is c_{PQ}.

The surface types analyzed here are radius r and height h cylinder x_c, and the ellipsoid x_e, with semiaxes s_x, s_y and s_z, given in (4.35):

$$x_c(u,v) = \begin{bmatrix} r\cos u \\ r\sin u \\ v \end{bmatrix}, \quad \begin{array}{c} 0 \le u \le 2\pi \\ -\dfrac{h}{2} \le v \le \dfrac{h}{2} \end{array} \qquad x_e(u,v) = \begin{bmatrix} s_x \cos v \cos u \\ s_y \cos v \sin u \\ s_z \sin v \end{bmatrix}, \quad \begin{array}{c} 0 \le u \le 2\pi \\ -\dfrac{\pi}{2} \le v \le \dfrac{\pi}{2} \end{array}$$

$$f_c(x) = x^2 + y^2 - r^2 = 0 \qquad\qquad f_e(x) = \left(\dfrac{x}{s_x}\right)^2 + \left(\dfrac{y}{s_y}\right)^2 + \left(\dfrac{z}{s_z}\right)^2 - 1 = 0$$

(4.35)

4.2.6 Static Optimization

After the determination of the muscle path, the muscle forces have to be turned into generalized forces through the muscle Jacobian Φ_q, by the principle of virtual work, to have included them in the equation of motion [16, 17, 24]. The simplest case is represented by a straight-line muscle connecting the bodies i and j through the attachment points A and B respectively, depicted in Figure 4.8, which the virtual work δW_m is written in (4.36):

$$\begin{cases} r_A = t_i + R_i \bar{u}_A \\ r_B = t_j + R_j \bar{u}_B \end{cases} \rightarrow \hat{l}_{AB} = \dfrac{r_B - r_A}{|r_B - r_A|} \rightarrow \delta W_m = -F_m \hat{l}_{AB}^T (\delta r_B - \delta r_A)$$

$$\delta W_m = F_m \left(\hat{l}_{AB}^T \begin{bmatrix} I & -R_i \tilde{\bar{u}}_A \bar{G}_i \end{bmatrix} \begin{bmatrix} \delta t_i \\ \delta \theta_i \end{bmatrix} - \hat{l}_{AB}^T \begin{bmatrix} I & -R_j \tilde{\bar{u}}_B \bar{G}_j \end{bmatrix} \begin{bmatrix} \delta t_j \\ \delta \theta_j \end{bmatrix} \right) \quad (4.36)$$

$$\delta W_m = F_m \left(\Phi_{q,i} \delta q_i + \Phi_{q,j} \delta q_j \right)$$

Multibody Biomechanics

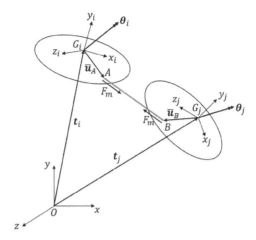

FIGURE 4.8 Straight-line muscle.

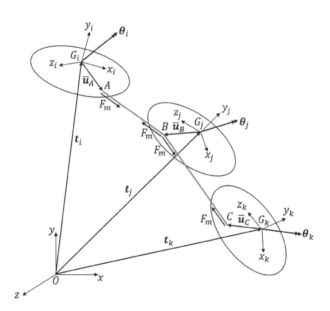

FIGURE 4.9 Muscle series.

The case of a more complex path muscle is modeled as a series of more straight-line muscles which share the same muscular force F_m. Considering the example in Figure 4.9, the work done by a muscle linking the bodies i and j, through the attachment points A and B, and the bodies j and k, through the points B and C, is written in the equation (4.37):

$$\begin{cases} r_A = t_i + R_i \bar{u}_A \\ r_B = t_j + R_j \bar{u}_B \\ r_C = t_k + R_k \bar{u}_C \end{cases} \rightarrow \begin{cases} \hat{l}_{AB} = \dfrac{r_B - r_A}{|r_B - r_A|} \\ \hat{l}_{BC} = \dfrac{r_C - r_B}{|r_C - r_B|} \end{cases} \rightarrow \delta W_m = -F_m \hat{l}_{AB}^T (\delta r_B - \delta r_A) - F_m \hat{l}_{BC}^T (\delta r_C - \delta r_B)$$

$$\delta W_m = F_m \left(\hat{l}_{AB}^T \begin{bmatrix} I & -R_i \tilde{\bar{u}}_A G_i \end{bmatrix} \begin{bmatrix} \delta t_i \\ \delta \theta_i \end{bmatrix} - \hat{l}_{AB}^T \begin{bmatrix} I & -R_j \tilde{\bar{u}}_B G_j \end{bmatrix} \begin{bmatrix} \delta t_j \\ \delta \theta_j \end{bmatrix} \right.$$

$$\left. + \hat{l}_{BC}^T \begin{bmatrix} I & -R_j \tilde{\bar{u}}_B G_j \end{bmatrix} \begin{bmatrix} \delta t_j \\ \delta \theta_j \end{bmatrix} - \hat{l}_{BC}^T \begin{bmatrix} I & -R_k \tilde{\bar{u}}_C G_k \end{bmatrix} \begin{bmatrix} \delta t_k \\ \delta \theta_k \end{bmatrix} \right)$$

$$\delta W_m = F_m \left[\Phi_{q,i,AB} \delta q_i + \left(\Phi_{q,j,AB} + \Phi_{q,j,BC} \right) \delta q_j + \Phi_{q,k,BC} \delta q_k \right]$$

(4.37)

The last case is represented by a muscle wrapped around a surface: since the wrapping surface is fixed to a body, the location t_w and the orientation θ_w of the surface are known and the muscle force acting on the surface is directly transferred to the related body; moreover, since there is no friction between the muscle path and the surface, the wrapped muscle doesn't share tangential force along the geodesic [34]. With reference to Figure 4.10, the work done by a muscle attached to the bodies i and j through the points A and B and wrapped around a surface fixed to the body w along the geodesic from P to Q is written in the equation (4.38):

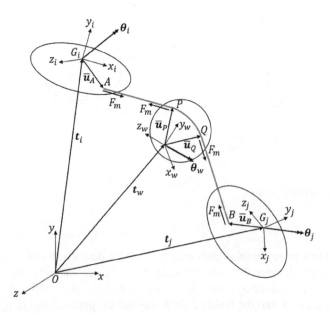

FIGURE 4.10 Wrapped muscle.

Multibody Biomechanics

$$\begin{cases} r_A = t_i + R_i \bar{u}_A \\ r_P = t_w + R_w \bar{u}_P \\ r_Q = t_w + R_w \bar{u}_Q \\ r_B = t_j + R_j \bar{u}_B \end{cases} \rightarrow \begin{cases} \hat{l}_{AP} = \dfrac{r_P - r_A}{|r_P - r_A|} = \hat{t}_P \\ \hat{l}_{BQ} = \dfrac{r_Q - r_B}{|r_Q - r_B|} = \hat{t}_Q \end{cases} \rightarrow \delta W_m = -F_m \hat{l}_{AP}^T (\delta r_P - \delta r_A) - F_m \hat{l}_{BQ}^T (\delta r_Q - \delta r_B)$$

$$\delta W_m = F_m \left(\hat{l}_{AP}^T \begin{bmatrix} I & -R_i \tilde{\bar{u}}_A G_i \end{bmatrix} \begin{bmatrix} \delta t_i \\ \delta \theta_i \end{bmatrix} - \hat{l}_{AP}^T \begin{bmatrix} I & -R_w \tilde{\bar{u}}_P G_w \end{bmatrix} \begin{bmatrix} \delta t_w \\ \delta \theta_w \end{bmatrix} \right.$$
$$\left. + \hat{l}_{BQ}^T \begin{bmatrix} I & -R_w \tilde{\bar{u}}_Q G_w \end{bmatrix} \begin{bmatrix} \delta t_w \\ \delta \theta_w \end{bmatrix} - \hat{l}_{BQ}^T \begin{bmatrix} I & -R_j \tilde{\bar{u}}_B G_j \end{bmatrix} \begin{bmatrix} \delta t_j \\ \delta \theta_j \end{bmatrix} \right)$$

$$\delta W_m = F_m \left[\Phi_{q,i,AP} \delta q_i + \left(\Phi_{q,w,AP} + \Phi_{q,w,BQ} \right) \delta q_w + \Phi_{q,j,BQ} \delta q_j \right]$$
(4.38)

Then, assembling the muscle Jacobian Φ_q and the muscle force vector F_m, the generalized muscle force Q_m can be used as internal force in the motion equations (4.25) instead of the constraint Jacobian part related to the rheonomic constraints, as reported in (4.39):

$$Q_m^T \delta q = F_m^T \Phi_q \delta q \rightarrow \delta q^T \left(M \ddot{q} - Q_v - Q_e - \Phi_q^T F_m + C_{q,s}^T \lambda_s + C_{q,b}^T \lambda_b \right) = 0 \quad (4.39)$$

By changing the orientation coordinates, the equation (4.40) is obtained by neglecting the constraint Jacobian part related to the unitary norm of the quaternions:

$$\Phi_{\bar{q}} = \Phi_q J_q \rightarrow \Phi_{\bar{q}}^T F_m - C_{q,s}^T \lambda_s = Q_c \quad (4.40)$$

Each muscle force $F_{m,i}$ depends on the muscle length $l_{m,i}$, the muscle deformation velocity $v_{m,i}$ and the pennation angle $\alpha_{p,i}$ through the Hill model: these quantities can be calculated through the equation (4.30) evaluating the musculotendon length $l_{mt,i}$ and deformation velocity $v_{mt,i}$. Analyzing each muscle series i, in general, it can be composed by n_s straight-line units (from A_j to B_j) and n_w wrapped units (from P_k to Q_k), so the musculotendon length $l_{mt,i}$ and deformation velocity $v_{mt,i}$ can be calculated as the sum of the individual contributions in the equation (4.41):

$$\begin{cases} l_{mt,i} = \sum_{j=1}^{n_s} |r_{B,j} - r_{A,j}| + \sum_{k=1}^{n_w} \int |c'_{PQ,k}| ds \\ v_{mt,i} = \sum_{j=1}^{n_s} (v_{B,j} - v_{A,j})^T \hat{l}_{AB,j} + \sum_{k=1}^{n_w} \left(v_{Q,k}^T \hat{t}_{Q,k} - v_{P,k}^T \hat{t}_{P,k} \right) \end{cases} \quad (4.41)$$

From the equation (4.29), each muscle force $F_{m,i}$ is written in the equation (4.42) as the sum of an active part $\bar{F}_{CE,i}$ multiplied by the activation level a_i and a passive part $\bar{F}_{PE,i}$, in order to relate the muscle force vector F_m to the activation vector a, the maximum active muscle force $\bar{F}_{CE}$ and the passive muscle force vector $\bar{F}_{PE}$:

$$\begin{cases} F_{m,i} = \left(a_i f_l(l_{m,i}) f_v(v_{m,i}) + f_{PE}(l_{m,i})\right) F_{0,i} \cos\alpha_{p,i} \\ \bar{F}_{CE,i} = f_l(l_{m,i}) f_v(v_{m,i}) F_{0,i} \cos\alpha_{p,i} \quad \rightarrow \quad F_{m,i} = a_i \bar{F}_{CE,i} + \bar{F}_{PE,i} \\ \bar{F}_{PE,i} = f_{PE}(l_{m,i}) F_{0,i} \cos\alpha_{p,i} \end{cases} \quad (4.42)$$

$$D_{CE} = diag\left(\bar{F}_{CE}\right) \quad \rightarrow \quad F_m = D_{CE} a + \bar{F}_{PE}$$

Substituting in (4.40), the unknown in the equation of motion (4.43) are the activation vector a and the Lagrange multipliers related to the scleronomic constraints λ_s, which definitely represent the joint reactions, by including the muscle activation Jacobian $\Phi_{\bar{q},CE}$ and the generalized passive muscle force vector Q_{PE}:

$$\begin{cases} \Phi_{\bar{q},CE} = D_{CE} \Phi_{\bar{q}} \\ Q_{PE} = \Phi_{\bar{q}}^T \bar{F}_{PE} \end{cases} \rightarrow \begin{bmatrix} \Phi_{\bar{q},CE}^T & -C_{\bar{q},s}^T \end{bmatrix} \begin{bmatrix} a \\ \lambda_s \end{bmatrix} = Q_c - Q_{PE} \quad (4.43)$$

The linear system (4.43) has more unknowns than equations due to the muscle redundancy; it was used in the static optimization problem to minimize the global muscle activation level (physiological criterion). However, if the muscle topology modeling is not accurate, the static optimization could fail, so the Lagrange multipliers associated with the rheonomic constraints λ_r have to be introduced in the equation (4.43), acting as residual actuators. Their action has to be minimized together with the muscle activations (bounded between 0 and 1), in order to ensure the optimization convergence while satisfying the motion equations, as reported in (4.44).

$$\begin{bmatrix} \Phi_{\bar{q},CE}^T & -C_{\bar{q},s}^T & -C_{\bar{q},r}^T \end{bmatrix} \begin{bmatrix} a \\ \lambda_s \\ \lambda_r \end{bmatrix} = Q_c - Q_{PE}$$

$$\begin{cases} A = \begin{bmatrix} \Phi_{\bar{q},CE}^T & -C_{\bar{q},s}^T & -C_{\bar{q},r}^T \end{bmatrix} \\ x = \begin{bmatrix} a \\ \lambda_s \\ \lambda_r \end{bmatrix} \quad \rightarrow \quad \begin{matrix} \min_x J(x) = a^T a + \lambda_r^T \lambda_r \\ Ax = b \\ 0 \leq a \leq 1 \end{matrix} \\ b = Q_c - Q_{PE} \end{cases} \quad (4.44)$$

4.3 RESULTS AND DISCUSSION

The described model was entirely developed in a Matlab environment. We considered the input data "arm26" available from the OpenSim commercial software [21]. The analyzed system is composed by ground, humerus, and forearm, linked by the

Multibody Biomechanics

shoulder and elbow. The musculoskeletal system is moved by six muscles: long triceps, lateral triceps, medial triceps, long biceps, short biceps, and brachialis. The wrapping surfaces considered were a cylinder fixed to the ground interacting with the long triceps, two ellipsoids fixed to the humerus interacting respectively with the long biceps and with the long triceps and a cylinder fixed to the humerus interacting with all the triceps on the back and with the brachialis on the front. In the following simulations, the upper limb is considered subjected only to gravity as the external action. The degrees of freedom are the shoulder and the elbow rotations; the analyzed kinematics is depicted in Figure 4.11 with respect to the elbow motion, from 0° to 90° during 1 second, while the shoulder substantially doesn't move.

Figure 4.12 shows the analyzed system with the body's mass centers, the reference frames, the muscles, and the wrapping surfaces in correspondence of four equally spaced instants, from the start to the end of the analyzed time period.

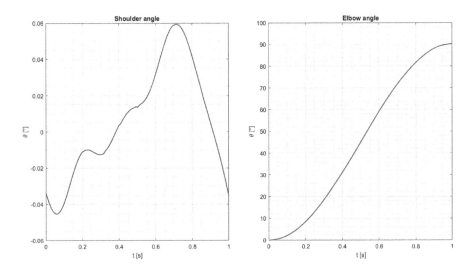

FIGURE 4.11 Arm26 degrees of freedom over time.

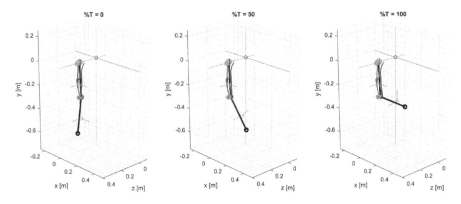

FIGURE 4.12 Kinematics first time instant.

The long biceps wrapped on the ellipsoid keep his path on the surface during the simulation due to the shoulder angle values (Figure 4.13).

Figure 4.14 shows the wrapping muscles on the cylinder close to the elbow in correspondence of four equally spaced time instants in which are clear both the brachialis wrapping on the cylinder front and the triceps wrapping on the cylinder back.

To propose a first validation of the developed model, a quantitative comparison is showed in Figure 4.15, considering the muscles' fiber length l_m with respect to time, calculated by the proposed model with those calculated by the OpenSim software.

Given that the comparison is very satisfactory, the unique noticeable difference is related to the wrapping muscles fiber length, probably due to a different wrapping algorithm considered by the OpenSim software. The time evolution of the muscles'

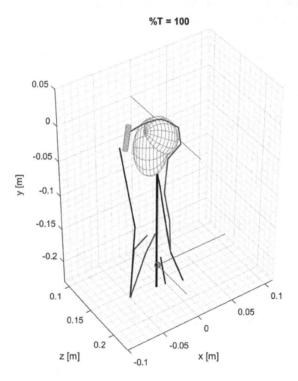

FIGURE 4.13 Shoulder wrapping.

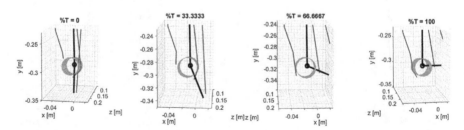

FIGURE 4.14 Elbow wrapping.

Multibody Biomechanics

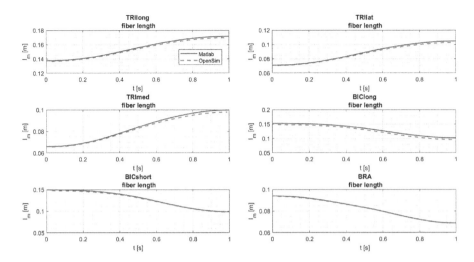

FIGURE 4.15 Muscles' fiber length comparison.

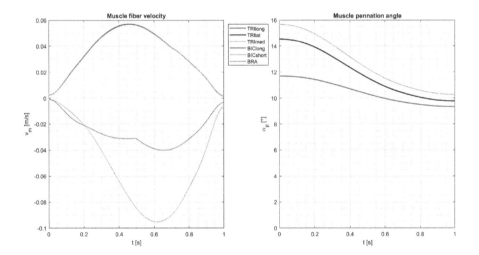

FIGURE 4.16 Muscles' fiber deformation velocity and pennation angle.

fiber deformation velocity v_m and pennation angle α_p are shown in Figure 4.16, in order to visualize the increase of the absolute values of the deformation velocity due to the wrapping of the triceps and the brachialis.

Results of the inverse dynamics are shown in Figure 4.17, in which the comparison between OpenSim and Matlab is made on the driving forces (rheonomic Lagrange multipliers λ_r). The inverse dynamics outputs result in a very satisfactory matching between the Matlab model and the OpenSim software.

The OpenSim "Static Optimization" tool doesn't take into account the passive muscle force. It allows us to choose between the physiological criterion by using the muscle's force-length-velocity relationships, or not. In the latter option, the muscular

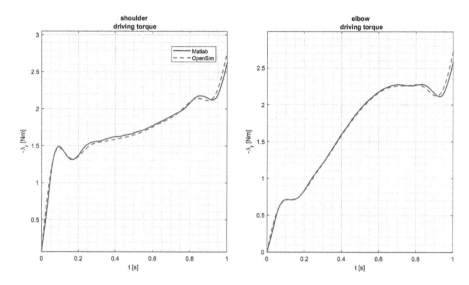

FIGURE 4.17 Inverse dynamics comparison.

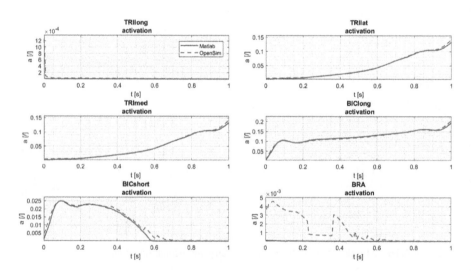

FIGURE 4.18 Static optimization activations without physiological criterion and passive forces.

activation a is intended as the ratio between the muscle force F_m and the maximum isometric force F_0, bounded between 0 and 1. In the configuration of the non-physiological criterion, the comparison of the muscles' activation is shown in Figure 4.18. The activations a, calculated by the Matlab model, are nearly in line with respect to the ones evaluated by OpenSim, which show some discontinuities.

The results obtained with the physiological criterion, but not considering the passive muscle forces, are showed in Figure 4.19, in terms of muscle activations a, and

Multibody Biomechanics

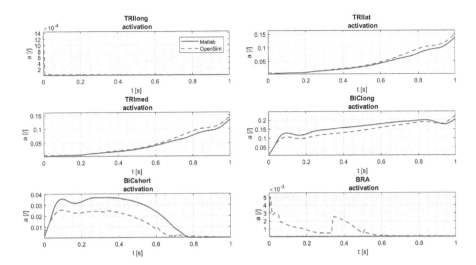

FIGURE 4.19 Muscle activations with physiological criterion and no passive forces.

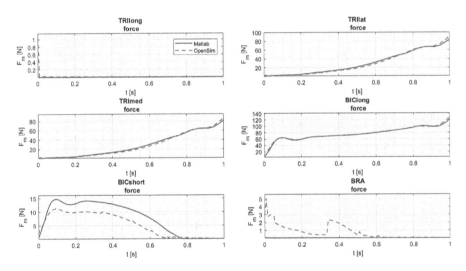

FIGURE 4.20 Muscle forces with physiological criterion and no passive forces.

in Figure 4.20, in terms of muscle forces F_m. In this configuration there are small underestimations and overestimation related to wrapping muscles.

The OpenSim "Computed Muscle Control" tool [35] allows us to evaluate the muscle activations also considering the passive muscle forces, by calculating through proportional–integral–derivative (PID) controllers the necessary muscle actions to obtain the minimum difference between the trajectories of the degrees of freedom simulated by the forward dynamics and the ones known by the inverse kinematics. The comparison results considering the muscle activation a and the muscle forces F_m

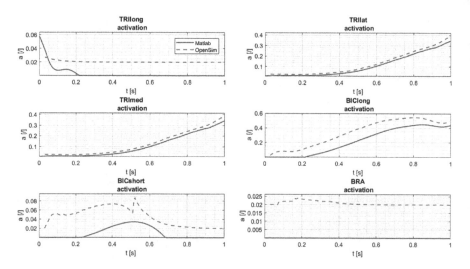

FIGURE 4.21 Muscle activations with physiological criterion and passive force.

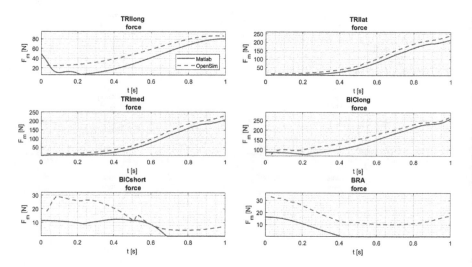

FIGURE 4.22 Muscle forces with physiological criterion and passive force.

are shown respectively in Figures 4.21 and 4.22. In this last configuration, which includes all the analyzed phenomena, despite the good qualitative match between the Matlab model and the OpenSim software, there are some discrepancies, probably due to the different static optimization criteria. Anyway, the muscles' force and activations are slightly underestimated.

Another interesting result is obtained regarding the residual actuators λ_{res} (the rheonomic Lagrange multipliers λ_r of the (4.44)), also provided by the OpenSim

Multibody Biomechanics

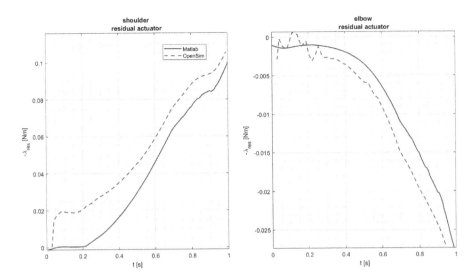

FIGURE 4.23 Residual actuators.

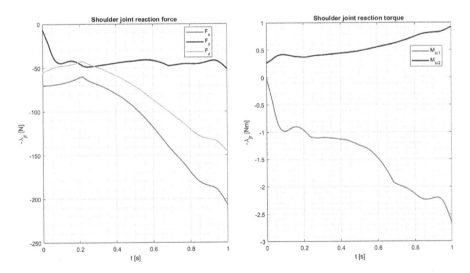

FIGURE 4.24 Shoulder joint reactions.

tools, in the analyzed configuration. With reference to Figure 4.23, the residual actuators show similar behavior, both quantitively and qualitatively.

Once the inverse dynamics problem of the musculoskeletal system was solved, the Matlab model provides the joint reactions. In Figures 4.24 and 4.25, the joint reactions λ_{jr} (the scleronomic Lagrange multipliers λ_s of the (4.44)) which act respectively on the shoulder and the elbow joints during the analyzed kinematics are shown.

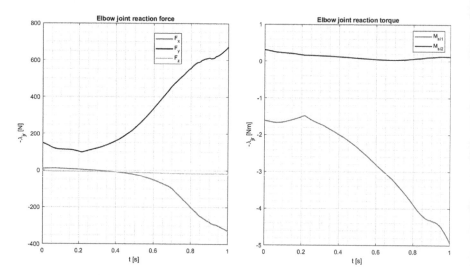

FIGURE 4.25 Elbow limb joint reactions.

4.4 CONCLUSIONS

This chapter aimed to show step by step the analytical development of a musculoskeletal multibody model, previously published by the same authors in a research paper, able to solve, in a classical formal approach, the inverse dynamics problem of the upper limb biomechanical system. The followed approach allows the system kinematical analysis, based on the evaluation of the constraints kinematical behavior. Subsequently, considering muscular actuators and including the external forces, the proposed approach makes possible to solve the inverse dynamic problem by evaluating the rheonomic Lagrange multipliers, related to the driving actions, which lead the system to move following the imposed kinematic. The description of the muscle topology is involved in the biomechanical analysis through the wrapped muscles modeling, obtained by an algorithm based on the calculus of the geodesic curves. The muscle paths are involved in the calculation of the muscle length, deformation velocity, and pennation angles, which, through the Hill muscle model, allows to calculate the muscles' passive forces and the muscle activations to be included in the motion equations. The static optimization and the solution of the inverse dynamics problem allow the evaluation of the muscle activation level and the joint reaction forces, useful in biomechanical analyses and in the optimization of the artificial joints structural and tribological design. The model's effectiveness was examined by its application on an upper limb model subjected to simple kinematics and gravity forces. All the input data are taken from the commercial software OpenSim, and the simulation results were compared with the ones provided by the same software, obtaining a very satisfactory matching. The only difference found was a small overestimation of the long biceps muscle fiber length, probably due to the different wrapping criteria used by OpenSim.

Multibody Biomechanics

In the framework of the limitations of the proposed model, due mainly to the necessity of a deeper validation considering more imposed kinematics and comparisons with experimental data, the proposed approach results as a suitable, open, and fully controllable tool for upper limb biomechanical analysis, and it represents a general procedure extendible to the analysis of others biomechanical systems like for example the lower limb.

LIST OF MAIN SYMBOLS

T	Topology matrix
q	Lagrangian coordinates
t	Translation vector
θ	Unit quaternion vector
$E, \bar{E}, G, \bar{G}$	Quaternion matrices
$\omega, \bar{\omega}, \dot{\omega}, \dot{\bar{\omega}}$	Angular velocity and acceleration in the floating reference frame and in the ground one
R	Rotation matrix
$\bar{u}$	Local position vector
r	Position vector in the ground reference frame
n_B, n_{dof}, n_c	Number of bodies, degrees of freedom and constraints
C	Constraint equations
Cq	Constraint Jacobian
$\hat{v}$	Rotation axis unit vector
q_{dof}	Degrees of freedom vector
M	Mass matrix
Q	Generalized force
F_e	External force vector in the ground reference frame
λ	Lagrange multipliers
Jq	Coordinate change matrix
l_t	Tendon length
l_m	Muscle fiber length
v_m	Muscle fiber deformation velocity
w_m	Muscle width
α_p	Muscle fiber pennation angle
F_{CE}	Muscle contractile element force
F_{PE}	Muscle passive element force
F_m	Muscle force
l_0, α_0	Optimal muscle fiber length and the related pennation angle
F_0	Maximum isometric force
l_{mt}, v_{mt}	Musculotendon length and deformation velocity
$x(u,v), f(x)$	Surfaces' parametric and implicit equations
s	Curvilinear coordinate
c	Curve
$\hat{t}, \hat{n}, \hat{b}$	Tangent, normal, and binormal unit vectors
Φq	Muscle Jacobian
a	Muscle activation vector
λ_r, λ_s	Lagrange multipliers related to the rheonomic constraints (or residual actuators) and to the scleronomic constraints (or joint reactions)

REFERENCES

1. A. Ruggiero e A. Sicilia, "A mixed elasto-hydrodynamic lubrication model for wear calculation in artificial hip joints," *Lubricants*, vol. 8, n. 7, p. 72, 2020.
2. A. Ruggiero e A. Sicilia, "Lubrication modeling and wear calculation in artificial hip joint during the gait," *Tribology International*, vol. 142, p. 105993, 2020.
3. A. Ruggiero, A. Sicilia e S. Affatato, "In silico total hip replacement wear testing in the framework of ISO 14242-3 accounting for mixed elasto-hydrodynamic lubrication effects," *Wear*, p. 203420, 2020.
4. J. Hu, Z. Chen, H. Xin, Q. Zhang e Z. Jin, "Musculoskeletal multibody dynamics simulation of the contact mechanics and kinematics of a natural knee joint during a walking cycle," *Proceedings of the Institution of Mechanical Engineers, Part H: Journal of Engineering in Medicine*, vol. 232, n. 5, pp. 508–519, 2018.
5. P. A. Varady, U. Glitsch e P. Augat, "Loads in the hip joint during physically demanding occupational tasks: A motion analysis study," *Journal of Biomechanics*, vol. 48, n. 12, pp. 3227–3233, 2015.
6. A. Ruggiero, R. D'Amato e N. Ungureanu, "Musculoskeletal multibody simulations for the optimal tribological design of human prostheses: the case of the ankle joint," *Materials Science and Engineering*, vol. 749, n. 1, p. 012008, 2020.
7. A. P. Stylianou, T. M. Guess e M. Kia, "Multibody muscle driven model of an instrumented prosthetic knee during squat and toe rise motions," *Journal of Biomechanical Engineering*, vol. 135, n. 4, 2013.
8. A. Ruggiero, M. Merola e S. Affatato, "On the biotribology of total knee replacement: A new roughness measurements protocol on in vivo condyles considering the dynamic loading from musculoskeletal multibody model," *Measurement*, vol. 112, pp. 22–28, 2017.
9. S. Affatato, M. Merola e A. Ruggiero, "Development of a novel in silico model to investigate the influence of radial clearance on the acetabular cup contact pressure in hip implants," *Materials*, vol. 11, n. 8, p. 1282, 2018.
10. A. Ruggiero, M. Merola e S. Affatato, "Finite element simulations of hard-on-soft hip joint prosthesis accounting for dynamic loads calculated from a musculoskeletal model during walking," *Materials*, vol. 11, n. 4, p. 574, 2018.
11. G. Bergmann, A. Bender, J. Dymke, G. Duda e P. Damm, "Standardized loads acting in hip implants," *PloS one*, vol. 11, n. 5, p. e0155612, 2016.
12. J.-P. Kassi, M. O. Heller, U. Stoeckle, C. Perka e G. N. Duda, "Stair climbing is more critical than walking in pre-clinical assessment of primary stability in cementless THA in vitro," *Journal of Biomechanics*, vol. 38, n. 5, pp. 1143–1154, 2005.
13. P. Westerhoff, F. Graichen, A. Bender, A. Halder, A. Beier, A. Rohlmann e G. Bergmann, "In vivo measurement of shoulder joint loads during activities of daily living," *Journal of Biomechanics*, vol. 42, n. 12, pp. 1840–1849, 2009.
14. M. Nordin e V. H. Frankel, *Basic biomechanics of the musculoskeletal system*, Lippincott Williams & Wilkins, Philadelphia, PA, 2001.
15. U. Trinler e R. Baker, "Estimated landmark calibration of biomechanical models for inverse kinematics," *Medical Engineering & Physics*, vol. 51, pp. 79–83, 2018.
16. M. T. Silva, A. F. Pereira e J. M. Martins, "An efficient muscle fatigue model for forward and inverse dynamic analysis of human movements," *Procedia IUTAM*, vol. 2, pp. 262–274, 2011.
17. M. P. Silva e J. A. Ambrosio, "Solution of redundant muscle forces in human locomotion with multibody dynamics and optimization tools," *Mechanics Based Design of Structures and Machines: An International Journal*, vol. 31, n. 3, pp. 381–411, 2003.

18. N. Curtis, "Craniofacial biomechanics: an overview of recent multibody modelling studies," *Journal of Anatomy*, vol. 218, n. 1, pp. 16–25, 2011.
19. S. Duprey, A. Naaim, F. Moissenet, M. Begon e L. Cheze, "Kinematic models of the upper limb joints for multibody kinematics optimisation: An overview," *Journal of Biomechanics*, vol. 62, pp. 87–94, 2017.
20. K. Huynh, I. Gibson, B. Jagdish e W. Lu, "Development and validation of a discretised multi-body spine model in LifeMOD for biodynamic behaviour simulation," *Computer Methods in Biomechanics and Biomedical Engineering*, vol. 18, n. 2, pp. 175–184, 2015.
21. A. Ruggiero, e A. Sicilia. A novel explicit analytical multibody approach for the analysis of upper limb dynamics and joint reactions calculation considering muscle wrapping. *Applied Sciences*, vol. 10, n. 21, p. 7760, 2020.
22. A. Shabana, *Dynamics of multibody systems*, Cambridge University Press, 2020.
23. P. E. Nikravesh e G. Gim, "Systematic construction of the equations of motion for multibody systems containing closed kinematic loops," *Journal of Mechanical Design*, vol. 115, n. 1, pp. 143–149, 1993.
24. H. Oliveira, "Inverse Dynamic Analysis of the Human Locomotion Apparatus for Gait," Instituto Superior Técnico, Lisbon, 2016.
25. K. Jovanovic, J. Vranic e N. Miljkovic, "Hill's and Huxley's muscle models: Tools for simulations in biomechanics," *Serbian Journal of Electrical Engineering*, vol. 12, n. 1, pp. 53–67, 2015.
26. M. Millard, T. Uchida, A. Seth e S. L. Delp, "Flexing computational muscle: modeling and simulation of musculotendon dynamics," *Journal of Biomechanical Engineering*, vol. 135, n. 2, 2013.
27. F. Romero e F. Alonso, "A comparison among different Hill-type contraction dynamics formulations for muscle force estimation," *Mechanical Sciences*, vol. 7, n. 1, p. 19, 2016.
28. C. John, "Complete Description of the Thelen 2003 Muscle Model," *OpenSim Documentation*, 2011. https://simtk-confluence.stanford.edu/display/OpenSim/Thelen+2003+Muscle+Model.
29. D. G. Thelen, "Adjustment of muscle mechanics model parameters to simulate dynamic contractions in older adults," *Journal of Biomechanical Engineering*, vol. 125, n. 1, pp. 70–77, 2003.
30. M. Hada, D. Yamada e T. Tsuji, "An analysis of equivalent impedance characteristics by modeling the human musculoskeletal structure as a multibody system," *Proceedings of the ECCOMAS Thematic Conference*, pp. 1–20, 2007.
31. F. Gao, M. Damsgaard, J. Rasmussen e S. T. Christensen, "Computational method for muscle-path representation in musculoskeletal models," *Biological Cybernetics*, vol. 87, n. 3, pp. 199–210, 2002.
32. O. Zarifi e I. Stavness, "Muscle wrapping on arbitrary meshes with the heat method," *Computer Methods in Biomechanics and Biomedical Engineering*, vol. 20, n. 2, pp. 119–129, 2017.
33. I. Stavness, M. Sherman e S. Delp, "A general approach to muscle wrapping over multiple surfaces," 2012.
34. A. Scholz, I. Stavness, M. Sherman, S. Delp e A. Kecskemethy, "Improved muscle wrapping algorithms using explicit path-error Jacobians," *Computational Kinematics*, pp. 395–403, 2014.
35. D. G. Thelen, F. C. Anderson e S. L. Delp, "Generating dynamic simulations of movement using computed muscle control," *Journal of Biomechanics*, vol. 36, n. 3, pp. 321–328, 2003.

5 Metal-Organic Frameworks-Polymer Composites for Practical Applications
Compatibility, Processability, and Biotribology Studies

J. A. Sánchez-Fernández
Centro de Investigación en Química Aplicada Satillo, México

Rodrigo Cué-Sampedro and Domingo Ricardo Flores-Hernandez
Tecnologico de Monterrey, Escuela de Ingeniería y Ciencias, Monterrey, México

CONTENTS

- 5.1 Tribology 124
- 5.2 Biotribology 124
- 5.3 Tribology Testing of Biomaterials 126
- 5.4 Active Agents 127
  - 5.4.1 Small Molecules 127
  - 5.4.2 Proteins 128
- 5.5 New Concepts to Overcome Challenges in Medical Applications of MOFs 129
  - 5.5.1 Properties of Nanoscale Coordination Polymers in Biomedicine 129
  - 5.5.2 Therapeutic Strategies 130
  - 5.5.3 Composites and Bio-Based Therapeutics 131
- 5.6 Key Requirements for Medical Application of MOF .. 132
  - 5.6.1 Non-toxicity and Stability 132
- 5.7 Multitasking and Multifunctional MOF Materials in Biomedicine 133
  - 5.7.1 Biomaterials and MOF for Medical Application 134
    - 5.7.1.1 Materials and MOF for Implants 134

5.8   Ceramics Biomedical Materials (Bioceramics) 135
5.9   Tribological Properties of Materials for Biomedical Applications 135
    5.9.1   Biofunctional Coatings on Biomaterials 136
    5.9.2   Biolubricants and Lubricants with MOF 137
5.10 Perspective and Outlook 139
References 139

5.1   TRIBOLOGY

Tribology was officially defined in 1966 by the UK Department of Education and Science

Report as the "science and technology of interacting surfaces in relative motion and the practices related thereto" [1]. Success of tribology research depends on the ability of wear measurement in relative motion. It includes the study and application of the principles of friction, lubrication, and wear. It is an interdisciplinary subject involving principles and draws upon several academic areas, including physics, chemistry, materials science, and engineering. Great attention is focused on studying metal/metal and metal/ceramic contact tribology. However, polymer components are increasingly replacing metals in structures, housings, flexures, and bearings, particularly in automotive weight reduction applications. As their friction and wear mechanisms, polymer tribology is more complex than for metal and less well understood. Whereas there are well-established "Laws of Friction" for the tribology of metal and ceramic contacts in relative motion, polymer/metal contacts generally do not follow these laws. The reasons for this are several, including the relative softness of polymers compared to metals, their much lower thermal conductivities associated with heat generation in contacts, and significantly lower melting points. Polymer tribology differs from metal/ceramic tribology because polymer/metal or polymer/polymer contact is predominantly elastic; it also provides the possible development of metals and alloys, ceramics, and polymer-based materials used in implants and other medical devices, Table 5.1.

5.2   BIOTRIBOLOGY

The word biotribology was firstly used and defined by Dowson in 1970 as those aspects of tribology concerned with biological systems. Currently, biotribology is one of the most exciting and rapidly growing areas of tribology [12]. Biotribology has been one of the most studied and active research areas in the field of tribology. Increasingly, biotribology research is contributing significant scientific, social, and healthcare benefits; the opportunities are considerable [13]. The human body possesses a wide variety of sliding and frictional interfaces, mainly in the joints. Medical devices are heavily regulated because of their intended uses in human beings. The friction between the eyelids and eyeball, and skin friction, also fall under the scope of tribology. Hence, a separate domain, called biotribology, has been developed to deal with the application of tribological principles, such as friction, wear, and lubrication between interacting surfaces in relative motion, to medical and biological systems. In Figure 5.1 are presented some of the most representative

TABLE 5.1
Tribological Properties of Materials for Biomedical Applications

Material	Application	Tribological Improvement	Reference
UHMWPE, PTFE, PEG, PMMA	Jaw and joint bone implants, tubular devices	Wear and corrosion resistance, low coefficient of friction	[2–5]
Stainless steel, titanium alloys, titanium aluminum vanadium alloy, cobalt chromium alloy, cobalt chromium molybdenum alloy	Complete joint replacement	Wear and corrosion resistance	[2, 3, 5]
Al_2O_3, ZrO_2, Si_3N_4, SiC, B_4C, quartz, bioglass (Na_2O-$CaOSiO_2$-P_2O_5), crystalline hydroxyapatite ($Ca10(PO_4)_6(OH)_2$)	Bone–joint coating, orthopedic, and dental surgeries	Wear and corrosion resistance and mechanical	[2, 6–8]
Two or more biofunctional materials	Improve mechanical properties, biodegradability, cells interaction, reduce toxicity of metallic materials, drug delivery	wear and corrosion resistance, low coefficient of friction	[3, 9]
Natural: bovine serum, water, physiological saline lubrication, mucins Synthetic: PEG, PEG-DOPA-Lysine, pAA-graft-PEG copolymer	Tissue contacting medical devices	Wear and corrosion resistance, low coefficient of friction	[10, 11]

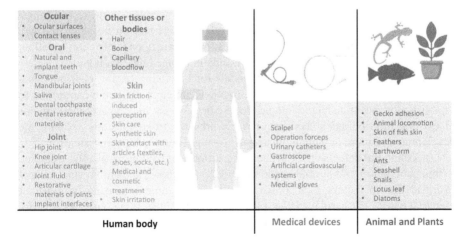

FIGURE 5.1 Representative investigations involving biotribology.

investigations involving biotribology and the diverse subjects this research is focused on. Even though biotribology comprises several topics, it is possible to categorize it into biotribology of the human body, medical devices, and animals and plants.

5.3 TRIBOLOGY TESTING OF BIOMATERIALS

Mechanical integrity and wear resistance of a biomaterial are vital for long-term implantable devices, such as total joint replacements, which need to function effectively. Allowed wear rates for such a system are significantly more sensitive to various factors. Ongoing efforts have been made to evaluate materials' durability, partly done through tribological testing [14]. Laboratory tests are necessary to help optimize the biomaterial performance, among which nanotribometer testing can be very significant for extended wear testing. Tribometry represents an area of tribology that encompasses means and methods of measuring: friction forces in contact zones, wear of tribosystem elements, temperature, surface roughness, contact surface sizes, and contact strain [3].

Friction and wear play an important role in determining the performance of biomaterials. It is noted that a majority of the tribological tests involving biomaterial combinations are subjected to standard reciprocating motion like real contact conditions prevalent in the human body. The wear of a sample is measured either through the conventional weight loss technique or directly from the instrument using a displacement transducer. The friction force is recorded with the help of a load cell, and the coefficient of friction is obtained by dividing the friction force by the normal force exerted by the counter body [15]. Many established tribological setups and characterization protocols are commonly used to investigate the friction and wear properties of artificial materials. The standard tribotesting configurations, namely ball-on-disk, pin-on-disk, block-on-disk, and three-ball-on-plate configuration [16], are employed to evaluate the tribological characteristics of biomedical materials, including metals and alloys, ultra-high molecular weight polyethylene (UHMWPE), ceramics, among others. Either the ambient temperature or the human body temperature (about 37°C) is selected as the working temperature of the tests. Using a mini traction machine-like test apparatus within a steel-ball on polymer disk has been used to study the effects of load and substrate elasticity on the friction of rolling sliding, lubricated, compliant contact for evaluating some lubricant liquids [17].

It is not easy to set up simulation models for laboratory testing of tribological systems concerning a human body. Investigations are currently being carried out to establish more accurate methodologies for predicting wear in complex environments of existing biotribological systems. These works would significantly enhance the development of more durable biomaterials for application in human systems.

Osteochondral defects on the articulating surfaces of the knee typically occur due to traumatic injuries, abnormalities in the subchondral bone, and chronic mechanical overload due to factors such as severe joint misalignments and the removal of meniscal tissue. The cartilage layer, integrated into the underlying bone, is primarily responsible for the biotribological function of osteochondral grafts in the natural joint environment and the subsequent maintenance or disruption of the biotribology in the surrounding and opposing cartilage surfaces [18]. Whereas replacing defective parts is often possible in technical settings, biological materials present in the human body need to show excellent performance and wear resistance for several decades. Indeed, many biological tissues show very low friction and wear. Furthermore, Lieleg and his team of researchers [19] conducted experiments with various materials relevant to the field of biotribology, including articular cartilage as probing material. The tribological measuring system comprises a measuring head and a bottom plate, both mounted into a commercial shear oscillatory rheometer.

Since there is no commercially available equipment for investigating the tribological behavior of soft contact lenses (SCLs), some researchers have investigated the tribological behavior using a new technique as an alternative to conventional tribometers based on the technique called dynamic oscillating tribometer [20]. In this context, a particular test machine was developed to be used as a tribometer, which operates as an oscillator with horizontal vibration movement and can be modeled as a vibratory mass-spring-damper mechanical system. The friction assessment method is based on evaluating the free damping vibration movement of the mass-spring system induced by an initial non-equilibrium condition [21].

Tyurin et al. have studied data control and acquisition and processing it in a laboratory of biotribology. The authors created a method of calculating the transfer of action by tribocontact, do it at each frequency level. The research approaches applied on a "pin-on-disk" fixture were similar to those used in input-output systems, with additional measurement channels by which the dynamics of friction processes and wear in real time [22].

5.4 ACTIVE AGENTS

5.4.1 SMALL MOLECULES

The high strength and high resistance to crack propagation of the materials make them suitable for safety-critical applications and load-bearing structural applications in, for example, the aerospace, automobile, microelectronics, and sporting industries. Similar structural gradients can be introduced in gradient nanostructured (GNS) ceramics and ceramic composites for applications as dental and orthopedic implants [23]. However, to tribologists, specialists in the physical and chemical phenomena associated with friction, wear, and lubrication, these interfacial processes take center stage. Putterman's research group in the University of California physics department demonstrated that the everyday act of unrolling commercial tape – simply peeling a strip of it from the underlying roll – causes friction-based events that lead to the emission of light and flashes of X-rays [24]. By peeling pressure-sensitive adhesive tape is an example of tribocharging and triboluminescence: the emission of visible light. Tape provides an interesting example of these phenomena because it has been claimed that the van der Waals interaction provides the fundamental energy that holds tape to a surface for deformable solids, this true area of contact depends strongly on the pressure applied and on the surface forces in a crucial arrangement [25]. Tribocharging of insulators involves the statistical mechanical transfer of mobile ions between surfaces as they are separated adiabatically. A competing theory proposes that a charged double layer is formed by electron transfer across the interface of different surfaces in contact [24].

Nevertheless, repeated frictional forces can cause these particles to agglomerate, reducing a lubricant's effectiveness. A team of researchers tried using them as lubricant additives to discover that crumpled graphene balls don't stick together. Results of tribology tests, in which a steel pin was dragged across a steel plate, show a reduction of friction and wear. The test includes a standard poly(α-olefin) oil containing crumpled graphene balls [26].

The mechanism of energy dissipation in inert molecular or atomic layers moving on substrates is crucial for understanding and manipulating the tribological properties of lubricated interfaces. Here, the van der Waals interactions result from: (1) the electrostatic force between two permanent dipoles; (2) the inductive force between a permanent dipole and an induced dipole; and (3) the dispersion force between two spontaneously induced dipoles. The first two dipole-dipole interactions can be well treated by the density functional theory (DFT). The last one, also called the London dispersion force, associates the correlated fluctuations between electrons on two sides [27, 28].

5.4.2 Proteins

In synovial joints such as the knee, hip and shoulder, articular cartilage functions foremost for load-supporting and load transferring between bones. Synovial fluid (SF) contains the molecules hyaluronan (HA), proteoglycan four that is encoded by the PRG4 gene, also known as lubricin, superficial zone protein, and surface-active phospholipids (SAPL), each of which interacts with and adsorbs to the articular surface. Such molecules are all ideally positioned to contribute to boundary lubrication [29].

Hyaluronan, among other roles, gives rise to the shear-thinning properties of SF, critical to fluid film lubrication in articulating joints [30]. Matrix molecules present at the articular cartilage surface, primarily collagen II, can form molecular associations with a superficial zone protein (SZP) [31] and hyaluronan in SF. Collagen II is the most abundant collagen in articular cartilage and forms extended fibrils creating a structure linked to proteoglycans and other collagens [32, 33]. Another fibril forming protein essential for matrix formation is the glycoprotein fibronectin, which consists of two disulfide bound subunits of approximately 250 kDa. Further, fibronectin aids extracellular matrix formation by interacting with a range of components, including collagen, to arrange the extracellular matrix network [34]. The distribution of proteoglycan along the fibril requires co-assembly of collagen and proteoglycan before fibril assembly. A well-defined understanding of the tribology of cartilages can provide design criteria for tissue engineering. Using that understanding to engineer clinically applicable implants should be the aim of cartilage researchers [35].

Important advancements in preclinical and clinical studies have been achieved. Thus, several different fields branch from surface science, for example, tribology, which studies the interaction between two moving solid surfaces, friction, and lubricants. Surface wettability describes the properties and characteristics which govern the behavior between a liquid and a solid surface. Specifically, surface wettability is a crucial consideration in scaffold creation, promoting proper cell adhesion, and supporting the knowledge for medical manufacturing devices [36].

5.5 NEW CONCEPTS TO OVERCOME CHALLENGES IN MEDICAL APPLICATIONS OF MOFs

5.5.1 Properties of Nanoscale Coordination Polymers in Biomedicine

Metal-organic frameworks (MOFs) are hybrid nanoporous coordinated materials with two- or three-dimensional (2D/3D) topologies assembled by the coordination of metal ions/secondary building units (SBUs) with organic linkers [37, 38]. Those materials, including covalent organic frameworks (COFs) [39, 40] porous organic polymers (POPs) [41], and related sophisticated architectures have been the subject of extensive research for many applications. They share the common features of having supramolecular structures assembled from metal nodes and organic linkers to form a nanoporous crystalline lattice.

Liu et al. [42] describe the classification of porous materials according to pore width, following the International Union of Pure and Applied Chemistry Convention, how a microporous material with less than 2 mm, mesoporous materials with internal pore width into the range from 2 to 50 nm while for macroporous materials, the internal width of pores reaches over 50 nm. In order to achieve a mesoporosity-containing hierarchy of MOFs, there arises many novel synthetic strategies and structure design. MOFs are known to have valences of 3 to 24; COFs are limited to the lower valences of 3 and 4, principally owing to the heavy reliance of organic chemistry on sp^2 and sp^3 hybridization. COFs are made by connecting preformed trigonal-planar, square-planar, and tetrahedral organic building units with low valency linkages [43].

Thanks to advancements and developments in medicine, some studies in porphyrin-based MOFs present a promising opportunity for biomedical applications due to the highly active frameworks and improved performance [38].

Heteroatom-containing MOF precursors, such as nitrogen-rich zeolitic imidazolate frameworks (ZIFs) [44], can be used to prepare nanostructures doped with heteroatoms (for example, nitrogen, sulfur, boron, and phosphorus). This approach can result in the modification of the electronic and geometric structures, provide more active sites, and facilitate host-guest interactions while controlling the morphology of these nanostructures. For combinational phototherapy of photodynamic therapy (PDT) and photothermal therapy (PTT), a MOF was synthesized by carbonization of a zeolitic imidazolate framework (ZIF-8), where mesoporous-silica was used to prevent the aggregation of nanospheres during the high-temperature pyrolysis. The zinc and nitrogen co-doped carbons (Zn-N-C) can be used as stable photosensitizers to generate $^1O_2$ via electronic transfer from the conjugated p-bond of a porphyrin-like structure to molecular oxygen. Lee and Gaharwar focus on the recent development of light-responsive inorganic nanomaterials for biomedical applications, including PTT, PDT, drug delivery, and regenerative medicine [45].

Controlling the macroscopic structural features is not straightforward, given that the synthetic repertoire available is currently confined to molecular chemists. From studies based on Begum et al. [46], the key contents on the polymerization of monomers loaded inside the confined channels of MOF assemblies, thereby controlling the macromolecular growth process through the highly ordered geometry of the MOF nano spaces, the post-synthesis copolymerization of preorganized organic ligands in MOF, and self-polymerization of the immobilized homopolymerizable ligands in MOF without the need for guest molecules to form polymeric interwoven molecular architectures. However, nanoscale metal-organic frameworks (NMOFs) and nanoscale coordination polymers (NCPs), as a highly porous material composed of metal ions/clusters and organic ligands, provide novel opportunities for biological and medical applications [47]. NMOFs and NCPs can have diverse properties due to their molecular nature. By taking advantage of the tailorable properties of NMOFs and NCPs, cargo loading can be much more efficient than conventional nanoparticles to allow for higher therapeutics agent loadings without sacrificing the beneficial physicochemical properties of NMOFs and NCPs [48].

5.5.2 Therapeutic Strategies

Surface forces govern the outcome of a significant number of physical processes; colloidal stability, adhesion, wettability, boundary lubrication, or capillarity can all be better described if the different surface forces involved are correctly considered. In this order of ideas, Giasson and Drummond's group has observed the shear-induced normal forces, which can be large enough to entrain a fluid film that separates the surfaces of contact, driving the dynamic system from conditions of boundary to hydrodynamic lubrication. To illustrate the potential of their work, they studied the response of a compliant microgel-based coating under compression and shear to investigate the coupling between normal and tangential motion and forces. Understanding the tribology of compliant surfaces may be crucial in several different circumstances, from engineering to many aspects of biotribology (e.g., ocular tribology or mammalian joints) [49].

Biotribology is useful in a range of areas, including arthroplasty, a surgical procedure necessary to prevent bone surfaces from constantly sliding against each other and causing wear and friction to occur at the contact interface, resulting in harmful responses. Such responses may include thinning of the hip cartilage, potentially leading to a total hip replacement. A significant number of hip replacements can be classified according to their geometry (structure and dimensions) and materials [50]. Friction properties at the cellular level are important not only in normal biological functions such as respiration, cell adhesion, and cell migration but also in pathology and implants. Those frictional forces play a crucial role in the safety and life span of devices and vascular stents [51].

At the cellular scale, biotribological properties, such as friction coefficients of vascular smooth muscle cells (VSMCs), have been investigated and shown to be influenced by cytoskeletal depolymerization and cellular cross-linking agents such as glutaraldehyde [52].

Creating a device that reduces the amount of friction would increase the ease of implantation. These interactions between cells and devices are 3D in terms of cellular organization but have often been investigated through 2D modeling and culture approaches. In this context, the possible differences between 2D and 3D biotribology yield comparable results. While many systems have been studied in a 2D environment, advances in 3D methods now allow more researchers to study human and non-human systems with approaches that more closely resemble their native environments, regardless of the environment or whether the biological system is human or non-human [53].

5.5.3 Composites and Bio-Based Therapeutics

Many organic ligands within NMOFs/NCPs may provide therapeutic functions by themselves, such as chemotherapeutic prodrugs, photosensitizers, and fluorescent dyes. Application of NMOFs is being made in various biomedical and clinical applications of sensing and imaging of various body diseases. On the other hand, certain types of inorganic metal ions as the coordination centers may offer imaging contrast for magnetic resonance imaging (MRI), computed tomography (CT) imaging, and single-photon emission computed tomography (SPECT) imaging [47, 54]. The healthcare field offers targeted applications for MOF-based composites such as controlled drug release and antibacterial materials. For example, the controlled release of nitric oxide (NO) is critical in the biomedical field because of its bioactivity in antiplatelet aggregation and its antibacterial and anti-inflammatory effects [55].

A series of bioactive Zr-MOF-based composites embedded with aptamer strands (509-MOF@Apt), in which 509-MOF is constructed based on the ligand 4′,4‴,4′′′′-nitrilotris[1,1′-biphenyl]-4-carboxylic acid (H_3NBB) [56]. Zr-MOFs has shown exceptional stability and great potential biomedical applications for the low toxicity of Zr. Further, Zr-MOFs present a high affinity to phosphate groups of biomolecules [57], which have been used to immobilize DNA probes selectively, and for the specificity to phosphate recognition via fluorescence [58].

Interest in MOFs has moved beyond purely academic to engineering processes and new applications, opening new opportunities in various industries, including biomedicals.

A group of researchers directed by Barbaud synthesized racemic α,α,β-trisubstituted β-lactones biodegradable biopolyesters (Figure 5.2), showing great potential for biomedical applications. Using different groups during the synthesis of these b-lactones allows a tailored synthesis of poly((R,S)-3,3-dimethylmalic acid) (PDMMLA) derivatives [59]. Belibel et al. evaluated the PDMMLA used as cardiovascular stents coating [60].

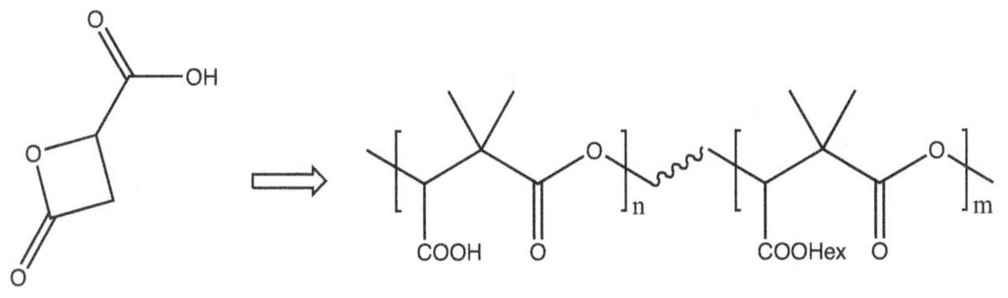

FIGURE 5.2 Synthesis of PDMMLA polymers through a retinopathy of prematurity (ROP) of the b-lactones [59].

5.6 KEY REQUIREMENTS FOR MEDICAL APPLICATION OF MOF

5.6.1 Non-toxicity and Stability

Various MOFs have been developed and prepared by scientists with different physicochemical properties because of their large linkers and metal ions/clusters. MOFs are dependent on the inorganic SBUs and the geometry of the organic linkers. High valency metal ion-based MOFs, such as Zr-MOFs, Fe-MOFs, and Cr-MOFs, are more stable and show excellent acid or base resistance than those of transition metal-based MOFs according to the hard–soft–acid–base (HSAB) theory [61]. Usually, as the lengths of the ligands increase, the synthesis steps of the ligands increase, indicating a more complex synthesis procedure. However, when the size of the rigid ligands increases, the solubility becomes poorer, which may lead to a lower yield of MOFs [62]. Also, the development of MOF materials comprising green and non-toxic ligand. Metal–insulator–metal (MIM) [63].

Biomaterials are divided into three main categories, known as synthetic, semi-synthetic, and natural polymers. This latter performs better in mimicking the extracellular matrix (ECM) and interaction with tissues, mainly due to the high similarity with tissue surroundings [64]. The pursuit of blood-compatible materials challenges nearly every aspect of materials design, including composition, mechanical properties, structure across multiple length scales, tribology, surface physical chemistry, and biochemical functionalization [65]. The most significant drawbacks and the modification strategies of natural and synthetic polymeric biomaterials have been described.

It is difficult to envisage MOF structures with stabilities that greatly exceed the thermal, mechanical, and chemical stabilities of the most robust existing MOFs. Mechanical stability has a crucial role if compacted forms of MOFs, such as pellets, are required in industrial processes [66, 67]. The synthesis parameters of MOFs (e.g., time, temperature, and heating rate), modifies the surface, ligand modulation, control of solvation during crystal growth, and physical grinding methods. These can be categorized into bottom-up and top-down methods and linked to the kinetics of MOF formation and the homogeneity of their size distribution and crystallinity. Likewise, the versatility of the surfactant-assisted method has led to the production of nanosized MOFs that both exhibit high monodispersity and colloidal stability. This feature is extremely attractive for catalytic studies and biomedical applications [68].

Moreover, the high and regular porosity and the unique combination of well-dispersed metal sites also have great relevance [69]. Engineering the morphologies, structures, and properties of the MOF-derived nanostructures are helpful to improve their performance. For example, fluorescent carbon nanodots, which can be produced directly from MOFs, are attractive for bioimaging and biosensing applications [70].

Some studies indicate that ZIF-8 coatings not only protect denaturing solvents and heat, but the nucleation and growth of the crystalline lattice do not alter the secondary or tertiary structure of protein and protein ensembles [71].

Samadian et al. [72] specify the principal properties a biomaterial must have to be biocompatible as well as non-toxic, mainly inherent to relations between the molecular structures and physicochemical as well as biological features of biomaterial, the effect of interfacial interactions between biological systems and biomaterial function, whit the controlled structural conversion of biomacromolecules together with the suitable engineering for stimulating specific cellular response for tuning of cell/tissue bioadhesive property. Recently, the evaluation of the protein corona on the toxicity of MOF-1s with the plasma proteins showed reduced toxicity at both concentrations (10 and 100% plasma). This decrease in MOF-1 toxicity could be due to masking the factors affecting the toxicity of these nanostructures, such as structural and chemical properties and the lack of direct contact of the nanoparticle surface with the cell surfaces [73]. Rosi and his research group created an anionic bio-MOF-1 constructed from zinc-adeninate and biphenyldicarboxylate and loaded the bio-MOF-1 with cationic procainamide hydrochloride at a loading amount of 0.22 g procainamide/g bio-MOF-1. Introducing biphenyldicarboxylic acid to reactions between adenine and zinc acetate dihydrate in dimethylformamide (DMF) yielded a single crystalline material formulated as $Zn_8(ad)_4(BPDC)_6O \cdot 2Me_2NH_2$, 8DMF, 11H$_2$O, heretofore referred to as bio-MOF-1 (ad= adeninate; BPDC = biphenyldicarboxylate) [74]. In the same context, a bio-MOF-1 coating was successfully fabricated on the surface of AZ31B Mg alloy [75].

Nanoscale MOFs (NMOFs) are intrinsically biodegradable because of their relatively labile metal–ligand bonds. The degradation profile of NMOFs should be considered a relevant parameter in the optimization and design to achieve desired therapeutic, imaging, or sensing functions. The improvement in the stability of NMOFs promotes the physiological environment, especially should be addressed before their successful applications in drug delivery, imaging, and sensing. Mostly when NMOFs are utilized as nanosensors for intracellular detection. The potential of NMOFs in biomedical applications depends on their cytotoxicity and general toxicity when applied in vivo [48]. Despite the clear societal and industrial interest of MOFs, there is still a lack of factual information about nanoMOF's in vivo toxicity [76].

The current state of biomedical applications of MOFs depends on the voids between the nanoparticles that can assist diffusion of selectively methylene blue (MB) molecules and consequently enhance the storage capacity. For example, based on the elemental analyses, ZIF-8 sodalite cages are only partially occupied and can be used for controlled release of the anticancer agent 5-fluorouracil [77].

5.7 MULTITASKING AND MULTIFUNCTIONAL MOF MATERIALS IN BIOMEDICINE

One of the primary testing challenges for biotribology is the minimal opportunity to test biological materials in a living being. Research is increasingly focused on obtaining a clearer tribological picture of the biological interface.

Due to the hydrogen bonds between hyaluronic acid (HA) and zeolitic imidazolate framework-8 (ZIF-8) and the high-stress transfer property of ZIF-8, HA/ZIF-8 has shown improved mechanical properties. Antibacterial characteristics and cell adhesion on HA-modified films are also improved [78]. Simple materials for biomedical applications are rarely used. The final fabricated, sterilized, and biocompatible form of a material used in bio-devices is biomaterial. Thus, biocompatibility is a relevant need to be focused on first. Each artificial implant demands performance requirements based on the physical properties of that biomaterial.

These requirements can be categorized according to mechanical performance, mechanical durability, and physical properties [79].

On the other hand, the hierarchical MOF structures, including atoms, building blocks, unit cells, crystallites, assemblies, and superstructures, are quite like the multilevel arrangement of proteins, which contain primary, secondary, tertiary, and quaternary structures. These superstructures contain precisely defined modules designed to execute specific tasks in sequence [80]. These materials are used to make very high-performance products with polymers of natural origin, such as some hydrogels for making many medical devices.

NanoMOFs for biomedical applications are still in the preclinical stage. Some Fe, Zn, and Cu-based nanoMOFs have shown good prospects due to their low toxicity and high therapeutic effect. Kim et al. reported that, due to their very small sizes and good biocompatibility, nanoMOFs had been widely investigated in biomedicine. Hyaluronic acid-nanoMOF (HA-nanoMOF) system loaded with anticancer drug doxorubicin (Dox) is highly efficient for cancer therapy. This approach is one step closer to precision medicine, providing multifunctional capabilities, including cancer-targeting, on-site drug release, and PDT [81].

5.7.1 Biomaterials and MOF for Medical Application

The medical device industry's growth demands numerous novel materials and biomaterials, scaffolds, and technologies to be used for orthopedic applications. Research is increasingly focused on obtaining a clearer tribological picture of a biological interface. For instance, the aim of biotribologists is to evaluate biological systems and understand how they function with efficiency, providing an increased understanding of their normal and their pathologic states. Biocompatibility is a prime requisite for materials to be used as an orthopedic implant [12].

5.7.1.1 Materials and MOF for Implants

A biomaterial is defined as any systemically, pharmacologically, inert substances, or combination of substances utilized for implantation within or incorporation in the living system to supplement or replace living tissue or organ function. Shape memory materials, also known as smart materials, are characterized by the unique property to recover the shape in response to external stimuli. The two most crucial and widely used shape memory materials are shape memory alloys (SMAs) and shape memory polymers (SMP). In general, all materials used for the fabrication of an implant should exhibit several properties that do not change over a long period of contact with the biological environment must be tested to demonstrate its biocompatibility. The SMAs that are widely used for knee and hip joint implants are Ni-Ti (55 nitinol) are investigated due to good corrosion, fatigue [82, 83].

The critical factor in periprosthetic osteolysis depends on the response to polyethylene wear particles released by orthopedic implants [84]. On the other hand, another study aimed at simultaneously enhancing wear resistance and mechanical performance of UHMWPE bearings by cross-linking the UHMWPE before melt processing followed by structural manipulation [85]. Another study evaluated the influence of prolonged artificial aging on oxidation resistance and the subsequent wear behavior of vitamin E-stabilized compared to standard and highly cross-linked, remelted polyethylene, and the degradation effect of third-body particles on cross-linked polyethylene (XLPE) inlays in total hip arthroplasty [86]. Applications of biological interfaces, which are predominantly soft, aqueous, and slippery, have also been studied. The origin of this slipperiness is thought to be linked to a high molecular weight surface gel layer. In the case of tear films, heavily glycosylated mucins act together to establish a viscoelastic hydrophilic gel. As a matter of engineering, a soft material may be anything with a modulus below 10 MPa; instead, to a biologist, it may be a material that is below one kPa. Developing opportunities for the measurement of friction over biological interfaces to assist in advancing medical devices (orthopedics, contact lenses, catheters, and implants) is greatly relevant [87].

5.8 CERAMICS BIOMEDICAL MATERIALS (BIOCERAMICS)

Bioceramics are inorganic materials that are bioactive to a specific function and biocompatible to the human body. The production process of bone generation begins with the bioactive element creating hydroxyl bonds, followed by the adsorption of calcium ions and solvated phosphate groups. A new family of glass (SiO_2–CaO–MgO–Na_2O–K_2O–P_2O_5) was used for deposition by the conventional enameling processes. Experiments showed that a critical range of silica content in the glass composition could be coated on the implant material to form apatite during the in-vitro test in simulated body fluid (SBF). Therefore, more silica content will make the glass biologically inactive, whereas less silica will make the glass largely soluble in SBF [79]. The advantages of hydroxyapatite nanowires are the abundant active sites on the surface, the magnetic nanoparticles, and MOF nanocrystals deposited on the surface, which avoids the tedious surface modification with organic linkers.

Further, the large specific surface area and relatively high MOF component content contribute to the improved capture efficiency and capture capacity. With these favorable characteristics, the magnetic metal–organic framework (mag-MOF) nanofibers show high selectivity, high detection sensitivity, desirable capture recovery, large capture capacity, and good repeatability. Moreover, some applications of mag-MOF nanofibers in the selective capture of phosphorylated peptides from practical biological specimens, including non-fat milk digest, human serum, and human saliva, have been demonstrated [88]. In additional context, an excellent example of methyl methacrylate (MMA) use is reported in a biological failure of a human femoral neck hydroxyapatite-coated titanium screw [89].

5.9 TRIBOLOGICAL PROPERTIES OF MATERIALS FOR BIOMEDICAL APPLICATIONS

Polymeric materials can be designed to emulate features of biological systems. The chemical composition and processing of these materials define their structural and mechanical properties, making them suitable for use in tissue engineering, implants, and prosthetic applications [90–92]. However, polymeric materials are often related to poor mechanical performance, such as low hardness and high wear rate; in order to address these drawbacks, polymeric materials can be combined with reinforcement materials to produce hybrid polymer matrix composites (HPMC). Moreover, their low manufacturing cost, high strength, and ease of fabrication make them suitable for biomaterials development in biomedical applications [93].

In its work, Chang et al. analyzed the tribological properties of ultra-high molecular weight polyethylene (UHMWPE) reinforce with zeolites prepared using hot compression molding for implant applications [94]. They compared the wear volume loss and coefficient of friction of pure UHMWPE and zeolite/UHMWPE composite with 10wt% and 20wt% of zeolite. An overall significant improvement of the tribological properties was obtained with the zeolite reinforcement. The wear volume loss was found to be less when zeolite concentrations were higher. The coefficient of friction was also reduced as the concentration of zeolite was increased.

Similarly, Yunus et al. compared the mechanical, corrosion, and tribological properties of HPMC materials with ceramic reinforcements [93]. Their work scope was to improve the modulus of elasticity, a critical material property when designing prosthetics. The polymer used was polyethylene (HDPE) reinforced with ceramic fillers such as titanium dioxide (TiO_2) and alumina (Al_2O_3). The reinforcements improved the tribological properties such as wear loss, coefficient of friction, and frictional forces. Their samples were submitted to various loads. While the pure HDPE presented increased wear loss as the loads were increased, this effect was diminished with the increase of alumina. Similarly, the frictional force was decreased with the increase of the ceramic reinforcements.

Besides HPMC, polymer science has taking advantage of the recent development of MOFs. This novel material possesses features such as high porosity, high surface area, and catalytic activity for developing bulk materials, membranes, and dispersed materials useful in biomedical applications [95]. While MOFs are crystalline and brittle porous solids, polymers are flexible and processable solids. Recently, studies have focused their attention on producing composites that hold the properties of each material. Impressive results showed that MOFs' presence influences polymers' structure, and polymers can modulate MOF's growth [96].

5.9.1 Biofunctional Coatings on Biomaterials

The success of integrating a biomaterial into a biological system depends on its incorporation into the surrounding tissues, where the interaction at the interface between both materials becomes critical. The physical and chemical properties of these materials must address various factors such as biocompatibility, osseointegration, corrosion resistance, controlled degradability, modulus of elasticity, and fatigue strength [97]. The development of novel nanomaterials and nanocomposites drives current materials to address high-performance biomaterials' requirements for biomedical applications. In this regard, incorporating these biofunctional materials into biomaterials can follow mechanical, chemical, and physical approaches [2, 98]. The association of biopolymers and MOFs is a nascent subject that still faces many challenges. Pairing "biopolymer-MOF" must be selected, optimized, and modeled to find the most successful hybrid combination. This relies primarily on a deeper understanding of the interactions occurring at the interface of the two phases [99].

Metal-Organic Frameworks-Polymer Composites

Typically, coatings can be classified as conversion coatings formed by specific reactions between the substrate and the environment and deposited coatings obtained by several techniques. Conversion coatings techniques can be obtained by ion implantation, anodization, heat treatment, and chemical conversion. These coatings are formed due to the interaction of metal dissolution and precipitation in aqueous systems. The nature of this approach led to a high level of adhesion [98].

5.9.2 BIOLUBRICANTS AND LUBRICANTS WITH MOF

With rising awareness of sustainability, current tribological research focuses on the development of sustainable and energy-efficient systems, which is called "green tribology" [100]. It includes investigations into complex fluids with anisotropic properties, e.g., mesogenic fluids, ionic liquids, and ionic liquid crystals (ILCs). ILC (Structure 5.1) is usually composed of cations with a long alkyl chain substituent and has shown its total potential for friction reduction [7]. Liquid crystals (LCs) are a further substance class of additives that have been shown to improve friction and optimize water as a lubricant [101]. For example, LCs are contained in the human SF and are essential for the excellent friction behavior of joints. Also, the lamellar LCs show lower coefficients of friction (COF) with a higher load-carrying capacity compared to the commercial lubricants. In the same context, low COF in a binary octyl-β-D-glucopyranoside (C8)/H$_2$O system with a concentration of 40% was already demonstrated [102, 103], Structure 5.2 presents a structure of octyl β-D-glucopyranoside or n-octyl glucoside. It was assumed that the interaction between the surface and the shear-induced molecular orientation is responsible for improving tribological properties.

STRUCTURE 5.1   IMIDAZOLIUM CATION

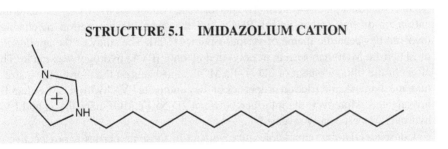

STRUCTURE 5.2   OCTYL β-D-GLUCOPYRANOSIDE

A nanolubricant of metallic silver nanoparticles was synthesized and suspended in polyethylene glycol (PEG). The nanolubricant exhibits excellent stability due to poly(vinyl pyrrolidone) used as the coating agent. PEG acts as both the solvent and reducing agent. The oxyethylene groups of PEG can form a crown ether-like structure in solution. Ag ions bind the cavities of crown ether. Results showed that the Ag particles, even at low concentration (4.5 mM), effectively reduce both the COF and wear. The water solubility, low volatility, natural lubricity, and non-toxicity of PEG make it a candidate lubricant for many applications [104]. In other research has been proposed emulsion microgel particles with stimuli-responsiveness to physiological enzyme and shear were proposed and have been realized, creating a novel biolubricant additive. In response to tribological shear and enzyme activity, some oil droplets are entrapped in the starch microgel particles to improve lubrication [105]. Lubricin-related friction regulation in soft eye tissues, where much lower forces are involved compared with knee joints, is related to dry eye disease and contact lens discomfort. The chemical structure of lubricin has inspired several chemists to synthesize new polymers that function just like lubricin to design new bio-based lubricants with ultra-low-friction coefficients [106]. In the same topic, the influence of protein concentration on the biotribological properties of the stem-cement interface was investigated using polished Ti6Al4V and bone cement, lubricated by protein solutions with different concentrations [107].

MOFs, as novel and innovative materials, have attracted considerable attention from the scientific community worldwide due to their large potential in diverse applications, especially for the adsorptive removal of endocrine-disrupting compounds (EDCs) into an aqueous system. The performance of several MOFs for the extermination of diverse categories of EDCs and the plausible adsorption mechanism involved has been the theme of various reviews [108]. The study of the application of 2D Ni-Fe MOF nanosheets in polyvinyl alcohol (PVA) hydrogel was made. The effect of the filling content of 2D Ni-Fe MOF nanosheets on the morphology, structure, mechanical, and friction properties of the composite PVA hydrogels was detailly investigated. Moreover, the interface between 2D Ni-Fe MOF nanosheets and PVA hydrogel was especially revealed.

Consequently, the remarkable improvement of those properties is prospective to provide a new direction for artificial articular cartilage [109]. In detail, it has been discussed to conventional MOFs materials. The micropores into MOFs are too small to adsorb lubricant macromolecules, and the compatibility between the embedded porous microstructures and the metallic/polymeric matrix remains a challenge. Mesoporous metal−organic frameworks (m-MOFs) may offer an efficient way to solve the problems due to their large specific surface area and high interfacial interaction with the matrix. Tribo-chemistry plays a major role in these lubrication regimes. Lubricants containing friction modifiers (FM) are used to reduce friction coefficient in light-load mixed lubrication regime or transition from hydrodynamic to mixed lubrication. Lubricants entrapped in benzene-1,3,5-tricarboxylate (BTC) ligand as the linkers (Cu-BTC) and m-MOFs as smart nanocontainers were synthesized and were incorporated into an epoxy resin (EP) matrix. Hence, a nanocomposite with a smart Cu-BTC container holds the promise of realizing extraordinary self-lubricating properties under stress stimuli [110]. MOFs with two or more metals such as heterogeneous inorganic nanoparticle@MOF can also be driven to the stage of bio-composites to enlarge the library of the prepared materials.

5.10 PERSPECTIVE AND OUTLOOK

The literature discussed here leaves no doubt that the extension of the MOFs into biomedical device applications is a highly active area of research. It is particularly noteworthy that several of the major challenges identified are the focus of vigorous research efforts. We emphasize points of the progress in structuring MOF-templated polymeric network materials; however, certain challenges remain, i.e., to act as whole supporting material, the scalability and processability that limit their practical that potential need to be addressed. From the perspective of synthetic planning and materials engineering at a molecular level, introducing modular building blocks with distinct ambitious features, for instance, switchability, chiral π-stacked conjugated molecular components like MOFs, will be of benefit. Common examples of medical devices include instruments, apparatus, appliances, and materials intended for use in human beings for diagnosis, prevention, monitoring, treatment, or alleviation of disease due to an injury or handicap, modification of the anatomy of a physiological process. Because of the nature of their applications, medical devices are heavily regulated. Hence, many medical devices involve moving parts, friction, and wear, factors that affect not only the functioning of these devices but also the potential to affect the natural tissues adversely.

Moreover, the system transits from the boundary to the hydrodynamic modes of lubrication, which is likely to trigger significant friction and wear reduction. Consequently, the use of MOFs, together with other materials such as synthetic and natural polymers, including biolubricants, must be biocompatible and non-toxic and accentuating the biotribological characteristics. Concluding, much remains to be done in the MOF-polymer-biotribology test conjunction.

REFERENCES

1. Hutchings I, Shipway P. *Trybology: Friction and Wear of Engineering Materials*. 2nd edition. Elsevier Ltd; 2017.
2. Rehman M, Madni A, Webster TJ. The era of biofunctional biomaterials in orthopedics: what does the future hold? *Expert Rev Med Dev.* [Internet]. 2018;15(3):193–204. Available from: http://dx.doi.org/10.1080/17434440.2018.1430569.
3. Zivić F, Babić M, Grujović N, Mitrović S. Tribometry of materials for bioengineering applications. *Tribol Ind.* 2010;32(1):25–32.
4. Buxadera-Palomero J, Calvo C, Torrent-Camarero S, Gil FJ, Mas-Moruno C, Canal C, et al. Biofunctional polyethylene glycol coatings on titanium: an in vitro-based comparison of functionalization methods. *Colloids Surfaces B Biointerfaces* [Internet]. 2017;152:367–375. Available from: http://dx.doi.org/10.1016/j.colsurfb.2017.01.042.
5. Uwais ZA, Hussein MA, Samad MA, Al-Aqeeli N. Surface modification of metallic biomaterials for better tribological properties: a review. *Arab J Sci Eng.* 2017;42(11):4493–4512.
6. Nath S, Sinha N, Basu B. Microstructure, mechanical and tribological properties of microwave sintered calcia-doped zirconia for biomedical applications. *Ceram Int.* 2008;34(6):1509–1520.

7. Avilés MD, Sánchez C, Pamies R, Sanes J, Bermúdez MD. Ionic liquid crystals in tribology. *Lubricants*. 2019;7(9):72.
8. Madhavasarma P, Veeraragavan P, Kumaravel S, Sridevi M. Studies on physiochemical modifications on biologically important hydroxyapatite materials and their characterization for medical applications. *Biophys Chem* [Internet]. 2020;267(September):106474. Available from: https://doi.org/10.1016/j.bpc.2020.106474.
9. Mishra A, Khobragade N, Sikdar K, Chakraborty S, Kumar SB, Roy D. Study of mechanical and tribological properties of Nanomica dispersed hydroxyapatite based composites for biomedical applications. *Adv Mater Sci Eng*. 2017;2017.
10. Chawla K, Lee S, Lee BP, Dalsin JL, Messersmith PB, Spencer ND. A novel low-friction surface for biomedical applications: modification of poly(dimethylsiloxane) (PDMS) with polyethylene glycol(PEG)-DOPA-lysine. *J Biomed Mater Res A*. 2009;90(3):742–749.
11. Andresen Eguiluz RC, Cook SG, Brown CN, Wu F, Pacifici NJ, Bonassar LJ, et al. Fibronectin mediates enhanced wear protection of lubricin during shear. *Biomacromolecules*. 2015;16(9):2884–2894.
12. Sahoo P, Das SK, Paulo Davim J. Tribology of materials for biomedical applications [Internet]. *Mechanical Behaviour of Biomaterials*. Elsevier Ltd.; 2019. 1–45. Available from: https://doi.org/10.1016/B978-0-08-102174-3.00001-2.
13. Zhou ZR, Jin ZM. Biotribology: recent progresses and future perspectives. *Biosurface and Biotribology*. 2015;1(1):3–24.
14. Zivic F. Nanotribometer area of application. *Tribol Ind*. 2007;29(3–4):29–34.
15. Choubey A, Basu B, Balasubramaniam R. Tribological behaviour of Ti-based alloys in simulated body fluid solution at fretting contacts. *Mater Sci Eng A*. 2004;379(1–2):234–239.
16. Taylor BL, Mills TB. Using a three-ball-on-plate configuration for soft tribology applications. *J Food Eng*. 2020;274(April):109838.
17. Myant C, Spikes HA, Stokes JR. Influence of load and elastic properties on the rolling and sliding friction of lubricated compliant contacts. *Tribol Int* [Internet]. 2010;43(1–2):55–63. Available from: http://dx.doi.org/10.1016/j.triboint.2009.04.034.
18. Bowland P, Ingham E, Jennings L, Fisher J. Review of the biomechanics and biotribology of osteochondral grafts used for surgical interventions in the knee. *Proc Inst Mech Eng Part H J Eng Med*. 2015;229(12):879–888.
19. Winkeljann B, Bussmann AB, Bauer MG, Lieleg O. Oscillatory tribology performed with a commercial shear rheometer. *Biotribology*. 2018;14(May):11–18.
20. Rigaud E, Perret-Liaudet JL, Belin M, Joly-Pottuz L, Martin JM. An original dynamic tribotest to discriminate friction and viscous damping. *Tribol Int*. 2010;43(1–2):320–329.
21. Carvalho AL, Vilhena LM, Ramalho A. Study of the frictional behavior of soft contact lenses by an innovative method. *Tribol Int*. 2021;153(September):3–9.
22. Tyurin A, Ganus G, Stepanov M, Ismailov G. Measurement instruments and software used in biotribology research laboratory. *Electr Control Commun Eng*. 2015;8(1):30–36.
23. Li X, Lu L, Li J, Zhang X, Gao H. Mechanical properties and deformation mechanisms of gradient nanostructured metals and alloys. *Nat Rev Mater* [Internet]. 2020;5(9):706–723. Available from: http://dx.doi.org/10.1038/s41578-020-0212-2.
24. Camara CG, Escobar J V., Hird JR, Putterman SJ. Correlation between nanosecond X-ray flashes and stick-slip friction in peeling tape. *Nature*. 2008;455(7216):1089–1092.
25. Gay C, Leibler L, Gay C, Leibler L, Letters R, Physical A. Theory of tackiness. *Phys Rev Lett*. 2016;82(5):936–939.
26. Dou X, Koltonow AR, He X, Jang HD, Wang Q, Chung YW, et al. Self-dispersed crumpled graphene balls in oil for friction and wear reduction. *Proc Natl Acad Sci U S A*. 2016;113(6):1528–1533.

27. Su G, Yang S, Jiang Y, Li J, Li S, Ren JC, et al. Modeling chemical reactions on surfaces: The roles of chemical bonding and van der Waals interactions. *Prog Surf Sci* [Internet]. 2019;94(4):100561. Available from: https://doi.org/10.1016/j.progsurf.2019.100561.
28. Yuan D, Zhang Y, Ho W, Wu R. Effects of van der Waals dispersion interactions in density functional studies of adsorption, catalysis, and tribology on metals. *J Phys Chem C*. 2020;124(31):16926–16942.
29. Schmidt TA, Gastelum NS, Nguyen QT, Schumacher BL, Sah RL. Boundary lubrication of articular cartilage: role of synovial fluid constituents. *Arthritis Rheum*. 2007;56(3):882–891.
30. Tamer TM. Hyaluronan and synovial joint: function, distribution and healing. *Interdiscip Toxicol*. 2013;6(3):111–125.
31. Flannery CR, Hughes CE, Schumacher BL, Tudor D, Aydelotte MB, Kuettner KE, et al. Articular cartilage superficial zone protein (SZP) is homologous to megakaryocyte stimulating factor precursor and is a multifunctional proteoglycan with potential growth-promoting, cytoprotective, and lubricating properties in cartilage metabolism. *Biochem Biophys Res Commun*. 1999;254(3):535–541.
32. Graham HK, Holmes DF, Watson RB, Kadler KE. Identification of collagen fibril fusion during vertebrate tendon morphogenesis. The process relies on unipolar fibrils and is regulated by collagen-proteoglycan interaction. *J Mol Biol*. 2000;295(4):891–902.
33. Flowers SA, Zieba A, Örnros J, Jin C, Rolfson O, Björkman LI, et al. Lubricin binds cartilage proteins, cartilage oligomeric matrix protein, fibronectin and collagen II at the cartilage surface. *Sci Rep*. 2017;7(1):1–11.
34. Kadler KE, Hill A, Canty-Laird EG. Collagen fibrillogenesis: fibronectin, integrins, and minor collagens as organizers and nucleators. *Curr Opin Cell Biol*. 2008;20(5):495–501.
35. Link JM, Salinas EY, Hu JC, Athanasiou KA. The tribology of cartilage: mechanisms, experimental techniques, and relevance to translational tissue engineering. *Clin Biomech* [Internet]. 2020;79(October):104880. Available from: https://doi.org/10.1016/j.clinbiomech.2019.10.016.
36. Villegas M, Zhang Y, Abu Jarad N, Soleymani L, Didar TF. Liquid-infused surfaces: a review of theory, design, and applications. *ACS Nano*. 2019;13(8):8517–8536.
37. Furukawa H, Cordova KE, O'Keeffe M, Yaghi OM. The chemistry and applications of metal-organic frameworks. *Science*. 2013;341(6149).
38. Chen J, Zhu Y, Kaskel S. Porphyrin-based metal–organic frameworks for biomedical applications. *Angew Chemie – Int Ed*. 2021;60(10):5010–5035.
39. Diercks CS, Yaghi OM. The atom, the molecule, and the covalent organic framework. *Science*. 2017;355(6328).
40. Haase F, Hirschle P, Freund R, Furukawa S, Ji Z, Wuttke S. Beyond frameworks: structuring reticular materials across nano-, meso-, and bulk regimes. *Angew Chemie – Int Ed*. 2020;59(50):22350–22370.
41. Lee JSM, Cooper AI. Advances in conjugated microporous polymers. *Chem Rev*. 2020;120(4):2171–2214.
42. Liu D, Zou D, Zhu H, Zhang J. Mesoporous metal–organic frameworks: synthetic strategies and emerging applications. *Small*. 2018;14(37):1–40.
43. Gropp C, Ma T, Hanikel N, Yaghi OM. Design of higher valency in covalent organic frameworks. *Science*. 2020;370(6515).
44. Wang B, Côté AP, Furukawa H, O'Keeffe M, Yaghi OM. Colossal cages in zeolitic imidazolate frameworks as selective carbon dioxide reservoirs. *Nature*. 2008;453(7192):207–211.
45. Lee HP, Gaharwar AK. Light-responsive inorganic biomaterials for biomedical applications. *Adv Sci*. 2020;7(17):2000863.

46. Begum S, Hassan Z, Bräse S, Tsotsalas M. Polymerization in MOF-confined nanospaces: tailored architectures, functions, and applications. *Langmuir.* 2020;36(36):10657–10673.
47. Zhu W, Zhao J, Chen Q, Liu Z. Nanoscale metal-organ frameworks and coordination polymers as theranostic platforms for cancer treatment. *Coord Chem Rev* [Internet]. 2019;398:113009. Available from: https://doi.org/10.1016/j.ccr.2019.07.006
48. He C, Liu D, Lin W. Nanomedicine applications of hybrid nanomaterials built from metal-ligand coordination bonds: nanoscale metal-organic frameworks and nanoscale coordination polymers. *Chem Rev.* 2015;115(19):11079–11108.
49. Vialar P, Merzeau P, Giasson S, Drummond C. Compliant surfaces under shear: elastohydrodynamic lift force. *Langmuir.* 2019;35(48):15605–15613.
50. Di Puccio F, Mattei L. Biotribology of artificial hip joints. *World J Orthop.* 2015;6(1):77–94.
51. Cobb JA, Dunn AC, Kwon J, Sarntinoranont M, Sawyer WG, Tran-Son-Tay R. A novel method for low load friction testing on living cells. *Biotechnol Lett.* 2008;30(5):801–806.
52. Dean D, Hemmer J, Vertegel A, LaBerge M. Frictional behavior of individual vascular smooth muscle cells assessed by lateral force microscopy. *Materials (Basel).* 2010;3(9):4668–4680.
53. Warren KM, Islam MM, Leduc PR, Steward R. 2D and 3D Mechanobiology in human and nonhuman systems. *ACS Appl Mater Interfaces.* 2016;8(34):21869–21882.
54. Meng HM, Hu XX, Kong GZ, Yang C, Fu T, Li ZH, et al. Aptamer-functionalized nanoscale metal-organic frameworks for targeted photodynamic therapy. *Theranostics.* 2018;8(16):4332–4344.
55. Ma K, Idrees KB, Son FA, Maldonado R, Wasson MC, Zhang X, et al. Fiber composites of metal-organic frameworks. *Chem Mater.* 2020;32(17):7120–7140.
56. Zhang ZH, Duan FH, Tian JY, He JY, Yang LY, Zhao H, et al. Aptamer-embedded zirconium-based metal-organic framework composites prepared by de novo bio-inspired approach with enhanced biosensing for detecting trace analytes. *ACS Sensors.* 2017;2(7):982–989.
57. Zhang GY, Deng SY, Cai WR, Cosnier S, Zhang XJ, Shan D. Magnetic zirconium hexacyanoferrate (II) nanoparticle as tracing tag for electrochemical DNA Assay. *Anal Chem.* 2015;87(17):9093–9100.
58. Della Giustina G, Zambon A, Lamberti F, Elvassore N, Brusatin G. Straightforward micropatterning of oligonucleotides in microfluidics by novel spin-on ZrO_2 surfaces. *ACS Appl Mater Interfaces.* 2015;7(24):13280–13288.
59. Gholizadeh E, Belibel R, Bachelart T, Bounadji C, Barbaud C. Chemical grafting of cholesterol on monomer and PDMMLA polymers, a step towards the development of new polymers for biomedical applications. *RSC Adv.* 2020;10(54):32602–32608.
60. Belibel R, Sali S, Marinval N, Garcia-Sanchez A, Barbaud C, Hlawaty H. PDMMLA derivatives as a promising cardiovascular metallic stent coating: physicochemical and biological evaluation. *Mater Sci Eng C* [Internet]. 2020;117(June):111284. Available from: https://doi.org/10.1016/j.msec.2020.111284
61. Ryu UJ, Jee S, Rao PC, Shin J, Ko C, Yoon M, et al. Recent advances in process engineering and upcoming applications of metal–organic frameworks. *Coord Chem Rev* [Internet]. 2021;426:213544. Available from: https://doi.org/10.1016/j.ccr.2020.213544
62. Zhao N, Cai K, He H. The synthesis of metal-organic frameworks with template strategies. *Dalt Trans.* 2020;49(33):11467–11479.
63. Krishtab M, Stassen I, Stassin T, Cruz AJ, Okudur OO, Armini S, et al. Vapor-deposited zeolitic imidazolate frameworks as gap-filling ultra-low-k dielectrics. *Nat Commun.* 2019;10(1):1–9.

64. Abbasian M, Massoumi B, Mohammad-Rezaei R, Samadian H, Jaymand M. Scaffolding polymeric biomaterials: are naturally occurring biological macromolecules more appropriate for tissue engineering? *Int J Biol Macromol* [Internet]. 2019;134:673–694. Available from: https://doi.org/10.1016/j.ijbiomac.2019.04.197
65. Hedayati M, Neufeld MJ, Reynolds MM, Kipper MJ. The quest for blood-compatible materials: recent advances and future technologies. *Mater Sci Eng R Reports* [Internet]. 2019;138(March):118–152. Available from: https://doi.org/10.1016/j.mser.2019.06.002
66. Howarth AJ, Liu Y, Li P, Li Z, Wang TC, Hupp JT, et al. Chemical, thermal and mechanical stabilities of metal-organic frameworks. *Nat Rev Mater*. 2016;1(15018):1–15.
67. Wu H, Yildirim T, Zhou W. Exceptional mechanical stability of highly porous zirconium metal-organic framework UiO-66 and its important implications. *J Phys Chem Lett*. 2013;4(6):925–930.
68. Usman KAS, Maina JW, Seyedin S, Conato MT, Payawan LM, Dumée LF, et al. Downsizing metal–organic frameworks by bottom-up and top-down methods. *NPG Asia Mater*. 2020;12(1).
69. Simon-Yarza T, Mielcarek A, Couvreur P, Serre C. Nanoparticles of metal-organic frameworks: on the road to in vivo efficacy in biomedicine. *Adv Mater*. 2018;30(37):1–15.
70. Dang S, Zhu QL, Xu Q. Nanomaterials derived from metal-organic frameworks. *Nat Rev Mater*. 2017;3.
71. Luzuriaga MA, Welch RP, Dharmarwardana M, Benjamin CE, Li S, Shahrivarkevishahi A, et al. Enhanced stability and controlled delivery of MOF-encapsulated vaccines and their immunogenic response in vivo. *ACS Appl Mater Interfaces*. 2019;11(10):9740–9746.
72. Samadian H, Maleki H, Allahyari Z, Jaymand M. Natural polymers-based light-induced hydrogels: Promising biomaterials for biomedical applications. *Coord Chem Rev*. 2020;420.
73. Jafari S, Izadi Z, Alaei L, Jaymand M, Samadian H, Kashani V, et al. Human plasma protein corona decreases the toxicity of pillar-layer metal organic framework. *Sci Rep* [Internet]. 2020;10(1):1–14. Available from: https://doi.org/10.1038/s41598-020-71170-z
74. An J, Geib SJ, Rosi NL. Cation-triggered drug release from a porous zinc-adeninate metal-organic framework. *J Am Chem Soc*. 2009;131(24):8376–8377.
75. Liu W, Yan Z, Zhang Z, Zhang Y, Cai G, Li Z. Bioactive and anti-corrosive bio-MOF-1 coating on magnesium alloy for bone repair application. *J Alloys Compd*. 2019;788:705–711.
76. Baati T, Njim L, Neffati F, Kerkeni A, Bouttemi M, Gref R, et al. In depth analysis of the in vivo toxicity of nanoparticles of porous iron(iii) metal–organic frameworks. *Chem Sci*. 2013;4(4):1597–1607.
77. Li R, Ren X, Zhao J, Feng X, Jiang X, Fan X, et al. Polyoxometallates trapped in a zeolitic imidazolate framework leading to high uptake and selectivity of bioactive molecules. *J Mater Chem A*. 2014;2(7):2168–2173.
78. Feng S, Zhang X, Shi D, Wang Z. Zeolitic imidazolate framework-8 (ZIF-8) for drug delivery: a critical review. *Front Chem Sci Eng*. 2021;15(2):221–237.
79. Roy S. Functionally graded coatings on biomaterials: a critical review. *Mater Today Chem*. [Internet]. 2020;18:100375. Available from: https://doi.org/10.1016/j.mtchem.2020.100375
80. Feng L, Wang KY, Willman J, Zhou HC. Hierarchy in metal-organic frameworks. *ACS Cent Sci*. 2020;6(3):359–367.

81. Kim K, Lee S, Jin E, Palanikumar L, Lee JH, Kim JC, et al. MOF × biopolymer: collaborative combination of metal-organic framework and biopolymer for advanced anticancer therapy. *ACS Appl Mater Interfaces*. 2019;11(31):27512–27520.
82. Abitha H, Kavitha V, Gomathi B, Ramachandran B. A recent investigation on shape memory alloys and polymers based materials on bio artificial implants-hip and knee joint. *Mater Today Proc* [Internet]. 2020;33:4458–4466. Available from: https://doi.org/10.1016/j.matpr.2020.07.711
83. Sabahi N, Chen W, Wang CH, Kruzic JJ, Li X. A review on additive manufacturing of shape-memory materials for biomedical applications. *Jom* [Internet]. 2020;72(3):1229–1253. Available from: https://doi.org/10.1007/s11837-020-04013-x
84. Green TR, Fisher J, Stone M, Wroblewski BM, Ingham E. Polyethylene particles of a "critical size" are necessary for the induction of cytokines by macrophages in vitro. *Biomaterials*. 1998;19(24):2297–2302.
85. Huang YF, Zhang ZC, Xu JZ, Xu L, Zhong GJ, He BX, et al. Simultaneously improving wear resistance and mechanical performance of ultrahigh molecular weight polyethylene via cross-linking and structural manipulation. *Polymer (Guildf)* [Internet]. 2016;90:222–231. Available from: http://dx.doi.org/10.1016/j.polymer.2016.03.011
86. Grupp TM, Holderied M, Mulliez MA, Streller R, Jäger M, Blömer W, et al. Biotribology of a vitamin E-stabilized polyethylene for hip arthroplasty – influence of artificial ageing and third-body particles on wear. *Acta Biomater*. 2014;10(7):3068–3078.
87. Pitenis AA, Urueña JM, McGhee EO, Hart SM, Reale ER, Kim J, et al. Challenges and opportunities in soft tribology. *Tribol – Mater Surfaces Interfaces*. 2017;11(4):180–186.
88. Huan W, Xing M, Cheng C, Li J. Facile fabrication of magnetic metal-organic framework nanofibers for specific capture of phosphorylated peptides. *ACS Sustain Chem Eng*. 2019;7(2):2245–2254.
89. Maglio M, Salamanna F, Brogini S, Borsari V, Pagani S, Nicoli Aldini N, et al. Histological, histomorphometrical, and biomechanical studies of bone-implanted medical devices: hard resin embedding. *Biomed Res Int*. 2020;2020:1804630.
90. Ravichandran R, Sundarrajan S, Venugopal JR, Mukherjee S, Ramakrishna S. Advances in polymeric systems for tissue engineering and biomedical applications. *Macromol Biosci*. 2012;12(3):286–311.
91. Cruz RLJ, Ross MT, Powell SK, Woodruff MA. Advancements in soft-tissue prosthetics part B: the chemistry of imitating life. *Front Bioeng Biotechnol*. 2020;8(April):1–23.
92. Green JJ, Elisseeff JH. Mimicking biological functionality with polymers for biomedical applications. *Nature*. 2016;540(7633):386–394.
93. Yunus M, Alsoufi MS. Experimental investigations into the mechanical, tribological, and corrosion properties of hybrid polymer matrix composites comprising ceramic reinforcement for biomedical applications. *Int J Biomater*. 2018;2018:9283291.
94. Chang BP, Akil HM, Nasir RM. Mechanical and tribological properties of zeolite-reinforced UHMWPE composite for implant application. *Procedia Eng* [Internet]. 2013;68:88–94. Available from: http://dx.doi.org/10.1016/j.proeng.2013.12.152
95. Schmidt BVKJ. Metal-organic frameworks in polymer science: polymerization catalysis, polymerization environment, and hybrid materials. *Macromol Rapid Commun*. 2020;41(1):1900333.
96. Kalaj M, Bentz KC, Ayala S, Palomba JM, Barcus KS, Katayama Y, et al. MOF-polymer hybrid materials: from simple composites to tailored architectures. *Chem Rev*. 2020;120(16):8267–8302.
97. Mahapatro A. Bio-functional nano-coatings on metallic biomaterials. *Mater Sci Eng C*. 2015;55:227–251.

98. Hornberger H, Virtanen S, Boccaccini AR. Biomedical coatings on magnesium alloys – a review. *Acta Biomater* [Internet]. 2012;8(7):2442–2455. Available from: http://dx.doi.org/10.1016/j.actbio.2012.04.012

99. El Hankari S, Bousmina M, El Kadib A. Biopolymer@metal-organic framework hybrid materials: a critical survey. *Prog Mater Sci* [Internet]. 2019;106(November):100579. Available from: https://doi.org/10.1016/j.pmatsci.2019.100579

100. Anand A, Irfan Ul Haq M, Vohra K, Raina A, Wani MF. Role of green tribology in sustainability of mechanical systems: a state of the art survey. *Mater Today Proc* [Internet]. 2017;4(2):3659–3665. Available from: http://dx.doi.org/10.1016/j.matpr.2017.02.259

101. Amann T, Dold C, Kailer A. Complex fluids in tribology to reduce friction: mesogenic fluids, ionic liquids and ionic liquid crystals. *Tribol Int*. 2013;65:3–12.

102. Chen W, Amann T, Kailer A, Rühe J. Thin-film lubrication in the water/octyl β-d-glucopyranoside system: macroscopic and nanoscopic tribological behavior. *Langmuir*. 2019;35(22):7136–7145.

103. Chen W, Amann T, Kailer A, Rühe J. Macroscopic friction studies of alkylglucopyranosides as additives for water-based lubricants. *Lubricants*. 2020;8(1):11.

104. Ghaednia H, Hossain MS, Jackson RL. Tribological performance of silver nanoparticle–enhanced polyethylene glycol lubricants. *Tribol Trans*. 2016;59(4):585–592.

105. Torres O, Andablo-Reyes E, Murray BS, Sarkar A. Emulsion microgel particles as high-performance bio-lubricants. *ACS Appl Mater Interfaces*. 2018;10(32):26893–26905.

106. Bayer IS. Advances in tribology of lubricin and lubricin-like synthetic polymer nanostructures. *Lubricants*. 2018;6(2):30.

107. Zhang HY, Zhou M. The influence of protein concentration on the biotribological properties of the stem-cement interface. *Biomed Mater Eng*. 2014;24(1):173–179.

108. Aris AZ, Mohd Hir ZA, Razak MR. Metal-organic frameworks (MOFs) for the adsorptive removal of selected endocrine disrupting compounds (EDCs) from aqueous solution: a review. *Appl Mater Today* [Internet]. 2020;21:100796. *Available from*: https://doi.org/10.1016/j.apmt.2020.100796

109. Gao D-Y, Liu Z, Cheng Z-L. 2D Ni-Fe MOF nanosheets reinforced poly(vinyl alcohol) hydrogels with enhanced mechanical and tribological performance. *Colloids Surfaces A Physicochem Eng Asp* [Internet]. 2021;610(October 2020):125934. Available from: https://doi.org/10.1016/j.colsurfa.2020.125934

110. Zhang G, Xie G, Si L, Wen S, Guo D. Ultralow friction self-lubricating nanocomposites with mesoporous metal-organic frameworks as smart nanocontainers for lubricants. *ACS Appl Mater Interfaces*. 2017;9(43):38146–38152.

6 The Use of C.P. Titanium in Medical Friction Pairs

S. Ye. Sheykin
V. Bakul Institute for Superhard Materials of the National Academy of Sciences of Ukraine, Kyiv, Ukraine

I. M. Pohrelyuk and O. V. Tkachuk
Karpenko Physico-Mechanical Institute of the National Academy of Sciences of Ukraine, Lviv, Ukraine

CONTENTS

6.1 Introduction 147
6.2 Technology of Machining of Femoral Head of Hip Joint Replacement Prosthesis Made of C.P. Titanium 149
6.3 Aspects of Hip Joint Endoprosthesis Design 154
6.4 Surface Hardening of C.P. Titanium by Thermodiffusion Saturation with Nitrogen 156
6.5 Tribological Test Methods and Aspects of Selection of Working Fluid 163
6.6 Aspects of Selection of Technological Regime of TDN 167
6.7 Testing of Nitrided C.P. Titanium/UHMWPE Friction Pairs on Stand-Simulator of Biomechanical Human Movement 171
References 176

6.1 INTRODUCTION

Endoprosthetics of the human joints is an effective method of restoring the working capacity of a person in the case of incurable diseases or injuries. Today, the most common operation of bone surgery is a hip joint replacement. Annually, prosthetics of the hip joint are required for 500–1000 patients per 1 million people [1]. For every 3–4 primary operations, one revision is conducted.

The reason for the surgical revision operation can be negative phenomena associated with the insufficient biocompatibility of the applied materials with the tissues of the human body, loosening of the stem in the bone, wear of the elements of the endoprosthesis leading to its instability, etc. [1]. It may be noted that the durability of the endoprosthesis is the main criterion of its quality and is determined to a large extent by the service properties of the materials used, an important place among which is the wear resistance and tribological characteristics. Therefore, improving the service functions of endoprostheses is very important [2].

It should be noted that a material that fully meets all the requirements has not been created to date. Each material has its advantages and disadvantages, which are described in sufficient detail in the literature, e.g., [3, 4].

The articulation (friction pair) is the most important part of the endoprosthesis that determines its durability. In 1958 Charnley [5] identified the problem of creating a friction pair of the endoprosthesis as primarily a problem of a tribological nature. The researcher suggested using CoCrMo alloy for the femoral head material and ultrahigh molecular weight polyethylene (UHMWPE) for the acetabulum (liner) – Figure 6.1.

The articulation with such a combination of materials has received the title of the gold standard of endoprosthetics and is still the most widely used in orthopedic practice. According to a survey carried out in 35 hospitals in the USA (from 1999 to 2007), the CoCrMo/UHMW PE endoprosthesis is used in 55% of cases, while metal-on-metal and ceramic-on-ceramic in only 37 and 6%, respectively [5]. Such a joint can remain operative for 20 years or more. According to [3], the reserves of the wear resistance of the UHMWPE-metal pair have not been exhausted at this point. However, it should be noted that, when used in clinical practice, cases of granulomatous inflammation caused by the products of wear of UHMWPE are documented [4]. Today, various materials and their combinations are used for manufacturing the components of the replacement prosthesis. For femoral heads, the CoCrMo alloy, various types of ceramics, and less often titanium alloys are used, and for the acetabulum, UHMWPE, CoCrMo alloy, and ceramics are used. A significant share in the total volume is occupied by combinations of metal/UHMWPE and ceramics/UHMWPE. For the manufacturing of femoral heads, metals, i.e., CoCrMo alloy and Ti-6Al-4V titanium alloy, are normally used [3, 5]. However, from the point of view of biocompatibility, these materials are not the best [6] – Figure 6.2. In the figure, the relative corrosion resistance is expressed as a percentage of ideal biocompatibility, where commercially pure titanium (c.p. titanium) corresponds to $\approx$ 99%. The corrosion

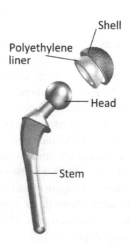

FIGURE 6.1 General view of the hip joint replacement prosthesis. (Source: Charnley 1961).

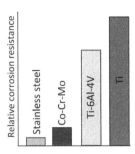

FIGURE 6.2 Relative corrosion resistance of various materials used for femoral heads. (Source: Nadeev 2015).

resistance is strictly related to biocompatibility with the human body, and low corrosion resistance can cause the release of carcinogens into living tissue and blood.

Apparently, from the biological point of view, among metals and alloys, the c.p. titanium is the best for manufacturing the endoprosthesis heads [1, 3, 5–8]. However, its main drawbacks, which hinder its use in endoprosthetics, are poor mechanical and tribological characteristics. However, because of the special features of the design (a compact form) and, considering that the UHMWPE component of the friction pair has a much lower elastic modulus, c.p. titanium can be reasonably used to manufacture spherical heads of hip joint endoprostheses, providing that the working surface is subjected to modification resulting to the optimal combination of the strength and adhesion inertness. Such a combination is possible by using nitriding as the modification method [9–12]. The methods of high-energy nitriding, especially magnetron sputtering, physical vapor deposition, provide the formation of surface nitride films without diffusion transition layer, which negatively affects the tribological characteristics of strengthened layers.

In our opinion, the technology of thermodiffusion nitriding (TDN) should be used to modify the working surface of such a critical part of the endoprosthesis as the femoral head [13, 14]. The method has advantages over others, e.g., the presence of a diffuse transitional layer between the thin surface layer of Ti-N compounds and the base material eliminates lapping and also ensures 100% reproducibility of the material features [15].

6.2 TECHNOLOGY OF MACHINING OF FEMORAL HEAD OF HIP JOINT REPLACEMENT PROSTHESIS MADE OF C.P. TITANIUM

The c.p. titanium can be successfully applied to manufacture parts of friction pairs dedicated to endoprosthesis; therefore, the development of the technology of machining especially femoral heads is an urgent task. It should be noted that up to now, such technology has not been created. The reason for this is the highly unsatisfactory machinability of c.p. titanium by abrasive methods. The increased tendency to "grasp" (this process occurs as a result of a deep pulling out of the material, transferring it from one friction surface to another) leads to the instability of the machining process and unsatisfactory quality of the treated surface for practically all structural and instrumental materials.

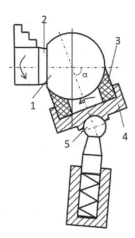

FIGURE 6.3 Scheme of free lapping.

The technological route of finishing process path of c.p. titanium should include preliminary precision machining operations aimed at obtaining product precision and operations whose purpose is to obtain surface roughness defined by Ra= 0.05 μm, which corresponds to ISO 7206-2-2005 (polishing).

The practice of manufacturing ceramic heads of endoprosthesis has shown that the free lapping (Figure 6.3) has proved to be quite effective in obtaining the required precision of the product [16]. Its advantage is that it does not require complex and costly equipment and may be implemented on a universal basis.

The tool (3) fixed in the clip (4) (which is supported by the hinge 5) is pressed at an angle (α) to the machined head (1) planted on the mandrel (2) mounted in the lathe chuck. A characteristic feature of the system is the low speed of the relative movement of the tool and the workpiece.

The main task of creating an abrasive tool for processing a workpiece from c.p. titanium is creating an abrasive composite, which avoids the accumulation and deterioration of surface quality of the surface to be processed.

The first part of the problem can be solved by applying a bond in the abrasive tool that holds the abrasive grains firmly.

The second part is solved by the creation of special abrasive composites. When using traditional abrasive composites, the vertices of cutting grains on the tool surface are at different heights. Therefore, only a small fraction of grains are in contact with the surface to be treated, which leads to their destruction with the separation of large fragments. As the abrasive grains are destroyed, the contact area of the bond and machined surface develops, which increases the probability of occurrence and development of "the focus of cutting."

To avoid the above-mentioned negative phenomena in the processing of titanium by possibly applying abrasive composites, their bond must be capable of reducing the modulus of elasticity when the mechanical load is increased on the abrasive grains [17].

An epoxy acrylate resin, filled with calcium carbonate powder, has the necessary property. When applied, the group of most protruding grains, without clumping, can be immersed in a bond to a greater depth, and the number of grains forming the base of the contact increases. In this case, the uniform wear of the massif of cutting grains occurs. This is not due to macro-scaling of the most protruding grains, but due to the microdestruction of a large number of cutting edges. With the optimum composition of the material, the clearance between the bond and surface being machined is stable and sufficient to prevent the "grasp." In addition, this property should help to increase the durability of the tool.

The tools (laps) based on the developed composite (Figure 6.4) have been tested in the processing of femoral heads made of c.p. titanium under laboratory conditions at the Institute for Superhard Materials of the National Academy of Sciences of Ukraine. The tool uses synthetic diamonds AC20 at 100% concentration. The tests were carried out at the processing of Ø28 mm femoral heads. As a lubricant, "Industrial-20" oil was used.

It has been experimentally established that the stable and safe operation of the tool based on the composite described above takes place at the rotation speed of the workpiece n = 1000 rpm.

Figure 6.5 shows the intensity of material removal during machining of the workpiece on the force of pressing by the tools with various grains.

It can be seen that the most intense wear (intensity of material removal) is provided by a tool with a grain size of 200/160. Its task is to eliminate the errors in the shape of the workpiece after turning.

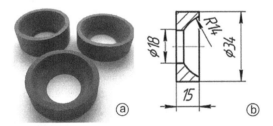

FIGURE 6.4 Laps for processing of titanium workpiece: (a) photographs of the tools; (b) technical drawing of the tool.

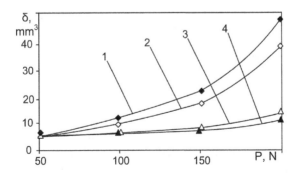

FIGURE 6.5 Dependence of the material removal on the force of pressing for different grains of diamonds: (1) 200/160; (2) 125/100; (3) 63/50; (4) 50/40.

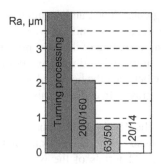

FIGURE 6.6 Dependence of the surface roughness on the granularity of synthetic diamond; the symbols 200/160 etc. – diamond grain size in the tool.

It has been experimentally established that the necessary condition for effective polishing of the working surface of the finished product (Ra 0.05 μm, ISO 7206-2:2011) is the roughness Ra = 0.25 μm after preliminary operations of precision machining (free lapping). This can be achieved by using smaller grain diamonds in the tools.

The roughness of the workpiece surface was measured using an interference profilometer. In Figure 6.6, the values of roughness of the processed surface of a femoral head are given in the sequence of applications of granularity of synthetic diamonds. The analyses performed using a scanning electron microscope (not included in the paper) did not reveal the coarse surface of the treated surface.

A polishing paste used to polish the heads was developed at the Institute for Superhard Materials of the National Academy of Sciences of Ukraine. The paste has an intense mechanical-chemical effect on the treated surface. It is based on an active complexing agent capable of selectively extracting titanium atoms from oxidized films on the surface; therefore, the process proceeds without the formation of defects in the deeper layers.

The mechanism of the influence of the complexing agent in the polishing paste on the intensity of the removal of allowance during the processing of titanium is associated with the peculiarities of the structure of the surface oxide film, which always exists, being self-replicating on the surface of the titanium in oxygen-containing media. Polishing waste analysis revealed that, in addition to microscopic polishing products, nanosized Ti_xO_y clusters are present. The presence of these particles is a direct consequence of the capture of the titanium atoms by the molecules of the complexing component on the boundary of the metal-paste contact. Due to the high energy of the Ti-O bond, metal titanium–oxygen clusters are removed from the surface of the metal, which are immobilized as part of multicore complex compounds.

Removing clusters of Ti_xO_y from the surface of the oxide film gives some porosity. One can assume that the intensity of the removal of allowance, as well as the roughness of the treated surface of titanium at the nanoscale level, will be related to the distribution of the surface pores of the equilibrium oxide film in dimension.

The appropriate distribution for c.p. titanium samples polished using paste with different complexing content was obtained by the Barrett–Joyner–Halenda (BJH) method. The results shown in Figure 6.7 correspond to small (1), optimal (2), and

The Use of C.P. Titanium in Medical Friction Pairs

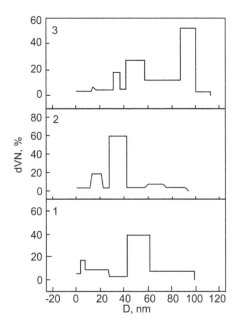

FIGURE 6.7 Distribution of the surface pores with small (1), optimal (2), and high content (3) of the complexing agent in the paste; dVV, % = is percentage of pores, and D, nm = is the size of the investigated area.

TABLE 6.1
Surface Roughness Parameters after Polishing; the Definitions of the Parameters Can be Found in ISO 25178-2:2012

Sq, μm	Ssk	Sku	Sp, μm	Sv, μm	Sz, μm	Sa, μm	Rz, μm	Ra, μm
0.0725	−1.66	9.85	0.243	0.62	0.863	0.524	0.2	0.04

high content of the complexing agent in the paste. The total porosity of the equilibrium oxide film for these three products corresponds to 1:1.8:1.6.

Thus, the use of a polishing paste with an optimal content of the complexing agent made it possible to form c.p. titanium polished surface with the highest efficiency. In this case, the roughness of the formed surface corresponds to the minimum size of the heterogeneities of the oxide film.

The results of measurements of the surface roughness parameters after polishing are given in Table 6.1. Figure 6.8 shows a photograph of the balls manufactured according to the developed technology.

It can be seen that the product also meets the requirements of the ISO 7206-2:2011 standard with respect to surface roughness.

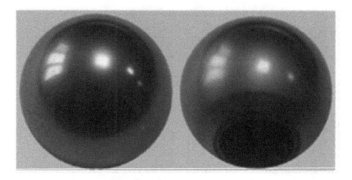

FIGURE 6.8 Femoral heads of endoprosthesis (c.p. titanium).

6.3 ASPECTS OF HIP JOINT ENDOPROSTHESIS DESIGN

The intensity of wear of hinged joints is largely determined by the load (contact pressure). So as to determine the main factors that influence the contact pressure in the joint, the finite element calculation for the case of a femoral (spherical) head from c.p. titanium and an acetabulum from UHMWPE has been performed. The problem was solved using dedicated software [18]. Figure 6.9 shows a diagram of the contact pressure in the joint at zero gap. The diagram shows that the largest values of the contact pressure are located along the axis of symmetry.

The dependence of the contact pressure on the forces and gap, which is well approximated by the static function (98% correlation), is obtained using Equation (6.1):

$$\sigma_{\max}(\delta, P) = a_1 + a_2 P^{a_3} + a_4 \delta^{a_5} + a_6 P^{a_3} \delta^{a_5} \qquad (6.1)$$

where: – maximum contact pressure [MPa]; P – load [N]; δ – radial clearance [mm], $a_1, a_2, \ldots$ – coefficient of approximation function [MPa], the values of which are given in Table 6.2, depending on the diameter of the femoral head.

Maximum contact pressure at zero gap is determined using Equation (6.2):

$$\sigma_{\max}(\delta, P) = 1.72 \frac{P}{D^2} \qquad (6.2)$$

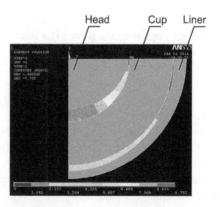

FIGURE 6.9 Distribution of contact pressures between the elements of the endoprosthesis.

TABLE 6.2
Coefficients of Approximation Function

D, mm	a_1, MPa	a_2, MPa	a_3, MPa	a_4, MPa	a_5, MPa	a_6, MPa
28	−0.90849	0.01122	0.81321	13.92142	0.72374	0.018412
38	−0.57037	0.00823	0.77824	8.19921	0.70792	0.017300
48	−0.53733	0.01074	0.69556	5.01997	0.67063	0.025249
58	−0.48997	0.01032	0.66045	3.78452	0.65636	0.025285

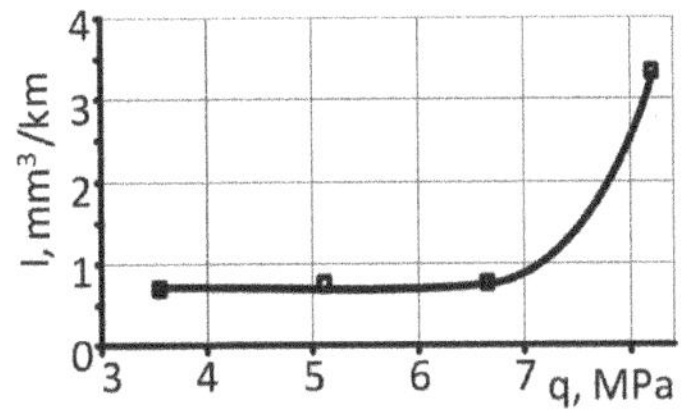

FIGURE 6.10 Dependence of the wear intensity (I) of UHMWPE on the contact pressure (q) in pairs with the nitrided sample of c.p. titanium; research performed using the ring-on-plane machine.

where: – maximum contact pressure [MPa]; P – load [N]; D – diameter of the sphere [mm]; 1.72 – coefficient obtained by statistical processing of data. The error of approximation of the calculated data is not more than 1%.

The analysis of Equations (6.1) and (6.2) shows that the increase in the diameter of the contact surfaces of the joints from 28 to 58 mm (ca. two times) leads to a decrease in the contact pressure by more than four times, and the increase in the gap leads to an increase in the contact pressure. Considering that the endoprosthesis should have a very high level of the reliability, the tests were also carried out for the "Nitrided c.p. titanium/UHMWPE" pair at higher contact pressures. The results are shown in Figure 6.10.

It can be seen that the increase of the contact pressure to values of ~6.5 MPa does not lead to a noticeable change in the wear intensity of the polyethylene sample. However, for high values of the contact pressure, the wear becomes catastrophic, which, in our opinion, is explained by the plasticity of the UHMWPE.

Based on the results obtained, one can formulate some practical recommendations regarding the choice of the size of the joint for a particular patient and the manufacturing of joints. These are as follows:

- The diameter of the femoral head and the acetabulum of the joints must be such that the contact pressure between the rubbing surfaces does not exceed 6.5 MPa. The desired diameter can be determined according to Equation (6.2).
- In the manufacturing of joints, it is necessary to provide the minimum possible clearance between the friction surfaces, that is, to manufacture parts with the highest possible accuracy.

6.4 SURFACE HARDENING OF C.P. TITANIUM BY THERMODIFFUSION SATURATION WITH NITROGEN

Thermodiffusion saturation of the samples of c.p. titanium was performed in the reaction chamber with a controlled nitrogen gas medium at 10^5 and 1 Pa in the temperature range of 650–950°C for 4–20 h. Subsequently, they were heated to the temperature of nitriding in a vacuum of 10 mPa to remove natural oxide films and exclude the formation of new films at the stage of heating [15, 19]. The rate of heating was 0.04°C/s. After the isothermal holding time, the samples were cooled within the furnace in a nitrogen atmosphere. The average cooling rate was 0.028°C/s.

The level of the near-surface hardening of c.p. titanium in the course of the TDN was achieved by varying temperature–time and gas–dynamic parameters of the saturation.

High-temperature nitriding at atmospheric pressure of nitrogen contributes to the formation of a nitrided layer, which contains the nitride zone and transition diffusion layer, i.e., a solid solution of nitrogen in α-titanium (regimes R1 and R2 in Table 6.3) [13]. According to the X-ray diffraction analysis, the nitride zone consists of δ-titanium nitride TiN_x and ε-titanium nitride Ti_2N. An increase of the intensity and number of reflections of the aforementioned nitride phases in diffraction patterns by

TABLE 6.3
Surface Roughness (Ra) and Surface Microhardness (H_μ) of c.p. Titanium after Nitriding

No	Regimes of nitriding	Ra, μm	$H_{0.49}$, GPa	$H_{0.98}$, GPa	ΔH*, GPa
R1	850°C, 8 h, $p_{N2} = 10^5$ Pa	1.50	18.8	13.2	5.6
R2	950°C, 8 h, $p_{N2} = 10^5$ Pa	6.56	22.5	18.4	4.1
R3	850°C, 6 h, $p_{N2} = 1$ Pa	–	10.7	9.8	0.9
R4	900°C, 4 h, $p_{N2} = 1$ Pa	–	8.9	6.4	2.5
R5	650°C, 5 h, $p_{N2} = 10^5$ Pa	0.10	4.5	4.3	0.2
R6	650°C, 20 h, $p_{N2} = 10^5$ Pa	0.10	8.7	6.2	2.5
R7	700°C, 5 h, $p_{N2} = 10^5$ Pa	0.11	7.5	6.2	1.3
R8	700°C, 20 h, $p_{N2} = 10^5$ Pa	0.17	12.6	8.8	3.8
R9	750°C, 5 h, $p_{N2} = 10^5$ Pa	0.13	12.0	8.6	3.4
R10	750°C, 20 h, $p_{N2} = 10^5$ Pa	0.33	17.0	14.0	3.0
R11	750°C, 10 h, $p_{N2} = 1$ Pa	0.13	8.2	6.5	1.7
R12	750°C, 20 h, $p_{N2} = 10^5$ Pa + 750°C, 4 h, 1 mPa	0.31	15.2	13.5	1.7
R13	750°C, 20 h, $p_{N2} = 10^5$ Pa + 750°C, 6 h, 1 mPa	0.29	12.3	11.7	0.6
R14	750°C, 20 h + 800°C, $p_{N2} = 10^5$ Pa	0.25	10.2	7.0	3.2
R15	650°C, 20 h + 800°C, $p_{N2} = 10^5$ Pa	0.37	16.7	14.3	2.4
R16	650°C, 20 h + 800°C, 0.5 h, $p_{N2} = 10^5$ Pa	0.18	9.0	6.9	2.1

* $\Delta H = H_{0.49} - H_{0.98}$.

increasing saturation temperature indicates on the intensification of the nitride formation on the titanium surface.

As the temperature increases from 850°C to 950°C, the curves of microhardness distribution on the cross-section of near-surface hardened layers shift to the higher hardness region, so that at a depth of about 30 μm the microhardness values differ more than by a factor of 4 (Figure 6.11).

The intensification of the nitride formation contributes to the microhardness increase of the c.p. titanium surface by 3.7 GPa and, in this case, ranges from 19 to 23 GPa (Table 6.3). Under these conditions, the microhardness gradient $\Delta H = H_{0.49} - H_{0.98}$ in a thin near-surface layer is 5.6 GPa and, as the saturation temperature increases, it somewhat decreases (Table 6.3).

With the intensification of the nitride formation, the characteristic surface relief of the nitride layer becomes more clearly and stronger (Figure 6.12), which negatively affects the nitrided surface quality. The profilometric analysis shows that by increasing the temperature the height of the surface profile Ra increases by a factor of 4 and the surface quality deteriorates by two accuracy degrees (Table 6.3).

The decrease of the nitrogen partial pressure to 1 Pa and the reduction of the isothermal holding time at nitriding decreases the surface hardening by a factor of 1.3–1.8 and substantially decreases the microhardness gradient, ΔH, see R3 and R4 in Table 6.3.

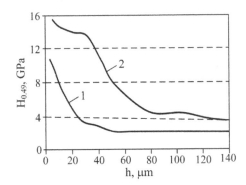

FIGURE 6.11 Microhardness distribution on the cross section of near-surface layers of c.p. titanium ($H_{0.49} = 1.8$ GPa) after nitriding for R1 (1), R2 (2) regimes, see Table 6.3.

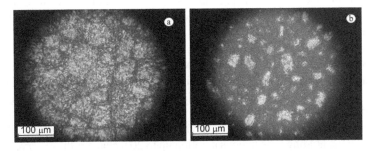

FIGURE 6.12 Surfaces of the c.p. titanium nitrided for R1 (a), R2 (b) regimes, see Table 6.3.

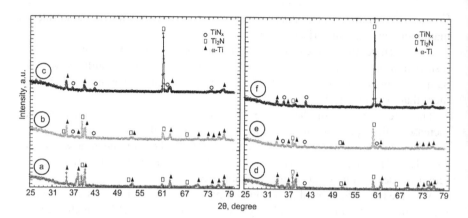

FIGURE 6.13 X-ray diffraction patterns of c.p. titanium after thermodiffusion nitriding: 650°C, 5 h (a); 650°C, 20 h (b); 700°C, 5 h (c); 700°C, 20 h (d); 750°C, 5 h (e); 750°C, 20 h; $p_{N2} = 10^5$ P (f).

The results of X-ray phase-diffraction analysis of the samples of c.p. titanium after low-temperature nitriding (see R5–R10 in Table 6.3) show that the saturation with nitrogen for the investigated temperature–time parameters guarantees the formation of a nitride zone formed by TiN$_x$ δ-nitride and Ti$_2$N ε-nitride (Figure 6.13). For the investigated temperature and time parameters, the thickness of the nitride zone does not exceed 1–3 μm. The characteristics of the nitride zone are estimated according to the results of X-ray diffraction and durometric analyses.

After the saturation of titanium mononitride for 5 h at a temperature of 650°C, TiN$_x$ was not recorded in the nitride zone. In the X-ray diffraction patterns, the Ti$_2$N phase is represented by the spectrum of the diffraction maxima (111), (220), (002), and (320) supplemented by the weak reflection (101) as a result of saturation at a temperature of 700°C.

After saturation at 750°C, the Ti$_2$N phase is identified only by the reference lines (111) and (002).

In the X-ray diffraction pattern of Ti$_2$N nitride, the lines (111) and (002) are predominant. The analysis of the intensities of the lines of Ti$_2$N phase shows that, as the temperature of saturation increases from 650 to 700°C, the predominant orientation of ε-nitride in the direction [111] becomes stronger (I(111)/I(002) changes from 2.95 to 3.03) and, after saturation at 750°C, a texture forms in the plane [002] (I(111)/I(002) is equal to 0.58).

In the X-ray diffraction pattern of the surface of nitrided titanium after saturation at temperatures of 700 and 750°C, the TiN$_x$ nitride is identified by the reference lines (111) and (200) and the phase is ordered in the direction [111], which is characteristic of materials with cubic structures [20], including cubic titanium mononitride. As the nitriding temperature increases from 700 to 750°C, the texture of TiN$_x$ in the direction [111] becomes weaker (I(111)/I(200) changes from 1.60 to 1.27). The increase in the holding time under saturation up to 20 h changes the observed tendencies in nitride formation. For instance, in the surface X-ray diffraction pattern, TiN$_x$

nitride is represented by the reference line (200) after saturation at 650°C, by the lines (111), (200), and (220) after saturation at 700°C, and by the lines (111) and (200) after saturation at 750°C. Note that, with an increase in the temperature, the predominant orientation in the direction [111] becomes stronger (I(111)/I(200) changes from 1.36 to 1.57).

The Ti$_2$N phase is represented by the spectrum of the diffraction maxima (111), (220), (002), (320), and (212) after nitriding at 650°C, by only the reference lines (111), (220), and (002) after nitriding at 700°C, and by the single line (002) of high relative intensity after nitriding at 750°C. Moreover, with increase in the saturation temperature, the predominant orientation of the ε-nitride in the direction [111] changes for the texture over the plane [002], which becomes substantially stronger after saturation at 750°C (I(111) I(002) decreases from 1.56 to 0.31 and 0.07 at temperatures of 650, 700, and 750°C, respectively).

The crystallographic orientations of the components of the formed nitride zone, namely, the TiN$_x$ and Ti$_2$N nitrides, as a result of holding for 20 h at investigated temperatures change as follows. For the TiN$_x$ nitride, after saturation at a temperature of 700°C, the texture in the direction [111] becomes weaker (I(111)/I(200) changes from 1.60 to 1.36), and after saturation at 750°C, on the contrary, becomes stronger (I(111)/I(002) changes from 1.27 to 1.57). As to the Ti$_2$N nitride, after saturation at a temperature of 650°C, the predominant orientation in the direction [111] becomes weaker (I(111)/I(002) changes from 2.95 to 1.56), after saturation at 700°C, the texture over the plane [002] was observed (I(111)/I(002) decreases from 3.03 to 0.31), which at 750°C becomes substantially stronger (I(111)/I(002) changes from 0.58 to 0.07). On the whole, the increase in the intensity and number of reflections of the nitride phases in X-ray diffraction patterns, the redistribution of their intensities with an increase in the temperature–time parameters of saturation is the evidence of intensification of nitride formation on the surface of titanium.

As nitride formation is activated, the topography of the surface, namely, wavy asperities that form a network (which obviously replicates the network of grain boundaries of the matrix of the nitrided material) typical of nitriding on the surface appears and becomes more pronounced (Figure 6.14). The formation of the surface relief negatively affects the quality of the nitrided surface. Under the general tendency to increase in the roughness, in view of saturation temperatures that are relatively low for nitriding of titanium [15], the standard deviation of the surface profile Ra corresponds to N3 and N4 of roughness N grade *ISO 1302:2002* (see Table 6.3). Only after holding for 20 h at a temperature of 750°C, the quality of the nitrided surface decreases by one grade.

At low-temperature nitriding (see R5–R10 in Table 6.3), a similar effect of variation of the surface hardening parameters is observed as at high-temperature nitriding (see R1–R4 in Table 6.3), which is accompanied by a decrease of the surface microhardness by a factor of 1.3–3.0 and the microhardness gradient, ΔH, by 0.3–2.8 GPa. The thickness of a nitride film, which consists of TiN$_x$ and Ti$_2$N, formed after nitriding in the temperature range of 650–750°C for 5–20 h, does not increase more than 3 μm. In this case, the depth of nitrided layer, assessed by the microhardness method as a distance, where the curve of the hardness variation passes to the horizontal segment corresponding to the core hardness, lies within 10–80 μm depending on the

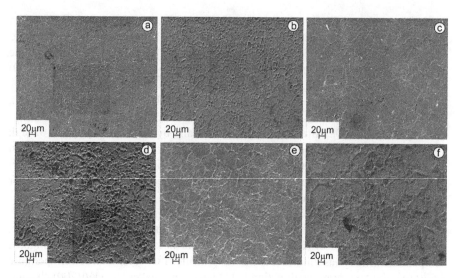

FIGURE 6.14 Surface of c.p. titanium after thermodiffusion nitriding: 650°C, 5 h (a); 650°C, 20 h (b); 700°C, 5 h (c); 700°C, 20 h (d); 750°C, 5 h (e); 750°C, 20 h; $p_{N2} = 10^5$ P (f).

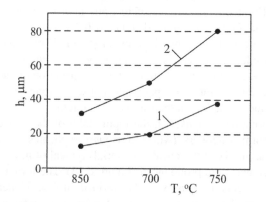

FIGURE 6.15 Dependence of the depth of the hardened c.p. titanium layer on the temperature of nitriding for 5 h (1), 20 h (2).

time-temperature parameters of nitriding (Figure 6.15). The depth of the diffusion layer, which is metallographically assessed as the size of a bright band with a decreased degree of etching, is lower by a factor of 1.5–3.3 (Figure 6.16).

The surface microhardness of c.p. titanium ranges from 4.5 to 17.0 GPa and increases with increasing parameters of nitriding in the given time-temperature range (Table 6.3). In this case, the microhardness gradient, ΔH, increases for 5 h of holding in nitrogen with increasing saturation temperature and, for 20 h increases only as the temperature increases from 650 to 750°C. At the further increase of nitriding temperature up to 750°C the ΔH decreases. The observed regularities of the surface microhardness variation illustrate the formation and growth of a thin nitride film on

The Use of C.P. Titanium in Medical Friction Pairs

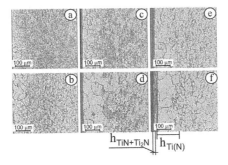

FIGURE 6.16 Microstructures of the near-surface layers of the c.p. titanium after nitriding at: 650°C (a, b), 700°C (c, d), 750°C (e, f) for 5 h (a, b, c), 20 h (d, e, f).

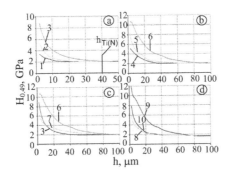

FIGURE 6.17 Microhardness distribution on the cross section of near-surface layers of c.p. titanium after nitriding for $p_{N2} = 10^5$ Pa: 650°C, 5 h (1); 700°C, 5 h (2); 750°C, 5 h (3); 650°C, 20 h (4); 700°C, 20 h (5); 750°C, 20 h (6); 750°C, 10 h (7); 750°C, 20 h + 800°C (8); 650°C, 20 h + 800°C (9); 650°C, 20 h + 800°C, 0.5 h (10).

the titanium surface and then, the formation of a gradient of properties in a thin surface layer.

As the saturation parameters increase, the microhardness distribution curves shift into the higher hardness region (Figure 6.17), while, with increasing saturation temperature from 650 to 700°C, the increment of hardness is not as noticeable as the temperature increase from 700 to 750°C for 5 h exposure (Figure 6.17a) and, especially, for 20 h one (Figure 6.17b).

To decrease the gradient of properties in a near-surface hardened layer of c.p. titanium and, hence, to increase the wear resistance, vacuum technology [15] was employed, in particular, nitriding was performed in a dynamic flow of nitrogen (1 Pa). After the TDN, additional vacuum annealing was used.

According to the X-ray diffraction analysis data, the decrease of the nitrogen partial pressure to 1 Pa decelerates the nitride formation on the titanium surface. The diffraction patterns of the nitrided sample surfaces exhibit no reflections of TiN_x hitride, while, the Ti_2N phase is represented only by two reference lines (111) and (002) with clearly defined orientation along the [002] plane. In this case, the relative intensity of the α-titanium line is high.

As the nitrogen partial pressure decreases, the quality of the nitrided surface increases, and its surface microhardness decreases (see R10, R11 in Table 6.3). The curves of microhardness distribution on the cross-section of near-surface hardened layers shift toward the regions of lower hardness at depth < 10 μm and of higher hardness at depth > 10 μm (Figure 6.17c, curves 6 and 7), resulting, therefore, in a more uniform hardness distribution in a diffusion layer. After 10 h of saturation at 750°C and partial pressure of nitrogen 1 Pa, the depth of the hardened layer of the c.p. titanium is about 60 μm.

Decrease of the gradient of the near-surface hardening due to the use of the additional vacuum annealing, which is part of the titanium surface treatment, caused by the dissociation of the surface nitride and nitrogen diffusion deep into titanium matrix, results in the improvement of the surface quality and decrease of the surface microhardness (see R12 and R13 in Table 6.3).

In addition to the surface microhardness, the ability of the hardened surface to resist the deformation due to mechanical loading was assessed by the H/E value obtained by the nanoindentation of titanium surfaces at the initial state and after nitriding. The load diagrams indicate that the work done by the Berkovich indenter against the material resistance of the nitrided sample is much larger than that of the sample without the surface treatment (Figure 6.18). The obtained H/E values are 0.03 for titanium without surface treatment and vary in the 0.047–0.060 range for nitrided titanium depending on the nitriding regime (Table 6.4). They correspond to the

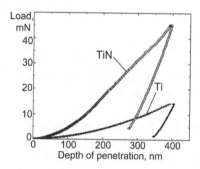

FIGURE 6.18 Load diagrams of untreated and nitrided c.p. titanium.

TABLE 6.4
Young Modulus (E) and Hardness (H) Defined at the Nanoindentation of the c.p. Titanium Surface after Nitriding

No	Regimes of Nitriding	E, GPa	H, GPa	H/E
1	Untreated	117	3.5	0.030
2	750°C, 5 h, $p_{N2} = 10^5$ Pa	257	13.8	0.054
3	750°C, 20 h, $p_{N2} = 10^5$ Pa	251	11.7	0.047
4	750°C, 10 h, $p_{N2} = 1$ Pa	211	12.7	0.060
5	750°C, 20 h, $p_{N2} = 10^5$ Pa + 750°C, 4 h, 1 mPa	261	12.7	0.049

values for metals and alloys (H/E < 0.04) and materials with hardened surfaces (H/E≈0.05–0.09), respectively [21].

Except for the isothermal nitriding, a step-by-step treatment was performed (R14-R16 in Table 6.3). At the first step of the isothermal saturation, the near-surface hardening was achieved. In contrast, at the second step through the temperature increase, not only the diffusion processes were activated, but the nitride formation was intensified as well. The best results of the near-surface hardening were achieved at the maximum difference between the temperatures at the first and second stages (150°C) (see R15 in Table 6.3 and Figure 6.17d). Under these conditions, the isothermal holding at the second stage impaired the efficiency of the near-surface hardening, i.e., the surface microhardness decreased by a factor of 1.9–2.1. The microhardness distribution curves in depth of the hardened layer shifted into the lower hardness region. In this case, the quality of the nitrided surface of the c.p. titanium improved, i.e., Ra was reduced by about 50% (R15 and R16 in Table 6.3).

6.5 TRIBOLOGICAL TEST METHODS AND ASPECTS OF SELECTION OF WORKING FLUID

The choice of working fluid for tribological testing and technological regimes of TDN were made based on the results of studies performed using a pendulum tribometer (Figure 6.19) and a ring-on-plane machine (Figure 6.20).

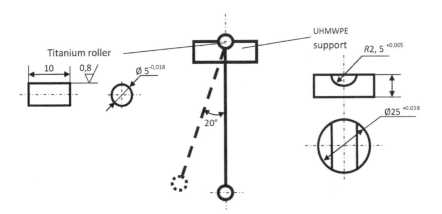

FIGURE 6.19 The tribosystem of a pendulum tribometer.

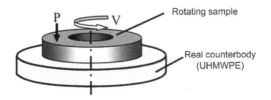

FIGURE 6.20 The ring-on-plane tribosystem.

The length of the pendulum (Figure 6.19) was 0.51 m, the weight of the load was 35.67 N, and the initial deviation angle was 20°. The coefficient of friction was estimated from Equation (6.1) [22]:

$$f = \frac{\Delta A}{4(n-1)r} \tag{6.3}$$

where: f – coefficient of friction; ΔA – decrease in amplitude of oscillations of the pendulum for a period [m]; r – radius of the roller of the friction support unit [m], n – number of oscillation cycles.

During the tests using the ring-on-plane machine (Figure 6.20), the rotating sample in the form of a ring was pressed against a stationary UHMWPE disk. The friction force and the normal force were measured with a strain gage dynamometer. By profiling, the cross-section area of the wear groove was determined. The sliding speed of the metal sample was v = 0.057 m/s and the contact pressure q = 3.54 MPa. The roughness of the working surface of the metallic sample was Ra = 0.8 μm, and for the UHMWPE disk (ISO 5834-2), Ra was 3 μm.

The tribological characteristics of the friction pair were estimated from the coefficient of friction f and the wear intensity I of the surgical component, expressed in [mm^3/km].

It must be kept in mind, however, that it is not always correct to determine the contact pressure by dividing the load by the contact area. Each interaction scheme can have its own characteristics, which leads to uneven distribution of normal stresses along the contact surface. Considering that the endoprosthesis friction unit should have a very high degree of reliability, it is necessary to make sure that this approach is correct. For this purpose, the pressure in the contact zone was calculated using a dedicated software package.

As a result, it was found that the uneven distribution of the contact pressure along the friction surface of the ring does not exceed 3%, which, in our case, is quite legitimate to determine the normal stresses on the contact surface by dividing the load by the area of the contact surface.

So as to obtain the correct results, it is necessary to strive to bring the conditions of the laboratory tests as close as possible to those of the friction in the natural joint. According to the classical provisions of tribology, the environment in which the rubbing parts interact largely determines the functional characteristics of the friction pair. According to [23], a third body forms between the surfaces of the rubbing bodies, whose properties are largely determined by the working medium. An ideal option would be to perform articulation tests in human synovial fluid, but it is impossible to obtain it in the volume necessary for the tests. According to ASTM F732-82, in the pin-on-plate tests, serum of bovine blood should be used as a working fluid. This is due to the fact that the synovial fluid is a blood serum (BS) transudate, i.e., they contain the same components which determine the frictional conditions in the human joint. Minor differences in their compositions affecting the friction conditions are practically negligible [22].

The tribological function of the synovial fluid is realized due to the presence of liquid-crystalline components (LC) as complex esters of cholesterol acids. LCs form on the friction surfaces and orientate as a structure consisting of a number of nematic layers, the intermolecular interaction of which is small. This structure is similar to the structure of layered solid lubricants. During friction, the shear is localized between the layers, providing low friction [22, 24]. It was found that the introduction of LC into the working liquid leads to a significant reduction in the friction of virtually all materials used in practice [13]. Thus, the use of the bovine blood synovial fluid (SF) as a working medium in the tribological tests of artificial joints makes it possible to obtain the most reliable information about its functional characteristics.

However, the disadvantage of the SF is the time-limited use. When tested at 37°C, it quickly loses its properties, which can cause errors and, in addition, can lead to clogging of the pipelines of the testing equipment. Taking this into account, as well as the fact that tests in simulator stands require a significant volume of the working fluid, the question of replacing SF with a working fluid that is adequate in terms of tribological properties and can maintain its properties during tests performed for a longer time is a topical task.

In [25], the results of tribological studies, using a pendulum tribometer and a drug containing chondroitin sulfate, which is part of the SF and performs a lubricating function, are presented. In the studies, joints of animals were used. As a result it has been established that the fluid containing chondroitin sulfate and natural SF are approximately equal in tribological efficiency – Figure 6.21.

Taking this into account, in order to study the possibility of replacing BS in tribological tests of medical friction pairs, studies were conducted on the tribological efficiency of the drug "Artiflex Chondro" (AC) produced by LLC Pharmaceutical Company "Zdorovie" in Kharkov, Ukraine. The drug is a 10% aqueous solution of chondroitin sulfate, produced from animal raw materials.

In the tests on the pendulum tribometer, the components of the c.p. titanium friction pair were used, whose surface was modified by TDN technology in various modes, which provided different surface microhardnesses: 12.6, 6.0, 5.5, and 5.2 GPa.

In the tests using the ring-on-plane machine, the following materials were used: a CoCrMo sample (HV 4.5 GPa), samples of c.p. titanium modified by ion-plasma thermocyclic nitriding (IPTN) (surface microhardness HV 6 GPa), and TDN (surface microhardness HV 4.9 GPa) [13].

The results of the tests of the AC drug using the pendulum tribometer and the ring-on-plane machine are shown in Figures 6.22 and 6.23, respectively.

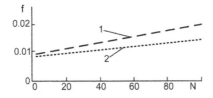

FIGURE 6.21 Dependence of the friction coefficient of the natural cartilage-cartilage pair on the number of oscillations of the pendulum tribometer when lubricated by: 1 – fluid containing chondroitin sulphate, 2 – synovial fluid (Source: Ermakov 2008).

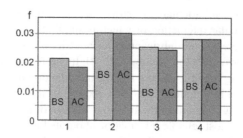

FIGURE 6.22 Friction coefficient during testing of pairs "c.p. titanium (TDN)/UHMWPE," lubricated with different media, using the pendulum tribometer: 1 – "c.p. titanium (HV 12.6 GPa)/UHMWPE", 2 – "c.p. titanium (HV 6.0 GPa)/UHMWPE," 3 – "c.p. titanium (HV 5.5 GPa)/UHMWPE," 4 – "c.p. titanium (HV 5.2 GPa)/UHMWPE"; BS – blood serum, AC – Artiflex Chondro.

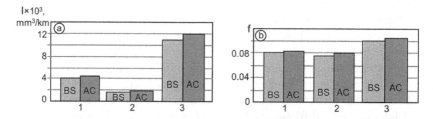

FIGURE 6.23 Wear intensity I (a) and friction coefficient f (b) during testing of pairs lubricated with different media, using the ring-on-plane machine: 1 – "c.p. titanium (IPTN)/UHMWPE," 2 – "c.p. titanium (TDN)/UHMWPE," 3 – CoCrMo/UHMWPE; BS – blood serum, AC – Artiflex Chondro.

It can be seen that the value of the friction coefficient (f) when using the drug AC and BS differ slightly. In testing using the pendulum tribometer, the maximum difference in f (14%) occurs when the titanium sample with a surface hardness of 12.6 GPa is used (Figure 6.22). Using the ring-on-plane machine, the differences in the values of the friction coefficient and the wear rate of the surgical component lubricated with the BS and AC do not exceed 5% and 4%, respectively (Figure 6.23).

Laboratory tests show that the AC product retains its properties in tribological tests 3 to 4 times longer than BS.

The differences in the values of the friction coefficient in the tests using the two methods can be a consequence of a significant difference, both in the dynamics of the tribometers and in the conditions of friction. Thus, the AC product can be successfully used in studies of tribological characteristics of friction pairs "CoCrMo/UHMWPE" and "Nitrided c.p. titanium/UHMWPE" using bench tribometers and simulator stands. Surgical components lubricated with the BS and AC do not exceed 5% and 4%, respectively (Figure 6.23). Laboratory tests show that the AC product retains its properties in tribological tests 3 to 4 times longer than BS. The differences in the values of the friction coefficient in the tests using the two methods can be a consequence of a significant difference, both in the dynamics of the tribometers and in the conditions of friction.

The Use of C.P. Titanium in Medical Friction Pairs 167

Thus, the AC product can be successfully used in studies of tribological characteristics of friction pairs "CoCrMo/UHMWPE" and "Nitrided c.p. titanium/UHMWPE" using bench tribometers and simulator stands.

6.6 ASPECTS OF SELECTION OF TECHNOLOGICAL REGIME OF TDN

The intensive wear of the UHMWPE component and the high friction coefficient of titanium after high-temperature nitriding in the nitrogen of the atmospheric pressure are caused by the impairment of the nitrided surface quality, whose roughness is the higher, the higher is the saturation temperature (Figure 6.12). Because of the aforesaid, in testing the samples nitrided according to regime R2 (950°C) the intensive wear of the UHMWPE component of the tribo-pair did not allow us to ensure the testing base; therefore, after the pair worked 472 m we had to terminate the experiment. The friction coefficient was fixed at 0.38.

The formation of the hardened surface layer in a dynamic nitrogen atmosphere (1 Pa) is favorable for decreasing the UHMWPE component wear in the tribo-pair, but the friction coefficient remains high (R3 in Table 6.5). Under these gas–dynamic conditions, an increase of the nitriding temperature of the titanium component essentially improves the tribological characteristics of the tribo-pair (R4 in Table 6.5).

At low-temperature nitriding in the nitrogen of atmospheric pressure, as the saturation temperature increases from 650 to 750°C, the specific wear of the UHMWPE component for 5 h holding time decreases by a factor of 1.7, while the friction coefficient decreases by a factor of 1.5 (R7 and R9 in Table 6.5).

In testing a Ti sample nitrided at 700°C for 5 h, vigorous heating of the working fluid (blood plasma) was observed. Though visible changes of the sample surface were not apparent (Figure 6.24), but due to the significant fluctuations of friction force, we failed to furnish the base of tests and correctly fix tribological characteristics. In friction of a sample nitrided at 750°C for 5 h, the working fluid was not heated. Despite the fact that, after friction at a base of 10 km the absence of the golden coloration inherent in TiN on a considerable part of the friction surface was observed (Figure 6.24c), the tribological characteristics of the pair remained stable.

The stability of the aforementioned characteristics was not violated after subsequent tests for 10 km as well, when the working liquid was changed, i.e., the blood plasma was replaced by Artiflex Chondro drug (Table 6.5). The basic acting substance of the Artiflex Chondro drug is chondroitin sulfate, which is an important structural component of cartilaginous tissue [26]. It is a component of the SF of joints and acts as a lubricant. During the tests, the heating of the working medium was not fixed.

As the temperature of the saturation in nitrogen of atmospheric pressure increases from 650 to 700°C and from 700 to 750°C at holding for 20 h, the specific wear of the UHMWPE component decreases by a factor of 2.4 and 6.8, respectively (Table 6.5). The friction coefficient decreases in the 0.22→0.16→0.07 row as the temperature increases in a row 650→700→750°C. With the temperature decrease from 700 to 750°C the friction coefficient decreases more essentially than from 650 to 700°C,

TABLE 6.5
Specific Wear of the UHMWPE Component (I) and a Friction Coefficient (f) of the Nitrided c.p. Titanium-UHMWPE Friction Pair in Blood Plasma

No	Friction pair c.p. titanium (nitriding regime R) /UHMWPE (according to Table 6.1)	I_s^*, mm/km (×10^3)	k mm^3/km·N (×10^3)	I, mm/ 1 mln. cycles	f	Friction path, km
0	c.p. titanium/UHMWPE	146.39	41.71	1.23	0.24	10
1	R1/UHMWPE	10.03	2.86	0.085	0.10	10
2	R2/UHMWPE	–	–	–	0.38	0.5
3	R3/UHMWPE	8.78	2.50	0.078	0.22	10
4	R4/UHMWPE	3.13	0.89	0.026	0.10	10
5	R5/UHMWPE	1.85	0.53	0.015	0.12	5
6	R6/UHMWPE	17.12	4.85	0.144	0.22	0.3
7	R7/UHMWPE	8.15	2.50	0.069	0.21	0.4
8	R8/UHMWPE	7.08	2.02	0.059	0.16	5
9	R9/UHMWPE	1.10/ 1.0***	0.31/ 0.28***	0.00045	0.08 /0.08***	10
10	R10/UHMWPE	1.03	0.28	0.0085	0.07	5
11	R11/UHMWPE	1.79	0.51	0.015	0.08	5
12	R12/UHMWPE	0.94	0.26	0.08	0.07	5
13	R13/UHMWPE	1.76	0.5	0.0145	0.10	5
14	R14/UHMWPE	1.19	0.34	0.010	0.08	5
15	R15/UHMWPE	0.69/ 0.41**	0.2/ 0.117**	0.006/ 0.004**	0.06/ 0.04**	200
16	R16/UHMWPE	3.32	0.94	0.028	0.07	5

k-wear factor in Archard's equation:
* the specific wear was determined as the wear of UHMWPE sample divided into the friction path –mm^3/km;
** The sample treated by the regime R15 was polished after thermodiffusion nitriding;
*** Values obtained in the working medium of Artiflex Chondro drug.

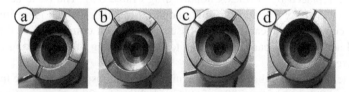

FIGURE 6.24 Surfaces of c.p. titanium nitrided at 650ºC (a), 700ºC (b) for 5 h; at 650ºC (c), 700ºC (d) for 20 h after friction in a pair with UHMWPE.

e.g., by a factor of 2.3 and 1.4, respectively. It should be noted that the test of the c.p. titanium samples with a 20 h nitriding was accompanied by heating of the working liquid irrespective of the nitriding temperature.

Additional vacuum annealing for 4 h after the thermodiffusion saturation of titanium with nitrogen reveals positive tendencies toward a change of characteristics of the tribo-pair (R12 and R13 in Table 6.5). Note that, in the case of annealing for 6 h, the UHMWPE-specific wear increases by a factor of 1.7 and its friction coefficient is raised from 0.07 to 0.10.

A decrease of the nitrogen partial pressure to 1 Pa in the saturation at 750°C and a reduction of the holding time from 20 to 10 h, as well as the step-by-step nitriding at the basic regime of 750°C and 20 h, results in reducing the tribological characteristics of the tribo-pair (R11 and R14 in Table 6.5). The intensity of the UHMWPE component wear increases by a factor of 1.7 and 1.2, respectively, while the friction coefficient changes from 0.07 to 0.08.

The step-by-step nitriding at the basic regime of 650°C for 20 h essentially reduces the specific wear of the UHMWPE component by a factor of about 25 (R15 in Table 6.5), while the friction coefficient decreases by a factor of 3.4. At the second stage of nitriding, the isothermal holding time slightly increases the friction coefficient from 0.06 to 0.07, but increases the wear of UHMWPE component by a factor of 4.8 (R16 in Table 6.5).

The additional polishing of the surface of the titanium component, after step-by-step nitriding, considerably improves the tribological characteristics of the friction pair (Table 6.5), especially in a basic regime 650°C for 20 h (R15 in Table 6.5). The wear decreases by a factor of 1.3 and the friction coefficient is 0.04. The surface of unpolished and polished c.p. titanium spheres are presented in Figure 6.25.

Figure 6.26 shows the views of UHMWPE samples after friction. The view of the wear groove on the UHMWPE surface after friction in a pair with unnitrided titanium component is presented in Figure 6.26a. The inclusions of titanium into the sample surface, which are the result of seizure of the titanium component with UHMWPE are clearly visible. The seizure is absent on the UHMWPE surface after friction in a pair with nitrided titanium components (Figure 6.26b). On the outer perimeter of the interface is the relevant roll. It is the result of the creep of UHMWPE.

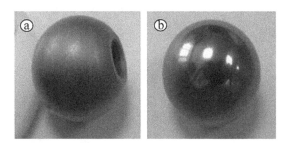

FIGURE 6.25 Surface of c.p. titanium spheres: unpolished (R_a = 0.2-0.5 μm) (a), polished (R_a = 0.04 μm) (b).

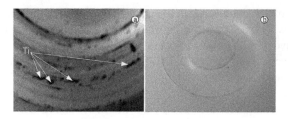

FIGURE 6.26 caption Sticking of titanium on the UHMWPE surface after friction in a pair with untreated titanium (a) and view of the wear groove on the UHMWPE surface after friction in a pair with nitrided titanium (b).

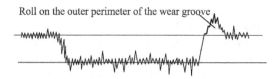

FIGURE 6.27 Profilogram of the cross-section of the wear groove.

Figure 6.27 shows an example of profilogram of the wear groove determined by profilograph VEI-Kalibr. The roll is clearly visible on the outer perimeter of the wear groove. It is the result of the creep of UHMWPE. The volume of roll is less than 10% of the volume of the wear groove.

The comparison of the efficiency of the implant materials indicated that nitrided c.p. titanium exceeds the stainless steel and CoCrMo (ISO 5832/4) as far as the friction coefficient and specific wear of the UHMWPE component of the tribo-pair are lower, and it is at the level of ZrO_2 zirconium ceramics (Figure 6.28). Its brittle fracture is completely eliminated at dynamic loading, the probability of which is always retained, when ceramic components are used. Note that, after a friction path of 200 km, the wear of the Ti component was not revealed.

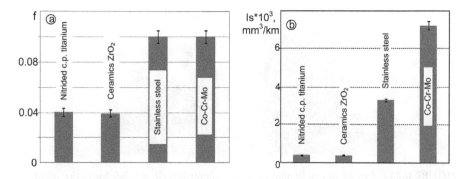

FIGURE 6.28 Friction coefficient in the friction pair of nitrided c.p. titanium (R15)/UHMWPE (a) and specific wear intensity of the UHMWPE component (b) during the tests on the ring-on-plane trybosystem.

Ceramics based on ZrO_2 in the tribological tests in a pair with UHMWPE showed good results [27]. It has a high hardness and strength. But this material has poor thermal stability, and clinical results of the use of ZrO_2 heads were worse than the aluminum oxide heads. This has led to the removal of ceramic ZrO_2 heads from sale in 2002 [28, 29].

6.7 TESTING OF NITRIDED C.P. TITANIUM/UHMWPE FRICTION PAIRS ON STAND-SIMULATOR OF BIOMECHANICAL HUMAN MOVEMENT

Testing friction pairs of endoprostheses is a difficult task. So as to obtain real data on the wear resistance of the friction pair, the endoprosthesis must be inserted into the human body and the condition monitored for several years. But it is possible to accelerate such research using the so-called stands-simulators, reproducing a complex kinematic system of human movements. These tests take several months. They were conducted at the Institute for Sustainable Technologies – National Research Institute, Tribology Department in Radom, Poland, on a T-24 stand-simulator (Figure 6.29).

The T-24 simulator is used to study the tribological characteristics of spherical kinematic systems of biomaterials that can be used in the elements of human hip arthroplasty. The kinematics of the device creates conditions that simulate the operation of complex spherical kinematic systems with three degrees of freedom. This

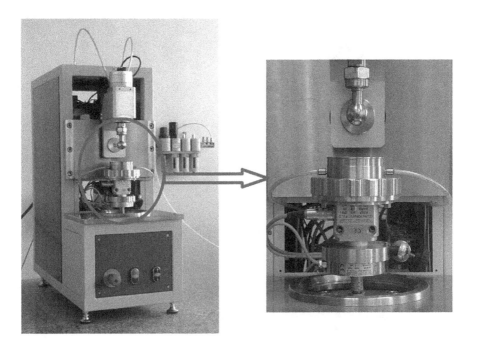

FIGURE 6.29 General view of a T-24 stand-simulator and its working part.

makes it possible to better reproduce the operating conditions of the joint than in friction machines, and thus to obtain more accurate data on the performance of tested materials in conditions close to real ones.

Comparative tribotechnical tests were performed for two friction pairs: a head made of pure titanium with UHMWPE (nitrided Ti/UHMWPE) and the most common in the practice of endoprosthesis friction pair CoCrMo/UHMWPE. Chemical composition of c.p. Ti and UHMWPE according to ASTM B256 and ASTM D4020 standards, respectively.

Figure 6.30 shows photographs of titanium (a) and CoCrMo (b) heads on mandrels and UHMWPE counterbody (c). SEM images of the surface of the heads (a – nitrided c.p. Ti, b – CoCrMo) before the tests are shown in Figure 6.31. It is seen that there are cavities on the surface of nitrided c.p. titanium, and a large number of scratches on the surface of CoCrMo. The surface roughness of the details (Sa) before the test is shown in Figure 6.32. It should be noted that the value of Sa is higher than the value of Ra specified in the international standard. This is due to the fact that according to the standard, measurements of Ra are performed on a line with a length of 0.08 mm, and Sa measurements were performed on the area with a side length of 1.2 × 1.2 mm.

According to the international standard ISO 14242-1, the limit values of technological parameters of the stand were set for tests and measurements of volume and gravimetric wear of UHMWPE cup were performed every million cycles.

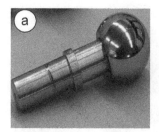 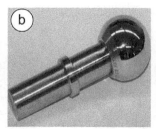 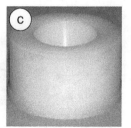

FIGURE 6.30 (a, b) Titanium and Co-Cr-Mo heads on mandrels accordingly; (c) UHMWPE counterbody.

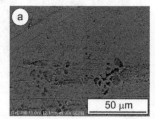 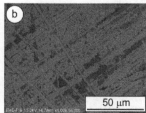

FIGURE 6.31 SEM images of surface of details: (a) nitrided c.p. titanium; (b) Co-Cr-Mo.

The Use of C.P. Titanium in Medical Friction Pairs

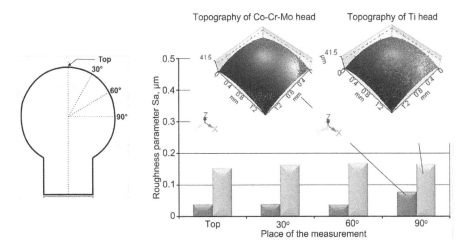

FIGURE 6.32 The surface roughness of Co-Cr-Mo and c.p. titanium heads before tests.

The basis for the working fluid used in the tests was chondroitin sulfate. To prepare it, chondroitin sulfate powder was stirred with distilled water and benzyl alcohol.

Figure 6.33 shows the values of the surface roughness of the heads during the tests obtained using an optical profilometer Talysurf CCI (Taylor Hobson, Leicester, UK). It is seen that there are local irregularities on the surface of both heads. On the surface of the CoCrMo head there are traces of the previous abrasive treatment, on the head of titanium cavities, which is probably a consequence of the formation of a modified layer in the process of TDN. It is seen that the values of the surface roughness of the titanium head slightly exceed the roughness of the CoCrMo head. The presence of roughness peaks can probably be explained by the presence of small cavities on the surface of the titanium.

After three million cycles, the surfaces of the heads were examined with a scanning electron microscope (Figure 6.34). The particles of polyethylene were observed on the surface of the CoCrMo head (Figure 6.34b).

The results of studies of volume and gravimetric wear of the UHMWPE cup in a friction pair are shown in Figures 6.35 and 6.36. Histograms of volume and gravimetric wear of the UHMWPE sample are shown in Figure 6.37.

It is seen that the wear of UHMWPE in the friction pair with CoCrMo in both cases of measurement is greater than in the friction pair with the titanium head. At the same time, the data scatter in the study of gravimetric wear is smaller than in the study of volume wear. According to this method, the wear rate of the UHMWPE cup paired with a titanium head is 1.28 mg/million cycles, compared with 4.26 mg/million cycles for a friction pair with CoCrMo, i.e., less than 3.3 times (Figure 6.37).

Thus, the developed technology of manufacturing a head of c.p. titanium allows obtaining a hinge joint Ti/UHMWPE, the resource of which exceeds the resource of the pair CoCrMo/UHMWPE.

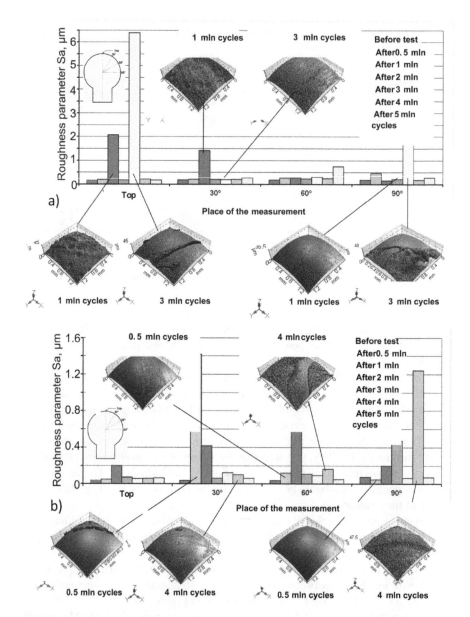

FIGURE 6.33 The surface roughness of c.p. titanium (a) and Co-Cr-Mo (b) heads.

The Use of C.P. Titanium in Medical Friction Pairs 175

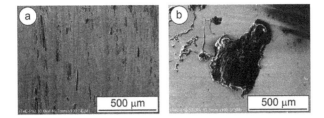

FIGURE 6.34 SEM images of the surfaces of the heads after three million cycles: titanium (a); Co-Cr-Mo (b).

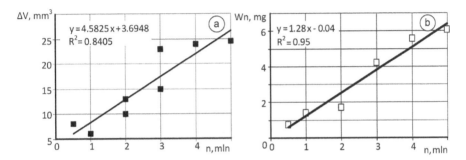

FIGURE 6.35 Volume (a) and gravimetric (b) wear of UHMWPE in pair with nitrided c.p. titanium head.

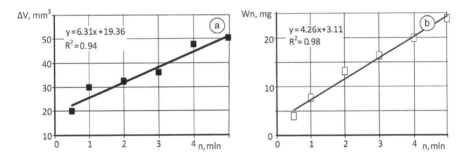

FIGURE 6.36 Volume (a) and gravimetric (b) wear of UHMWPE in pair with Co-Cr-Mo head.

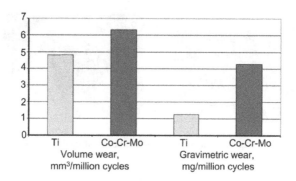

FIGURE 6.37 Volume and gravimetric wear of UHMWPE.

REFERENCES

1. Miletic, K. G., Taylor, T. N., Martin, E. T., Vaidya, R., and Kaye, K. S. 2014. Readmissions after diagnosis of surgical site infection following knee and hip arthroplasty. *Infect Control Hosp Epidemiol* 35:152–157.
2. Sheykin, S. E., Pohrelyuk, I. M., and Mamalis, A. G. 2014. On the effectiveness of commercially pure titanium-UHMWPE endoprosthetic friction pairs. *J Biol Phys Chem* 14:11–17.
3. Pinchuk, L. C., Nikolaev, V. I., Tsvetkova, E. A., and Goldade, V. A. 2006. *Tribology and biophysics of artificial joints*. Oxford: Elsevier.
4. Filippenko, V. A., and Tankut, A. V. 2009. Evolution of joint prosthetics problem. *Int Med J* 1:70–74.
5. Charnley, J. 1961. Arthroplasty of the hip. A new operation. *Lancet* 1:1129–1132.
6. Nadeev, A., and Ivannikov, S.V. 2015. *Endoprostheses of the hip joint in Russia: the construction philosophy, implant review, rational choice*. Knowledge Lab.
7. Kurtz, S. M. 2009. *Ultra high molecular weight polyethylene in total joint replacement and medical devices*. Burlington: Academic Press.
8. Sidambe, A. T. 2014. Biocompatibility of advanced manufactured titanium implants–a review. *Mater* 7:8168–8188.
9. Rahman, M., Reid, I., Duggan, P., Dowling, D. P., Hughes, G., and Hashmi, M. S. J. 2007. Structural and tribological properties of the plasma nitrided Ti-alloy biomaterials: Influence of the treatment temperature. *Surf Coat Tech* 201:4865–4872.
10. Manhabosco, T. M., Tamborim, S. M., dos Santos, C. B., and Muller, I. L. 2011. Tribological, electrochemical and tribo-electrochemical characterization of bare and nitrided Ti6Al4V in simulated body fluid solution. *Corros Sci* 53:1786–1793.
11. Kapzhinski, M. P., Kinast, E. J., and dos Santos, C. A. 2003. Near-surface composition and tribological behaviour of plasma nitrided titanium. *J Phys Appl Phys* 36:1858–1863.
12. Nolan, D., Huang, S. W., Leskovsek, V., and Braun, S. 2006. Sliding wear of titanium nitride thin films deposited on Ti-6Al-4V alloy by PVD and plasma nitriding processes. *Surf Coat Tech* 200:5698–5705.
13. Pohrelyuk, I. M., Sheykin, S. E., Dub, S. M. et al. 2016. Increasing of functionality of c.p. titanium/UHMWPE tribo-pairs by thermodiffusion nitriding of titanium component. *Biotribology* 7:38–45.

14. Sheykin, S. Ye., Pohreliuk, I.M., Iefrosinin, D.V., Rostotskiy I. Yu., and Sergach, D.A. 2015. The use of titanium in the friction units of artificial joints. *Sci Innov* 11:5–10.
15. Pohrelyuk, I., and Fedirko, V. 2012. Chemico-thermal treatment of titanium alloys – nitriding. In *Titanium alloys – towards achieving enhanced properties for diversified applications*, ed. A. K. M. Nurul Amin, 141–174. Rijeka: InTech.
16. Novikov, N. V., Rosenberg, O. A., and Gavlik, J. 2011. *Endoprostheses of the human joints: Materials and technologies*. Kyiv: ISM them. VN Bakul NAS of Ukraine.
17. Paschenko, Ye. A., Sheykin, S. Ye., and Iefrosinin, D. V. 2013. Tools for precision diamond machining of spherical heads of endoprostheses from pure titanium. *J Superhard Mater* 35:175–182.
18. Grushko, A. V., Sheykin, S. E., and Rostotskiy, I. Y. 2012. Contact pressure in hip endoprosthetic swivel joints. *J Frict Wear* 33:124–129.
19. Pohrelyuk, I. M., Sheikin, S. Ye., and Efrosinin, D. V. 2014. Surface hardening of VT1-0 titanium in the course of thermodiffusion saturation with nitrogen within the temperature range 650–750ºC. *Mater Sci* 50:70–79.
20. Hultman, L., Sundgren, J.-E., Greene, J. E., Bergstrom, D. B., and Petrov, I. 1995. High-flux low-energy (~20 eV) N^{+2} ion irradiation during TiN deposition by reactive magnetron sputtering: Effects on microstructure and preferred orientation. *J Appl Phys* 12:5395–5404.
21. http://obuch.com.ua/informatika/11247/index.html.
22. Ermakov, F. 2008. *Tribological physics of liquid crystals*. Gomel: IMMS of the National Academy of Sciences of Belarus.
23. Sheykin, S., Pohrelyuk, I., Rostotskyi, I., Iefrosinin, D., Tuszynski, W., Mankowska-Snopczynska, A. 2018. Tribological behavior of the friction pair "GRADE 2/ PE-UHMW" and the technology of the production of its spherical part made of GRADE 2. *Tribologia* 6:137–148.
24. Chernyakova, Yu. M., and Pinchuk, L. S. 2007. Synovial joint as a clever friction unit. *Frict Wear* 28:410–417.
25. Ermakov, S. F., and Beletsky, A. V. 2011. Tribological principles of blood serum preparations as a liquid crystalline medium for therapeutic correction of synovial joints. *Frict Wear* 32:65–71.
26. Ermakov, S. F., Beletskii, A. V., and Nikolaev, V. I. 2011. Tribological principles of developing medicinal preparations based on blood serum as a liquid crystalline medium for therapeutic correction of synovial joints. *J Frict Wear* 32:49–53.
27. Novikov, N. V., Rozenberg, O. A., and Gavlik, Y. 2011. *Endoprosthesis of human joints: materials and technologies* (in Russian). V. Kyiv: Bakul Institute for Superhard Materials of the NAS of Ukraine.
28. Oonishi, H. 2000. Clinical experience with ceramics in total hip replacement. *Clin Orthop* 379:77–84.
29. Santos, E. M., Vohra, S., Catledge, S. A., McClenny, M. D., Lemons, J., Moore, K. D. 2004. Examination of surface and material properties of explanted zirconia femoral heads, *J Arthroplasty* 19:30–34.

7 Electrochemical Techniques Applied to the Tribocorrosion Tests
Advantages and Limitations of Stationary and Non-Stationary Methods

J. A. C. Ponciano Gomes and C. D. R. Barros
Federal University of Rio de Janeiro, Rio de Janeiro

CONTENTS

7.1	Introduction	179
7.2	Tribocorrosion Simulation Devices	180
7.3	Electrochemical Techniques	193
7.4	Other Techniques and Concepts	202
7.5	Tribocorrosion Results	216
7.6	Methodology Proposal	220
	7.6.1 Step 1 – Physicochemical Characterization of the Environment/Solution	222
	7.6.2 Step 2 – Preliminary Electrochemical Assessment	223
	7.6.3 Step 3 – Tribocorrosion Tests	224
	7.6.4 Step 4 – Surface Analysis	226
References		227

7.1 INTRODUCTION

Tribocorrosion is a mechanically assisted corrosion process promoted by the conjoint action of mechanical removal of the material and electrochemical reactions occurring on a metal electrolyte interface. The main electrochemical reaction is basically the anodic dissolution of metallic components, followed by the release of metal ions to the environment. The intensity and morphology of tribocorrosion are influenced by the mechanical process, and the degradation is much more intense than the sum of isolate mechanical and electrochemical processes. Separation of elementary and synergic components is commonly based on the model prescribed by ASTM G 119-09 [1] standard and others. The direct assessment of the electrochemical parameters measured during the experimental simulation is a basic requirement to achieve a better understanding of the degradation mechanism.

Several experimental techniques are used to simulate tribocorrosion, assisted by electrochemical measurements. The objective is to understand the basic tribocorrosion mechanisms and select the best alternatives to avoid or control this degradation process. An overview of the experimental resources available is presented and discussed in the present work. The use of electrochemical methods is emphasized, and one integrated methodology is outlined and proposed.

7.2 TRIBOCORROSION SIMULATION DEVICES

The main device used to assess tribocorrosion is the tribometer, which is an experimental apparatus designed to simulate the wear produced by the relative motion occurring at the contact interface of two bodies. An electrochemical cell is connected to the material under test immersed in a corrosive environment. The cell is connected to a potentiostat or to a zero-resistance ammeter (ZRA), which allows monitoring in real time the electrochemical reactions occurring during the process.

The relative motion between the surfaces can occur through different contact modes. The main contact modes described in the literature are fretting, sliding, rolling, impingement and micro-abrasion [2–7]. The ASTM G 40-17 [2] standard contains the definition of the terminology to be used in tribocorrosion systems. Fretting is defined as the oscillatory motion between the contact surfaces of two bodies, within small amplitudes, commonly tangential. Sliding is described as the relative motion between two bodies occurring at one tangential contact plane. Rolling is the rotating motion of a ball, cylinder, or wheel, in a direction parallel to one plane of the surface, either in part or in the total contact area. Impingement is defined as the result of successive impacts of solid or liquid particles on a solid surface.

Different devices are designed, constructed, and used to simulate the different contact modes. For example, an indenter in linear reciprocating sliding with a sample, being the sample holder used as an electrochemical cell to promote a tribocorrosion simulation [8]. Micro-scale abrasion devices are also used to simulate wear-corrosion or erosion-corrosion, where the corrosive medium contains abrasive particles in suspension, called slurry, widely used in rolling contact mode [9–11].

The tribometer is more extensively used on evaluations under sliding and fretting contact modes. The movement can be rotational or linear and the direction can be unidirectional or reciprocating (alternate backward and forward movements). The associations of unidirectional rotational sliding and linear reciprocating fretting are the most used. Two standards describe these systems: Linearly Reciprocating Ball-on–Flat by ASTM G 133-05 [12] and rotational pin-on-disk by ASTM G 99-05 [13].

The standard ASTM G 133-05 [12] describes a linear reciprocating test where the counter body is a ball, a cylinder pin, or other spherical-ended specimen, positioned under a vertical load over a horizontal flat specimen. The standard enables varieties of this configuration. The counterbody is fixed in contact with the moving flat specimen, or the counterbody can move against the flat specimen. Consequently, the relative motion occurs under uniform vertical constant contact load (Figure 7.1). The motor used on the device is variable and the basic requirement is to impose a

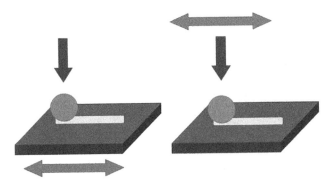

FIGURE 7.1 Schematic diagram of a linear reciprocating ball-on-flat specimen. (a) fixed counterbody ball and plate movement; (b) movement of counterbody ball with fixed plate.

TABLE 7.1
Main Parameters of Linear Reciprocating Tribometer Tests

Parameter	Unit
Normal Load	N
Ball/ Tip	mm (radius)
Stroke length	mm
Displacement amplitude	mm
Duration of test	s or min (time)/mm (curse distance)
Oscillation Frequency	Hertz/rpm
Ambient Humidity	%
Temperature	°C
Maximum Hertzian Contact stress	MPa

smooth and regular movement. The standard is of great importance for the definition of the parameters to be considered on tribocorrosion tests. The standard is flexible and different design criteria are allowed to construct the basic setup. However, the apparatus must permit the accurate determination of the parameters listed in Table 7.1, with their respective S.I. units.

The Hertzian contact pressure is calculated based on the applied normal load, the diameter of the counterbody (ball/tip), elastic modulus, and Poison coefficient of the materials in relative contact motion. This parameter is important since the contact surface is not a single point, but an area where tridimensional stresses are produced, including shear components, and where elastic and plastic deformation occurs during wear.

The same information is also obtained in the case of rotational pin-on-disk, as described by ASTM G 99-05 [13]. The differences, beyond the movement type, are the possibility of the plan or disk specimen remaining horizontally or vertically oriented in reference to the pin or ball counterbody. Consequently, the sliding paths can be a spherical hole or a circle. The parameters associated with the tests are the same

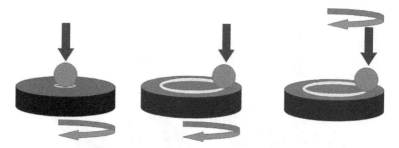

FIGURE 7.2 Schematic diagram of a sliding rotational ball-on-disk. (a) fixed counterbody ball at disk center with disk movement; (b) fixed counterbody ball at determined radius from disk center with disk movement (c) movement of counterbody ball at determined radius from disk center with fixed disk.

as mentioned in Table 7.1, with the additional information of the position of the counterbody. The ball or pin can be positioned at the center of the disk, resulting in a spherical hole wear area, or can be placed at a constant distance from the center, which means the formation of a radial wear track. The moving element can be the counterbody or the flat specimen (Figure 7.2).

One important experimental condition is the test duration, which can be converted to elapsed distance. In the case of rotational sliding, the distance is defined by the number of laps or cycles. Test time and distance are linked by the rotating speed selected. For the linear reciprocating device, one cycle corresponds to one back and forward movement. The cumulative cycles correspond to the wear distance and the test duration will be defined in a similar way. The tribometers use a revolution counter associated with the motor drive, having the ability to record the distance and stop the engine when the number of rotations or cycles is achieved. In some systems, the contact can be intermittent, depending on the test protocol adopted.

Another relevant parameter to be obtained is the coefficient of friction, calculated from the contact force measured during the test. The tribometer must be equipped with a load cell capable to continuously measure the friction force in both directions, backward and forward, in case of a bidirectional or reciprocating test. The friction force recorded is used to calculate the coefficient of friction (COF) in real time or by processing the data after the test (Figure 7.3). The final result of tribocorrosion tests is the wear volume loss, experimentally calculated after the tests using different surface analysis methods and integration methodologies to be addressed on further topics.

The tribometer in all configurations previously mentioned can simulate the wear phenomenon with or without the influence of lubrication at the contact surface. For tribocorrosion simulation, the process occurs in the presence of an electrolyte. The interface under test is positioned into an electrochemical cell containing the corrosive environment. This cell contains, in general, three electrodes connected to one potentiostat, an electronic instrument that measures and controls the electrochemical potentials and currents of one metal/electrolyte interface. Based on this information, corrosion intensity, morphology, and mechanisms can be investigated. When connected to the tribometer, fundamental information about tribocorrosion can be obtained during the tests.

Electrochemical Techniques Applied to the Tribocorrosion Tests 183

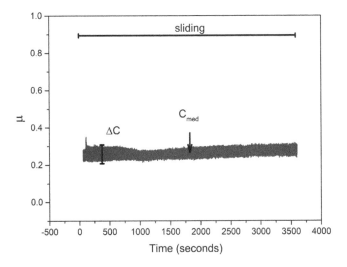

FIGURE 7.3 Coefficient of friction calculated from the load data registered during the tribocorrosion test.

The electrochemical cell associated with the potentiostat and tribometer (tribocorrosion cell) is a three-electrode system, containing a reference electrode (RE), a counter electrode (CE), and the material under investigation, referred to as working electrode (WE). The cell is made of inert materials, like nylon, glass, or polymers. The WE is the specimen submitted to the wear test, being the counterbody placed inside the cell attached by an inert supporting holder under the applied load. The counterbody holder is placed perpendicularly to the WE holding the pin or ball inside the electrochemical cell in contact with the flat material surface in the corrosive medium. On the external part of the cell, the counterbody holder is connected to the load cell. All the materials in contact with the electrolyte, except the electrodes, must be non-metallic or coated with a polymer. The electrodes connected to the potentiostat are the CE, RE, and WE, as shown in (Figure 7.4). The material used as CE is platinum, in general, and the RE is a standard reference electrode of different types.

The configurations presented in Figure 7.4 are extensively used by many authors [3, 14–29]. The electrochemical parameters obtained are basically *potential* and *current*. The potential can be measured and controlled by the potentiostat. When only measured, it corresponds to the potential difference between the WE and RE. This value is commonly referred to as open circuit potential (OCP) or corrosion potential (Ecorr). The connection between the pair of electrodes is of high impedance and no current flows between them. The measurement is very simple, but the correct interpretation of these parameters depends on other information, as will be further discussed.

The potentiostat is capable of measuring and controlling the electrochemical potential of the metal/electrolyte interface on the WE. To accomplish this potential control and measurement, the instrument needs a third electrode, which is the counter electrode, CE. Using the CE, the potentiostat can fix the OCP on a constant value and shift it to higher or lower values, imposing a controlled current flowing between

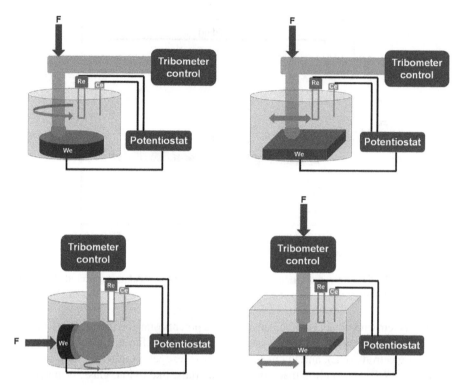

FIGURE 7.4 Schematic diagram of different tribometers with electrochemical cell.

WE and CE. This process is referred to as polarization; the shift to higher potential values is defined as anodic polarization, and to lower values is defined as cathodic polarization. The use of different polarization protocols permits the application of different electrochemical techniques, depending on the corrosion process under investigation, among them tribocorrosion, as will be described. It is important to point out that, despite the essential knowledge obtained about corrosion using the polarization methods, on real applied conditions the corrosion phenomenon occurs without the influence of an external polarization.

Another setup that can be used to perform electrochemical measurements during tribocorrosion is shown in Figure 7.5. One similar electrochemical cell containing one secondary electrode, which is electrically connected to the WE in order to establish a low impedance circuit. The instrument is an ammeter, referred to as ZRA, and can be used to measure the electrochemical current flowing between the electrodes [15, 16, 21, 29, 30]. The WE is the material against wear during the tribocorrosion test. In this setup, the ZRA quantifies the current flow between the worm and unworn areas. A third electrode can be used as a reference, and the electrochemical potential of the pair can be measured by using a high impedance voltmeter between the pair and RE.

The flexibility of the setup selected to construct the tribometer allows the emergence of new models, not described in standards, such as tribometers with conjugated movements or associated with other techniques. Among these is the use of a

Electrochemical Techniques Applied to the Tribocorrosion Tests

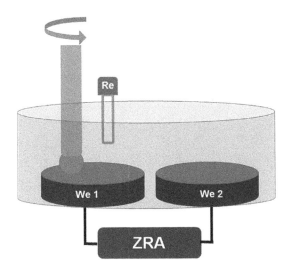

FIGURE 7.5 Schematic diagram of ZRA setup in electrochemical cell attached to tribometer.

cell with an incubator containing cell culture environments to identify degradation effects induced by wear products [31]. The innovation is the association of Raman and fluorescence techniques and one local confocal spectrometer attached to the tribometer, through a charge couple-device (CDD) camera. This configuration is capable of making in situ analysis of the contact surface area, characterizing the phase transformation of the warmed alloy [32]. An example of conjugated movements is the pin-on-plate reciprocates tribometer, where the stationary pin rotates while the plate moves to simulate tribocorrosion of CoCrMo pin and plate components of hip joints [27].

Other tribometers are developed with set-ups closer to the real condition, like the hip joint simulators, which includes the similar contact mode and geometry closer to the real for an acetabular cup and femoral head [33–35]. Among the first tribocorrosion studies with hip joint simulators, simulating flexion-extension movement, was the study published by Yan et al. 2009 [36] with CoCrMo femoral head and acetabular cups. Hua et al. [34] also performed wear tests using a biotribological hip joint simulator, but with the ability to simulate three pair of movements widely performed by hip joints in vivo: abduction-adduction, extension-flexion, and external-internal rotation, in assessments produced by UHMWPE acetabular cup and CoCrMo femoral head of real prostheses.

The tribometer device must be able to simulate, as close as possible, the contact condition that occurs in the real application under investigation. Therefore, countless different custom tribometer devices can be found in the literature. Besides, the standards related to the phenomenon only describe the basic device setup, making possible the necessary adaptations for each condition to be simulated, which is an advantage. However, the disadvantage is that different devices used to simulate the same condition can be found in literature, and the results cannot directly be compared. Some examples of the various tribometers and the corresponding systems present in the literature are shown in Table 7.2.

TABLE 7.2
References of Some of Various Tribometers Devices in the Literature

References	Tribometer	Counterbody	Parameters	Material	Medium	Techniques	Surface Analysis	Other Analysis and Comments
Barros et al. (2020a) [15]	Ball-on-disk Rotational unidirectional (ball in movement)	Alumina ball 4 mm Ø	Load: 2 N Frequency: 1 Hz Track radius: 4 mm Hertzian pressure contact: 814.5 MPa (NiCr) 998.7 MPa (Ti6Al4V) Duration time: 3600 s	Ti6Al4V NiCr	227 ppm F⁻ pH 5.5 12,300 ppm F⁻ pH 4	OCP during sliding Galvanic couple Coefficient of friction	Confocal	ZRA Thermodynamic analysis Wear volume total loss (confocal) Wear track profile Wear rate
Dalbert et al. (2010) [16]	Reciprocating motion tribometer	Corundum pin	Load: 10 N Frequency: 1 Hz Hertzian pressure contact: 405 MPa Number of cycles: 1000	AISI 430 Graphite (ZRA)	0.1 M Na_2SO_4 pH = 1.5, 6.5, 12.5	Galvanic couple OCP during sliding Current during sliding	Profilometer FE-SEM	ZRA Wear volume loss Wear track profile
Corne et al. (2019) [37]	Pin-on-plan fretting	Zirconia Ti6Al4V 20 mm Ø	Load: 127.5–80 N Frequency: 1 Hz Hertzian pressure contact: 80 MPa (finite element) Number of cycles: 57600 Time: 16 h Temperature 20°C	Ti grade 4 Ti6Al4V grade 5	Human saliva collected	Cathodic polarization OCP during fretting EIS during fretting Coefficient of friction	Optical profilometer SEM/EDS FEG TEM/STEM	Galvanic couple Wear volume loss (profilometer)

Dalmau Borrás et al. (2019) [38]	Ball-on-disk rotational sliding	Zirconia ball 6 mm Ø	Load: 5 N Frequency: 60 rpm Track radius: 1 mm Sliding velocity: 6.28 mm/s Hertzian pressure contact: 654 MPa (counterbody) 585 MPa (Ti) Time: 300–3600 s Temperature 37 °C	Ti grade 4	Artificial saliva pH 6.5	OCP during sliding Cathodic polarization+ sliding Anodic polarization + sliding Coefficient of friction	Optical microscopy Confocal FE-SEM FIB	Wear volume total loss (confocal) Zirconia profile
Simsek and Ozyurek (2019) [39]	Pin-on-disk rotational (ASTM G-99)	Stainless steel ball 8 mm Ø	Load: 10-20-30 N Sliding distance: 400-800-1200–1600 m Sliding speed: 1 ms^{-1} Temperature 37°C	Ti5Al2.5Fe Ti6Al4V 12 mm Ø	Body fluid pH 7.25	Preliminary Corrosion tests (OCP, Potentiodynamic polarization) Coefficient of friction	SEM/ EDS	Hardness Weight Loss (gravimetric) Wear rate
Pejaković et al. (2018) [40]	Ball-on-plate Linear reciprocating sliding (ball in movement)	Alumina ball 5 mm Ø	Load: 10 mN – 100 mN – 1 N Frequency: 1 Hz Length stroke: 1 mm Sliding velocity :2 mm/s Hertzian pressure contact : 90–430 Mpa Time: 1200 s Number of cycles: 1000 Temperature room	Ti6Al4V 1 cm^2	Artificial Seawater	Preliminary Corrosion tests (Cathodic polarization, OCP, Potentiodynamic polarization) OCP during sliding Anodic and cathodic potential applied during sliding Coefficient of friction	Confocal SEM/EDX	Wear volume loss (confocal) Ratio Corrosion/ Wear

(*Continued*)

TABLE 7.2 (Continued)

References	Tribometer	Counterbody	Parameters	Material	Medium	Techniques	Surface Analysis	Other Analysis and Comments
Sivakumar et al. (2017) [19]	Ball-on-flat Linear reciprocating fretting (ball in movement)	Alumina ball 8 mm Ø	Load: 3 N Frequency: 5 Hz Linear displacement amplitude: 180 µm Temperature 20°C	Ti c.p.	Ringer	Preliminary Corrosion tests (Potentiodynamic polarization, AC impedance) OCP during sliding Anodic potential applied during sliding Intermittent corrosion tests during sliding	Optical microscopy SEM XPS	Image J (fretted area dimensions) Wear track profile
Alves et al. (2015) [41]	Pin-on-disk Linear sliding reciprocating	Alumina ball 10 mm Ø	Load: 2 N Frequency: 2 Hz Linear displacement amplitude: 3 mm Time: 720 s Temperature 37 °C	Ti c.p. 1 cm^2	Artificial saliva Fusayama	OCP during sliding Coefficient of friction	XRD FE-SEM Confocal	Wear volume loss (confocal) Roughness (profilometer)
Li et al. (2015) [22]	Ball-on-plate Linear reciprocating sliding (ball in movement)	Ceramic ball 3 mm Ø	Load: 1-2-3-4 N Frequency: 20 Hz Linear displacement amplitude: 3 mm Temperature 25°C	316 L SS	Slurry of artificial saliva pH 5.7	Potentiodynamic polarization during wear test EIS during sliding Coefficient of friction	SEM	

Licausi et al. (2015) [42]	Ball-on-flat Linear reciprocating fretting (ball in movement)	Alumina ball 6 mm Ø SiC pin 2.8 mm Ø	Load: 3 N (alumina) 2–10 N (SiC) Frequency: 1 Hz Hertzian pressure contact: 830 MPa (alumina) 1410 MPa (SiC) Temperature 37°C	Ti6Al4V	Artificial saliva Fusayama Meyer	Preliminary Corrosion tests (OCP, Cathodic polarization) OCP during sliding Current during sliding Coefficient of friction	SEM Confocal	ZRA Wear volume loss (Confocal) Wear track profile Synergism interaction estimated
Souza et al. (2015) [23]	Ball-on-plate Linear reciprocating sliding	Alumina ball 10 mm Ø	Load: 0.5 N Frequency: 1 Hz Linear displacement amplitude: 3 mm Number of cycles: 1200 Temperature 37°C	Ti6Al4V 0.5 cm^2	Artificial saliva Fusayama	OCP during sliding Coefficient of friction	Optical microscopy SEM/EDX	Weight Loss (gravimetric)
Wimmer et al. (2015) [24]	Ball-on-disk rotational	Alumina ball 28 mm Ø	Load: 8–64 N Frequency: 1 Hz Cycles: 1800 Temperature 37 °C	CoCrMo 1.13 cm^2	Bovine calf serum diluted in simulated synovial fluid pH 6	OCP during sliding EIS before and after sliding Coefficient of friction	SEM/ EDS Light interferometer Raman	Wear volume loss (interferometer) Synergism interaction estimated
Holmes et al. (2014) [11]	Ball-on-plate Rotational unidirectional (ball in movement)	UHMVPE 31.75 mm Ø	Load: 0.5–4 N Frequency: 150 rpm Time: 0.5–3 h	316 L	Slurry of artificial saliva Fusayama and abrasive particles pH 5.7	Potentiodynamic polarization during wear test Coefficient of friction	SEM	Volume loss (scar diameter – SEM) Wear maps

(*Continued*)

TABLE 7.2 (Continued)

References	Tribometer	Counterbody	Parameters	Material	Medium	Techniques	Surface Analysis	Other Analysis and Comments
Espallargas et al. (2013) [30]	Ball-on-flat Linear reciprocating fretting (pin in movement)	SiC pin 1 cm Ø	Load: 10–20 N Frequency: 1 Hz Sliding distance 20 mm Linear speed : 72 m/h Hertzian contact pressure: 768–967 MPa	Super duplex UNS S32750 5.6 cm^2 2.8 cm^2	NaCl 3.4%	Preliminary Corrosion tests (OCP, (Potentiodynamic polarization) Galvanic measurements Current (ZRA)	Confocal	ZRA Evans diagram Wear volume loss (Confocal) Wear track profile Synergism interaction estimated
Swaminathan and Gilbert (2013) [43]	Pin-on-disk fretting (pin in movement)	Cone-shape pin 0.041–0.246 cm^2 CoCrMo Ti6Al4V	Load: 5 N Frequency: 0.1 – 1.25 – 2.5 Hz Nominal displacement: 50 μm Time: 5000 s	CoCrMo Ti6Al4V Disk 0.001– 0.011 cm^2	Phosphate Buffered saline solution pH 7.4	Potentiostat fretting with increment of potentials steps Coefficient of friction	SEM/ EDS	Galvanic couple
Dimah et al. (2012) [44]	Ball-on-disk rotational sliding (disk in movement)	Alumina ball 6 mm Ø	Load: 5 N Frequency: 60 rpm Track diameter: 6 mm Sliding velocity:20 mm/s Hertzian pressure contact: 950 MPa Temperature ambient	Ti c.p. Ti6Al4V 30 mm Ø	Phosphate Buffered solution Bovine Serum Albumin pH 7.4	Preliminary Corrosion tests (OCP, Potentiodynamic polarization) OCP during sliding Cathodic polarization+ sliding Polarization during sliding Intermittent corrosion tests during sliding Coefficient of friction	SEM (ball and disk) Optical microscopy Confocal	Hardness Wear loss (confocal) Wear Track profiles Synergism interaction estimated

Mathew et al. (2012) [25]	Pin-on-ball Oscillatory motion	Ceramic ball 28 mm Ø	Load: 20 N Frequency: 1.2 Hz Hertzian pressure contact: 372 MPa Number of cycles: 2000	Ti c.p. 12 mm Ø	Artificial saliva pH 3-6-9	Preliminary Corrosion tests (Potentiodynamic polarization) Current during sliding Coefficient of friction	SEM Light Interferometry	Thermodynamic analysis Synergism interaction estimated
Mathew et al. (2011) [5]	Pin-on-ball Oscillatory rotational motion (hip joint simulator)	Ceramic ball 28 mm Ø	Load: 16 N Frequency: 1 Hz Amplitude: 15^0 Hertzian pressure contact: 350 MPa Number of cycles: 1000	CoCrMo pin 12 mm Ø	2.4% NaCl Bovine calf serum	OCP during sliding Current during sliding Coefficient of friction	Profilometer	Weight loss (profilometer) Weight loss (metal in solution)
Kumar et al. (2010) [26]	Ball-on-flat Linear fretting reciprocating (ball in movement)	Alumina ball 8 mm Ø	Load: 3-5-7-10 N Frequency: 5–10 Hz Hertzian pressure contact: 500 MPa (3 N) – 1200 MPa (10 N) Fretting cycles: 1500 – 3000 – 4500 – 9000 – 18,000 – 36,000 Temperature 37 °C	Ti c.p. (grade 2) 20 mm Ø	Ringer pH 7.8	OCP during sliding Current during sliding Coefficient of friction	SEM/ EDX	Normalization of potential
Tekin and Malayoglu (2010) [45]	Ball-on-holder Linear reciprocating sliding (holder in movement)	Silicone nitride ball 12.7 mm Ø	Load: 49 N Frequency: 0.5 Hz Length distance: 20 mm Stroke length cycle: 10 mm Time: 45 min Temperature 24 °C	Hastelloy G35 Hastelloy C2000 Haynes 625	Dry NaCl 3.5%	OCP during sliding Potentiodynamic Polarization during sliding	SEM/ EDX Profilometer	Wear volume loss (Profilometer) Wear track profiles ICP-MS

(Continued)

TABLE 7.2 (Continued)

References	Tribometer	Counterbody	Parameters	Material	Medium	Techniques	Surface Analysis	Other Analysis and Comments
Yan et al. (2009) [36]	Friction hip joint simulator (flexion-extension)	CoCrMo	Load: 25-100–300 N Frequency: 1 Hz	CoCrMo	Bovine synovial fluid 25% Serum 0.3% NaCl	OCP during sliding	Contact profilometer	ICP-AES
Yan et al. (2008) [27]	Pin-on-plate Reciprocating (Stationary pin in rotational movement and plate in reciprocating movement)	CoCrMo 12 mm Ø	Load: 80 N Frequency: 1 Hz Stroke length distance: 20 mm Hertzian pressure contact: 112 MPa Time: 4h	CoCrMo Alumina	Newborn bovine calf serum +0.1% sodium azide	OCP during sliding Cathodic protection during sliding	Interferometer Optical microscope	Wear volume loss (Interferometer) ICP-AES
Berradja et al. (2006) [4]	Ball-on-plate rotational sliding unidirectional (pin in movement)	Corundum cylinder 7 mm Ø	Load: 5, 20 N Frequency: 6, 60, 120 rpm Radius : 8 mm Hertzian pressure contact: 96, 207 MPa Cycles: 2500 Temperature 25°C	AISL 304 25 mm Ø	0.5 M H_2SO_4 Ringer	OCP during sliding Electrochemical current and potential noise	–	Power spectral density (PSD)
Vieira et al. (2006) [28]	Ball-on-plate linear bidirectional (reciprocating) fretting (ball in movement)	Corundum balls 10 mm Ø	Load: 2 N Frequency: 1 Hz Displacement amplitude: 200 μm Fretting Cycles: 5000–10,000 Temperature 23°C (ambient)	Ti c.p. (grade 2) 1 cm^2	Artificial saliva+ inhibitors	OCP during sliding Current during sliding Electrochemical noise	Light microscopy with contrast Laser profilometer SEM/EDX	Roughness ZRA Wear volume (profilometer)

In addition to the differences of the device and other variations like contact mode, movement type, and which component is placed in movement, as observed in Table 7.2, the parameter values reported are within wide ranges. It is possible to find in the cited literature normal load in a range of 10 mN to 300 N, frequency from 0.5 to 20 Hz, maximum contact pressure from 80 to 1200 MPa, and the most varied ratio of ball and specimen.

7.3 ELECTROCHEMICAL TECHNIQUES

The basic resources available to perform electrochemical monitoring during tribocorrosion were already described. There is a high number of techniques and corresponding parameters that can be used, supported by the electrochemical potential and current measurements. The main electrochemical techniques are:

- Open circuit potential – follow-up time evolution of the electrode potential of the material under testing, by using a second RE. The instrument can be the potentiostat or one high impedance voltmeter. The method can be used on a real-time basis, before, during, and after sliding, for instance. No external polarization is required.
- Amperometry – follow-up the electrochemical current of the material under test at a constant potential imposed and controlled by the potentiostat. The WE is under external polarization promoted by the potentiostat and the use of a third electrode, CE, is necessary. The measured current flows between WE and CE.
- Anodic and cathodic polarization – correlation between variable electrochemical potential controlled by the potentiostat and the polarization current necessary to establish each potential. The electrochemical interface is fully controlled by external polarization and the potential can vary toward higher potentials (anodic polarization) or lower potentials (cathodic polarization). The scan rate for the controlled potential is fixed and defined in mV/s.
- Electrochemical impedance spectroscopy – EIS – is a low amplitude and variable frequency polarization method, which consists of a sinusoidal polarization in potential or current within a fixed frequency range. Correlation between the amplitude of the response signal (potential or current) and the phase angle defines the complex impedance of the interface at each frequency. Steady-state and linearity are basic requirements to make possible the valid interpretation of the electrochemical data. The impedance will be composed of a Real part (resistive) and an Imaginary part (capacitive or inductive), depending on the electrochemical interface. The so-called frequency response of the electrochemical interface will contain relevant information about the electrochemical processes occurring and/or passivation characteristics.
- Electrochemical noise – EN – a technique based on the interpretation of potential and current signals on time and frequency domains, obtained in real time by using one dedicated instrument – ZRA – designed to record spontaneous fluctuations of the electrochemical signals with high accuracy and high noise

rejection capability. Permit the acquisition of information about corrosion intensity, corrosion morphology, and corrosion mechanisms without the use of external polarization.

All electrochemical techniques listed are commonly used during tribocorrosion tests, mainly the potential and the current produced during the test. Each technique will provide different information with variable accuracy and consistency. Real-time measurement of current and potential reveals characteristic profiles of non-stationary processes, and the consistency of the obtained results will depend on the instrumentation used and on the characteristics of the setup. The use of stationary, or steady-state-based methods, like EIS, is limited by the localized and transient nature of tribocorrosion. However, this class of electrochemical techniques, like anodic polarization and EIS has fundamental importance to support the precise interpretation of the results.

Figure 7.6 shows one schematic example of OCP monitoring of passive material. The result corresponds to an unworn surface and the positive shift of OCP with time corresponds to the evolution of the passive state to more protective conditions. The potential difference is due to the aging of the passive film with the increment of the electrochemical potential gradient at the interface which major component is the potential difference across the film thickness. This inference can be confirmed by

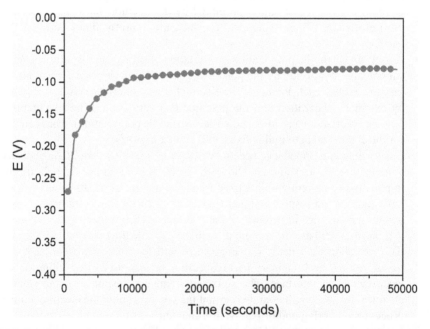

FIGURE 7.6 OCP evolution of an unworn, static metal/solution interface. Simple instrumentation and parameter that can be used to follow the build-up of passivation and the protective ability of the passive film formed. Data can be correlated with equilibrium thermodynamics information to confirm passive/active conditions on the same interface. Shift to higher values with time suggests the increment of the passivation quality in several systems.

anodic polarization and EIS. The amplitude of the OCP variation from the initial immersion to the steady-state condition is one parameter for further analysis. OCP shifts to lower values can be observed, which means probably a less protective condition with immersion time. Unable to provide kinetics information but make it possible for a thermodynamic analysis, which is relevant to support the assumption of passive or active conditions at the electrochemical interface.

The same material under anodic polarization is likely to exhibit one anodic potential range with extremely low values of current density, about 10^{-6} A/cm^2. At higher potentials, the material can exhibit localized corrosion susceptibility corresponding to an abrupt increment of the anodic current. One example of anodic polarization curves of passive materials susceptible and not susceptible to localized corrosion is shown in Figure 7.7. From EIS results, the existence of a stable passive condition will be confirmed by the capacitive behavior and very high polarization resistance, Rp – defined as the limit of the electrochemical impedance when the measurement frequency tends to zero. Figure 7.8 exhibits examples of Nyquist plots of EIS results.

The use of anodic and cathodic polarization during sliding is possible. However, the interpretation of the results is not evident. The correlation between potential and current during wear can be compared to the same information obtained with the static material. But the results will depend on the scan rate used and do not represent the spontaneous interactions among worn and unworn areas spontaneously occurring during tribocorrosion. Anodic polarization is a large amplitude signal technique and the correlation between the potential vs. current under tribocorrosion is not evident. The coupling of a mixed metal/electrolyte interface and scanning potential is not simple. In general, oscillating values are registered, depending on the scan rate and

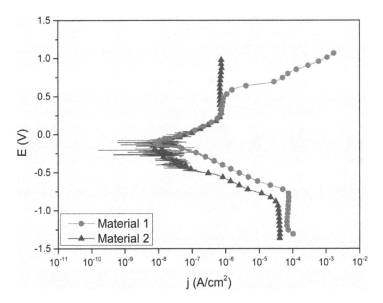

FIGURE 7.7 Anodic and polarization curves of passive metals, being material 1 susceptible to localized corrosion and material 2 do not susceptible to material corrosion.

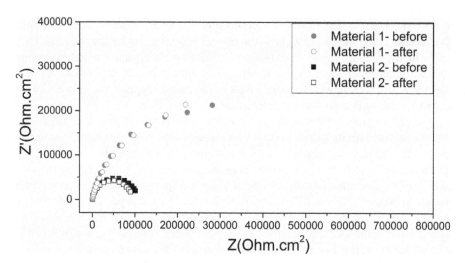

FIGURE 7.8 EIS Nyquist diagram of materials evaluated before and after.

on the dimensions of the WE used. For passive material, an increment of and oscillation of current under fixed potential is commonly observed during sliding.

The same limitation can be attributed to EIS data obtained under sliding. The process cannot be presumed as stationary and the validation of the impedance data is also not evident. Steady-state conditions and linearity are basic requirements for the proper use and interpretation of EIS, a low amplitude alternating current (AC) polarization method. Stable potentials and currents are not registered during tribocorrosion. The technique consists of imposing a sinusoidal potential perturbation to the WE. In the present case, it means to add a low amplitude potential to an already perturbed interface. The result corresponds to the frequency response of metastable and mixed electrochemical interface. Even in the case of a good definition is the impedance plot, the interpretation is not simple. The result corresponds to the frequency response of metastable and mixed electrochemical interface. Another remarkable point is the fact that the tribocorrosion process is heterogeneous or localized. Data obtained from the global WE surface cannot directly express the intensity of the corrosion damage. Besides that, when the corrosion morphology is localized, the basic theory behind anodic dissolution processes cannot be directly used, such as uniform corrosion rates derived from Stern Geary equations. In the same way, weight loss measurements are not indicative of the phenomenon, despite the guidelines of ASTM G 119-09. Worn and unworn areas coupled in the same surface produces a non-stationary process. The degradation is localized and the interpretation of the electrochemical response of the material under tribocorrosion deserves close attention and complementary information is necessary. The total anodic current can be measured, but the concept of current density is ambiguous. For passive materials, an increment of averaged values and oscillation of current at fixed potential is observed. Another aspect to be revised is the inference of corrosion rate based on anodic and cathodic polarization tests of passive materials, based on the same Stern Geary equation. For passive material, an increment of amplitude and oscillation of current under fixed potential is observed. The current produced from the worn surface cannot be separate from the intact surface. In summary, the direct use of the Faraday law under tribocorrosion condition is theoretically incorrect, due to the passive condition and the mixed nature of the metal/solution interface.

The use of EIS without disregarding the basic assumptions behind impedance theory – steady-state and linearity – can drive to misinterpretation of the results. EIS and Polarization are powerful techniques to investigate and establish the electrochemical behavior and corrosion resistance of the static or unworn surface. However, the use of both techniques during sliding deserves more discussion, and the limitations for the correct interpretation of the data must be taken into account.

Considering that the oscillating potential is a consequence of interaction between worn and unworn regions, the oscillations express the transient nature of the competitive process between passivation and depassivation. Kinetics and thermodynamic information can be estimated from the potential and current registered during tribocorrosion. Examples of potential and current profiles obtained from tribocorrosion tests are shown in Figure 7.9. Some parameters are easy to determine and interpret, such as the OCP decay produced by sliding, average current during sliding, amplitude of current and potential oscillations during sliding and OCP recovery after the interruption of sliding, as shown in Figures 7.10 and 7.11.

OCP evolution of an unworn, static metal/solution interface is easy to measure. Simple instrumentation and parameters can be used to follow the build-up of passivation and the protective ability of the passive film formed. Data can be correlated with equilibrium thermodynamics information to confirm passive/active conditions on the same interface. Shift to higher values with time suggests the increment of the passivation quality in several systems. Current can be measured under controlled potential by the potentiostat or the spontaneous current flowing through the ZRA.

Among the electrochemical methods, electrochemical noise (EN) – emerges as the most appropriate to be used for tribocorrosion monitoring. Based on the acquisition of potential and current without the imposition of external polarization, can provide information about the kinetics of competitive processes of depassivation and passivation occurring at the interface. The use depends on the selection of adequate instrumentation, avoiding aliasing, and interference of spurious noise. Interpretation is possible from the processing of the signals in real time or after the experiments.

For the interpretation of EN, it is assumed that the signal fluctuations are spontaneously produced by the tribocorrosion phenomenon. Care must be taken to acquire the data, using the proper frequency of acquisition and spurious noise rejection. The instrumentation necessary to achieve collect consistent data must be designed to comply with the intensity and kinetics of the mechanically assisted electrochemical process. Several authors use the ZRA to get the data and post-processing methods to interpret the results based on the conversion to the frequency domain by Fast Fourier transform (FFT) or statistically based analysis, depending on the non-stationary nature of the electrochemical noise. ZRA measurements are, hence, the best tool and comply with the stochastic characteristic of tribocorrosion. Power spectral density can be a powerful representation of the current and potential signals in the frequency domain. The characteristic frequency of the depassivation and passivation process can be identified under some particular conditions. The accurate definition of

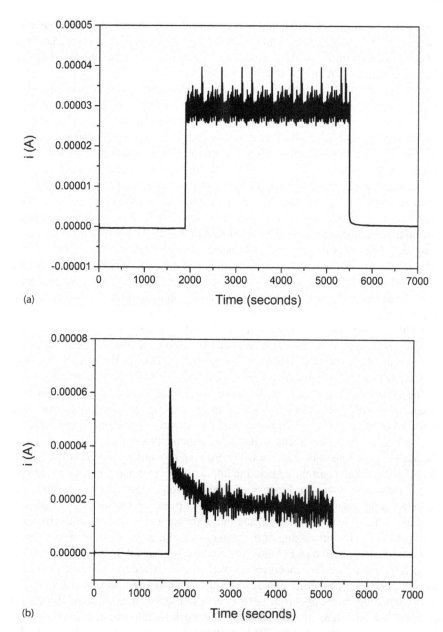

FIGURE 7.9 (a) Current measured during the experimental cycle of a tribocorrosion test. Oscillating current during sliding. Five higher amplitude spikes of current during sliding and zero slope of the averaged current. Data can be registered by one potentiostat or ZRA, depending on the setup used. Analysis can be made on time and frequency domain. (b) Current measured during the experimental cycle of a tribocorrosion test. High amplitude current registered right after the sliding start. Oscillating current during sliding. Data can be registered by one potentiostat or ZRA, depending on the setup used.

Electrochemical Techniques Applied to the Tribocorrosion Tests 199

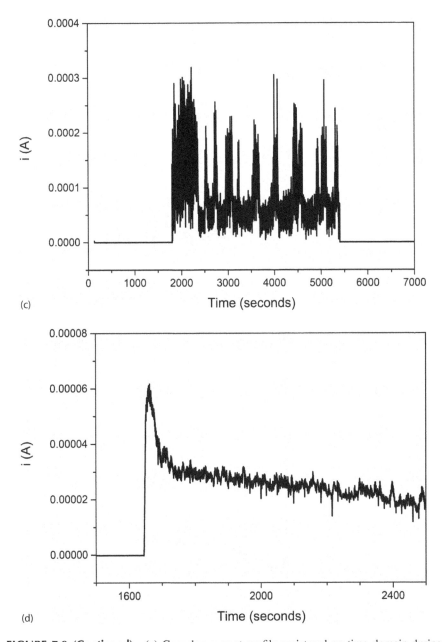

FIGURE 7.9 (Continued) (c) Complex current profile registered on time domain during tribocorrosion test. Variable signal envelopes and undefined average values during sliding, containing spikes. Statistical analysis in time domain recommended. Data can be registered by one potentiostat or ZRA, depending on the setup used. (d) Current signal registered on time domain during tribocorrosion test with a negative slope of the averaged signal after sliding, suggesting the attenuation of damage.

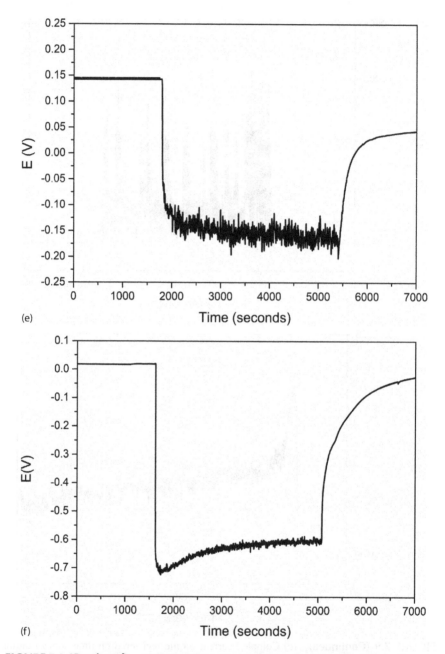

(e)

(f)

FIGURE 7.9 (Continued) (e) Potential signal registered on time domain during tribocorrosion with negative slope of the averaged signal during sliding, suggesting the increment of damage. (f) Potential signal registered on time domain during tribocorrosion with positive slope of the averaged signal during sliding, suggesting repassivation trend.

Electrochemical Techniques Applied to the Tribocorrosion Tests 201

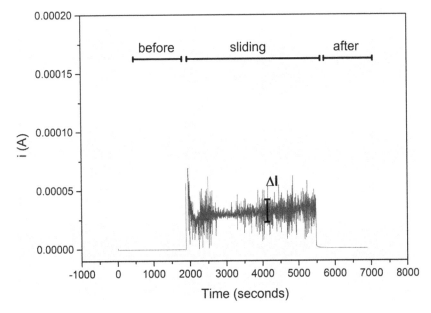

FIGURE 7.10 Characteristic current vs time profile registered during tribocorrosion tests. One parameter commonly used for analysis is the amplitude of oscillation, delta I (ΔI).

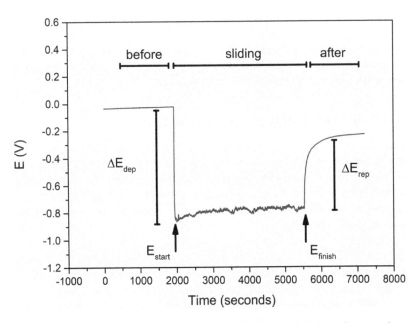

FIGURE 7.11 Characteristic potential vs time profile registered during tribocorrosion tests. Characteristics values are shown in the figure.

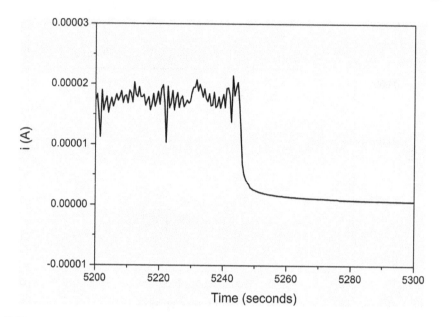

FIGURE 7.12 Current signal registered on time domain during tribocorrosion right after the interruption of sliding. Current relaxation can be used to assess the repassivation kinetics of the system, or time constant, depending on the accuracy of the data acquisition system used and characteristics of the tribometer.

transients, as indicated in Figure 7.12, can be used to assess the repassivation kinetics of the system, or time constant, depending on the accuracy of the data acquisition system used and the characteristics of the tribometer.

7.4 OTHER TECHNIQUES AND CONCEPTS

Surface analysis techniques have essential importance in tribocorrosion investigation. The volume of material removed and the morphology of the wear track are the major outputs of the tribocorrosion tests. The surface characterization will inform roughness, wear track profile and shape, counterbody profile after the test, and wear track topography. Other additional resources will inform the composition of the components of the surface. The techniques used for the analysis of the worn and unworn surfaces are:

- Chemical analysis by Raman spectroscopy – the Raman spectroscopy uses a light scattering to obtain the spectra of molecular vibrations, being widely used to characterize coatings and films, to discover inhomogeneity, local strain, lack of crystallinity, but with restrictions analysis to pure metals.
- X-ray excited photoelectron spectroscopy (XPS) – the XPS is a more sensitive technique widely used to characterize the chemical composition, the stoichiometry, of the sample surface, to analyze oxide films, identifying the elements or compounds present in the analyzed samples.

- X-ray diffraction (XRD) – the XRD is a technique to characterize the oxidized surface through a spectrum to obtain the crystallography parameters of samples, as phase, residual stress, structure, and lattice parameters, for example, if the material is amorphous or polycrystalline.
- Optical microscopy – the optical microscopy is a light microscopy that uses the principle of refraction and a system of lenses to obtain magnified images.
- Scanning electron microscopy (SEM) SEM utilizes a beam of focused electrons to scan the topography of solids objects. The emitted electrons interact with the atoms of the solid object resulting in an acquisition of signals from backscattered electrons (BSE) and secondary electrons (SE).
- Semi-quantitative chemical analysis by dispersive energy spectroscopy (EDX) – the dispersive energy spectroscopy (EDX) is a technique to detect chemical elements, where the X-ray emitted from a specimen is measured by an energy-dispersive spectrometer and the element composition is obtained based on each element presents an electromagnetic emission spectrum with a specific set of peak positions. The EDX is generally used in association with SEM, and allow constructing an element map distribution of the surface analyzed.
- Field emission scanning electron microscopic (FE-SEM) — FE-SEM is a microscopy similar to SEM, where the electrons emission is provided by a field emission cathode gun. Compared to SEM, FE-SEM can produce images with a higher resolution and less electrostatic distortion.
- Rugosimeter – the rugosimeter, or roughness tester, or roughness meter is a portable device able to obtain the surface texture information of the sample, where deviations from the nominal surfaces form a three-dimensional texture composed by the waviness height, peaks, valleys, and the waviness distances between peaks or valleys. The obtained texture can be described by the roughness parameters calculated from the obtained profiles.
- Contact and no-contact profilometer – the profilometer is an instrument that uses a light (no-contact) or a probe (contact) to obtain the texture information of sample, by scanning a single point, a line, or an area. The profilometer presents a better resolution than the rugosimeter, being able to perform a three-dimensional scan.
- Scanning atomic microscope (AFM) – the scanning atomic microscope (AFM) is a scanning probe microscopy where a probe in a cantilever uses the Van der Waals, capillary, electrostatic, or electromagnetic forces, to mapping the topography of a surface through the deflections of the cantilever. The technique allows obtaining the topography and texture of a surface.
- Light interferometer – the interferometer is a no-contact optical technique that uses a two-light beam and an interference pattern formed when these two beams are superposed. The photodetector integrates the different wavelengths and records the signal domain. The variation of the wave frequency of the record signal are used to reconstruct the three-dimensional structure's image.
- Laser confocal microscopy – the laser confocal microscopy is an optical scanning technique that uses a laser and a spatial pinhole to scan a X and Y axis of a focal plane for obtain images. It enables the reconstruction of three-dimensional structures from the conjugation of the focal plane images obtained at X and Y axis from different sections of the Z axis.

The physic characterization of the surface, before and after the test, mainly the wormed surfaces, can be made with photomicrographs obtained by using optical microscopy and SEM. In the wormed areas the obtained images enable identification of the wear track morphology, areas of plastic deformation, delamination, cracks, presence of adhesive particles or debris, localized dissolution, corrosion products, presence of adhesive third bodies, the incidence of micro-abrasion, and the boundaries of the wormed areas.

The detailed analysis of surface morphology on the contact area is important to support the understanding of possible predominant wear mechanism types, such as oxidative, adhesive, abrasive, or fatigue wear [24, 40].

Other surface parameters and material properties can be obtained from the worn and unworn surfaces, as roughness and hardness. The roughness parameters can be obtained by rugosimeter, profilometer, atomic force microscopy (AFM), light interferometer, and confocal microscopy. The profile roughness parameters are described in ISO 4287:1997 and the area roughness parameters in ISO 25178-2:2012, being the most applied the arithmetical roughness value (Ra – profile, Sa – area). The hardness can be obtained from microhardness tests. In the literature, it is possible to find hardness analysis comparing data obtained inside and outside the wear track to assess the work-hardening effect produced during sliding [44–49].

The light interferometer, profilometer and confocal microscopy laser techniques, in addition to the aforementioned resources, allow obtaining the wear track profile with respective parameters of width and depth, wear track length, and total wear volume loss. These data are essential to calculate the wear rate and the synergism interactions.

Although the standards list the surface analyzes techniques, there is no indication of mandatory methods or even standardization of the protocols to be followed. Therefore different sets of surface analyzes can be found for tribocorrosion assessments reports, some of them shown as literature examples in Table 7.3. The only recommendation is expressed in ASTM G 99-05, where the lower sensitivity resolution of 2.5 µm is preconized for the surface analysis selected.

Examples of bidimensional wear track profile obtained with confocal laser analysis are shown in Figures 7.13 and 7.14. The definition of the perpendicular profile of the wear track is the first step to measure the volume loss and complement the characterization of the wear track morphology. The technique is widely used after tribocorrosion tests of different materials under several conditions of corrosive solution composition, lubrication, and loading. The profiles in Figures 7.13 and 7.14 show an example of two dissimilar materials tested under the same tribocorrosion same conditions (Figure 7.13) and another example of the same material after tested under different load conditions (Figure 7.14).

The integration or convolution of similar profiles obtained at the different positions of the wear path will inform the total wear volume loss. In the case of obtaining the volume loss, the ASTM G 133-05 standard suggests the use of average track length, width, and depth of cross-section profiles to calculating the volume loss of linear reciprocating tribocorrosion tests. The profile analysis technique suggested by the standard is a profilometer. However, the document does not inform the minimum

TABLE 7.3
References of Some of Surface Analysis in the Literature

References	Counterbody	Material	Surface Analysis	Objective Output Parameters
Barros et al. (2020a) [15]	Alumina ball	Ti6Al4V NiCr	Confocal	Volume loss Wear track profile Wear track section 3D
Dalbert et al. (2010) [16]	Corundum pin	AISI 430 Graphite (ZRA)	Profilometer FE-SEM	Wear volume loss Wear track profile Wear track morphology
Corne et al. (2019) [37]	Zirconia Ti6Al4V	Ti gr. 4 Ti6Al4V gr.5	Optical profilometer SEM EDS FEG TEM/STEM	Volume loss Wear track profile Roughness Surface morphology Element map Cross-section wear area
Dalmau Borrás et al. (2019) [38]	Zirconia ball	Ti grade 4	Confocal FE-SEM FIB	Volume loss Wear morphology Wear track profile in perpendicular to the obtained by FE-SEM
Liamas et al. (2019) [49]	Alumina ball	Ti c.p.	SEM Nanoindenter Confocal AFM	Wear track morphology Hardness Volume total loss Wear track profile
Simsek and Ozyurek (2019) [39]	Stainless steel ball	Ti5Al2.5Fe Ti6Al4V	Microhardness indenter Density device XRD SEM EDS Analytical balance	Hardness Density Phase, lattice parameters Microstructure Element concentration Weight Loss (gravimetric)
Alves et al. (2018) [48]	Alumina ball	Ti	SEM EDS Profilometer Nanoindentation system	Surface morphology Chemical analysis Volume loss Wear track profile Hardness
Pejaković et al. (2018) [40]	Alumina ball	Ti6Al4V	Confocal SEM EDX	Volume loss Surface morphology Oxide in wear track
Bruschi et al. (2018) [33]	CoCrMo	Ti6Al4V	Optical profilometer with confocal objective	Roughness area Volume loss

(Continued)

TABLE 7.3 (*Continued*)

References	Counterbody	Material	Surface Analysis	Objective Output Parameters
Sivakumar et al. (2017) [19]	Alumina ball	Ti c.p.	XPS Profilometer SEM-EDX	Oxid film Roughness Wear surface morphology Wear track profile/ depth Wear debris Elements map
Zhao et al. (2016) [50]	Alumina ball	Ti SS316 CoCrMo	XRD Vickers identer SEM Confocal	Microstructure Hardness Coating Wear track morphology Volume loss Wear track profile
Alves et al. (2015) [41]	Alumina ball	Ti c.p.	XRD FE-SEM Confocal	Film characterization Wear track morphology Volume loss
Licausi et al. (2015) [42]	Alumina ball SiC pin	Ti6Al4V	Confocal SEM	Volume loss Wear track topography
Souza et al. (2015) [23]	Alumina ball	Ti6Al4V	Optical microscopy SEM Analytical balance	Wear track topography Weight Loss (gravimetric)
Wimmer et al. (2015) [24]	Alumina ball	CoCrMo	Light interferometer SEM EDS Confocal Raman	Surface topography Volume loss Surface morphology Surface layer Tribofilm
Butt et al. (2015) [51]	Alumina ball	Ti6Al4V disk	Light interferometry SEM	Wear track profile (depth, width, length) Volume loss Surface morphology
Holmes et al. (2014) [11]	UHMVPE	316L	SEM	Wear track morphology
Puppulin et al. (2014) [32]	zirconia	alumina	Raman confocal with a CCD camera FEG-SEM	Bands of zirconia and alumina Surface morphology
Espallargas et al. (2013) [30]	SiC	Super duplex UNS S32750	Confocal SEM	Volume loss Wear track profile (width, length) Wear track topography

(*Continued*)

TABLE 7.3 (*Continued*)

References	Counterbody	Material	Surface Analysis	Objective Output Parameters
Dimah et al. (2012) [44]	Alumina ball	Ti c.p. Ti6Al4V	Vickers indenter Optical microscopy Confocal SEM	Hardness Metallography Wear track morphology Volume loss Wear track profiles Wear track morphology
Mathew et al. (2012) [25]	Ceramic ball	Ti c.p.	SEM Light Interferometry	Wear track morphology Wear track morphology
Mathew et al. (2011) [5]	Ceramic ball	CoCrMo pin	Profilometer ICP-MS	Weight loss Weight loss (ions released)
Kumar et al. (2010) [26]	Alumina ball	Ti c.p. (gr. 2)	SEM EDX	Surface morphology Chemical analysis
Tekin and Malayoglu (2010) [45]	Silicon nitride ball	Hastelloy G35 Hastelloy C2000 Haynes 625	XRD EDX SEM Profilometer Microhardness indenter ICP-OES	Chemical Composition Oxygen content wear track Wear track morphology Volume loss Wear track profiles Hardness Ions Released
Yan et al. (2009) [36]	CoCrMo	CoCrMo	Contact profilometer	ICP-AES
Yan et al. (2008) [27]	CoCrMo	CoCrMo	Light Interferometer Optical microscopy ICP-AES	Volume loss Surface morphology Ions released
Vieira et al. (2006) [28]	Corundum balls	Ti c.p. (gr.2)	Laser profilometer SEM	Volume loss Wear track morphology

number of measures or their position to be considered. The absence of a protocol guiding to detail the methodology to perform the measurements and integrate the data leads to finding several forms used to obtain the profiles and estimate the volumes. Averages obtained from three to five random or equidistant measures, single measures, and even measures of one single profile section are used to estimate the total wear volume.

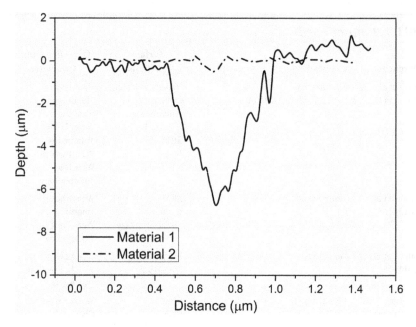

FIGURE 7.13 Bidimensional wear track profile of two dissimilar materials evaluated under same tribocorrosion conditions and environment.

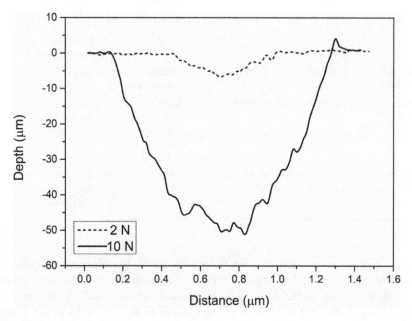

FIGURE 7.14 Bidimensional wear track profile of a materials evaluated under different load conditions in same environment.

Among the studies reported, some examples can be mentioned, illustrating this variety. Examples related to the lack of information about the position of the cross-section profile measured are in the study made by Liamas et al. [49] using a confocal laser, and Butt et al. [51], using light interferometry. In both studies, it was not cited if it was a single or an average of measures, and the latter converted the width and length in volume loss considering an ellipse area.

Another example is the option for equidistant measures. The study of Zhao et al. [50] using a confocal obtained profile measures in three points along the stroke length, at one-fourth, one-half, and three-quarter positions. The average area of them, a bidimensional integration, was multiplied by the stroke length to obtain the volume loss. Another example of using a defined position is on the study provided by Sivakumar et al. [19], considering a selected region in the middle of the wear track, assumed to be the deepest point, used to calculate the volume loss by polynomial order fit, although the measure did not represent the total volume loss of the entire track.

In the group of studies using an average of three to five random measures, Dimah et al. [44] use confocal microscopy to quantify the volume loss based on the average of three profiles, while Dalmau Borrás et al. [38] use the same method based on the average of five measurements. Alves et al. [41] used a 2D profilometer to obtain the wear track profile, being the average of three measures of width and depth used to calculate the volume loss by multiplying by the wear track length. Corne et al. [37] used a profilometer to measure five lengths of 1.1 mm and extrapolated them to estimate the volume loss. Some of the studies carried out repetitions of these three to five cross-section profile data. Espallargas et al. [30] and Licausi et al. [42] quantified the volume loss by the average of three width and depth profiles cross-section of the wear track, measured twice times each one, multiplied by the length of the wear track, being the values obtained by confocal technique.

Since not all assessments are in linear sliding and for some assessments where the gravimetric weight loss is not possible, mainly because the volume is too small, other techniques to obtain the volume loss are found in the literature. One of the techniques is the use of the Archad's law equation, as cited by Holmes et al. [11], where the volume loss was obtained by multiplying the COF, the load applied, and the length of sliding and then divided by hardness. Other techniques use integral or polynomials calculations from 3D reconstructions of the wear track, obtained mainly with a profilometer, interferometer, or confocal microscope. Examples of volume loss calculated from 3D reconstructions obtained through a confocal microscope can be found in the works of Pejaković et al. [40], and Barros et al. [15]. The former obtained the volume loss by 3D wear track measured using the flat surface as a reference. For the latter, the volume loss was obtained by polynomial integration of profile below the flat surface, using computational resources provided by the software of the confocal microscope, as shown in Figures 7.15 and 7.16, performed by Barros et al. [15].

During the tribocorrosion tests, two bodies are put in contact, the test specimen and the counterbody. Consequently, both can be subjected to wear degradation. Therefore, the wear produced on the components can be calculated according to ASTM G 99-05, ASTM G 133-05. In the case of the ball, wear loss corresponding to

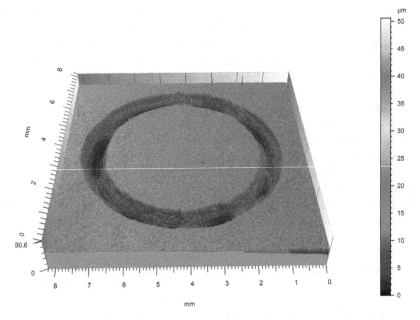

FIGURE 7.15 Three-dimensional reconstruction of wear track obtained by confocal microscope.

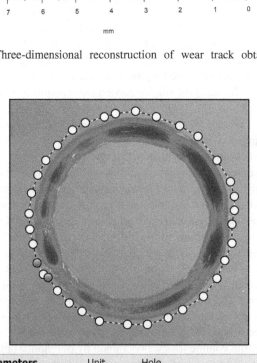

Parameters	Unit	Hole
Surface	mm²	18.9
Volume	µm³	123454184
Max. depth/height	µm	24.9
Mean depth/height	µm	6.55

FIGURE 7.16 Polynomial integration of profile below the flat surface provided by the software of the confocal microscope to obtain the volume loss.

only a few abrasions marks are considered as not measurable. Wear resulting in a flat region in the ball is considered relevant and ASTM G 133-05 recommends the use of the average value of maximum and minimum diameters as the effective diameter of the ball. For a ball with a not entirely flat surface at the contact wear area, the volume loss can be obtained by other techniques as informed in the ASTM G 99-05 and ASTM G 133-05. Although, the standards did not inform the possible techniques, only describes the use of photomicrographs and surfaces analysis.

For the test specimen, the volume loss could be determined by gravimetric measurements by the difference of weight before and after the tests and converted in volume, or by the metrological techniques when the weight loss is too small. An example of the possible techniques, for a weight loss too small, is the use of the profilometer.

Beyond the total volume loss, methods for the calculation of the contribution of each component comprising the phenomenon of tribocorrosion – mechanical, electrochemical, and synergist – are addressed on the standards. The mechanical wear, the electrochemical dissolution, and the interaction due to the synergism can be quantified as preconized by ASTM G 119-09, according to the equation:

$$T = W_0 + C_0 + S \quad (7.1)$$

where: T is the total mass loss of the specimen (flat or disk), W_0 is the material loss by wear, without corrosion contribution, C_0 is the material loss by corrosion, without wear contribution, and S is the synergistic component. S is assumed to be the sum of the wear contribution to corrosion (ΔWc) and the corrosion contribution to wear (ΔCw). This is represented in the following equations:

$$S = \Delta W_C + \Delta C_W \quad (7.2)$$

$$\Delta W_C = W_T - W_0 \quad (7.3)$$

$$\Delta C_W = C_T - C_0 \quad (7.4)$$

where W_t is the total component of wear, comprehending the sum of the component of wear and the wear contribution in corrosion, and C_T is s the total component of corrosion, comprehending the sum of the component of corrosion and the corrosion contribution in wear.

The determination of each component, the standard ASTM G 119-09 recommend the following guide of experimental procedures:

1. Wear test at the OCP condition to obtain the total material loss (T).
2. Corrosion test with wear. Linear polarization resistance and potentiodynamic polarization curves to obtain the polarization resistance (Rp) and Tafel constants, (βa, βc), used to calculate the corrosion current density (i_{corr}) based on the Faraday's law, that be converted in penetrating rate, which is equal to the total component of corrosion (C_T).

3. Similar wear test under cathodic polarization at one-volt cathodic, where the corrosion component is zero, to obtain the material loss only by wear (W_0).
4. Another similar corrosion test, as described in 2, but without wear, being the penetration rate equivalent to the component of the material loss only by corrosion (C_0).

Some indications of ASTM G 119-09 standards deserve more detailed discussion and analysis. The use of data obtained from gravimetric tests can be a drawback. Weight loss measurements are extensively used for materials under active dissolution and uniform corrosion. Materials under tribocorrosion investigation are in general passive alloys, e.g., biomaterials. The method depends on using an analytical balance and ASTM G 99-05 recommends an analytical balance with a sensitivity of 0.1 mg. For the assessment of weight loss of passive alloys, it is possible that the total loss achieved would be lower than the minimum accuracy of the balance. Another drawback is the wear-corrosion morphology, which is localized. One basic assumption made for the estimation of the corrosion rate using gravimetric methods is that the corrosion process is uniform. Even in the case of using a more sensitive balance – e.g., a microbalance which is 100 times more sensitive – and more aggressive wear and corrosion conditions, the weakness of the method related to the localized damage morphology remains. The best option becomes the determination of the volume loss by the surface as already described and considered in ASTM G 133-05.

Another point related to the guideline for experiments of the ASTM G 119-09 standard that deserves discussion is the use of cathodic protection. Cathodic polarization can suppress the anodic dissolution and set to zero the contribution of the corrosion component. However, the reason for using the applied one-volt cathodic potential is not clear. Under cathodic conditions, two relevant possibilities must be considered. The first is the hydrogen reduction on the WE surface. Detrimental effects on the mechanical behavior of several materials are well known and reported. Another point is the possible deterioration of the environment of the test by the potential imposed. Both aspects should consider the thermodynamic stability analysis of the solution, especially when complex environments containing organic molecules are used. For choosing an adequate cathodic potential value to be applied, the first point to be considered is the analysis of the Pourbaix diagram of the material. The second point is related to solution stability, which may be determined through the experimental oxyreduction curves obtained through the potentiodynamic polarization of an inert platinum electrode as the WE. The range between the higher anodic potential limit, where the oxidation of the solution occurs, and the lower cathodic potential limit, where the reduction of the solution occurs, is the stability domain of the solution.

Considering the two aspects mentioned, the most adequate cathodic potential to be applied will be a potential on the immunity domain of the material and above the hydrogen reduction potential using the Pourbaix diagram as reference. This potential must be within the electrochemical stability domain of the corrosive solution used, defined by the redox curve.

The use of one-volt cathodic for all materials and in all solutions, as a way of making the corrosion component almost zero, obtaining pure wear component, should be then revised. An alternative, not described in the standard, to obtain the wear component with corrosion almost zero would be to perform the tribocorrosion test in distilled water at OCP. However, it is important to have in mind that the physicochemical properties of the test solution could differ from those of distilled water, such as viscosity, which could affect lubrication conditions and consequently the wear mechanism. Therefore, the most appropriate would be to find a suitable potential to be applied for a condition where corrosion would be almost zero based on the thermodynamic of the material and the stability of the solution. An example of this thermodynamic analysis for titanium is presented in Figures 7.17 and 7.18.

The Pourbaix or E × pH diagrams are the representation of an electrochemical system established for pure metallic materials in aqueous environments. The thermodynamic stability and equilibrium conditions for metal and ions are represented as functions of the electrochemical potential and pH. The diagrams are based on Nernst equations, resulting in the thermodynamics analysis showing the pH-potential domains corresponding to corrosion, protection, and immunity of the metal [52–55].

In the primary study, the authors evaluated the OCP of Ti6Al4V in different combinations of fluoride concentration and pH. The electrolytes were the NaCl 0.9% with the combined concentrations of fluoride and pH of 227 ppm F⁻ pH 5.5, 227 ppm F⁻ pH 4.0, 2270 ppm F⁻ pH 5.5, 2270 ppm F⁻ pH 4.0, 12,300 ppm F⁻ pH 5.5 and 12,300 ppm F⁻ pH 4.0. The coordinates of pH and free corrosion potential for each combined medium obtained from these evaluations were inserted in an adapted E × pH diagram of the Ti–H$_2$O system, as seen in the adapted plotted diagram reproduced in Figure 7.17.

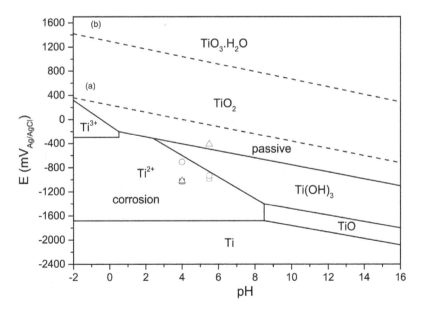

FIGURE 7.17 Adapted plotted E x pH diagram of Ti-H$_2$O system with the coordinate of free corrosion potential of titanium in each coordinates of pH combined with fluoride content.

Analyzing the results, it can be observed that only for the solution combination of 227 ppm F⁻ pH 5.5, the titanium alloys remained in the passive domain, being the others in the corrosion domain. Based on this, if a tribocorrosion assessment is carried out for the titanium alloy in this solution following the procedures preconized in the ASTM G 119-09 standard, the procedure of applying one-volt cathodic will take the alloy to the corrosion domain instead of the objective of almost zero corrosion disposal on the standard procedure. Even for a non-passive condition of alloy, since the standard is not well recommended for passive. For example, in a solution with combined 2270 ppm F⁻ pH 5.5, when applying one-volt cathodic the alloy will not achieve the immunity domain retained in the corrosion domain, being not in coherence with the stipulated by the standard. Furthermore, the corrosion products could influence from lubrication, and therefore friction coefficient, to wear mechanisms, such as the performance of these corrosion products as the third body.

The oxyreduction curves (redox curves) is an evaluation with great importance not commonly considered. Although the Pourbaix diagram presents the represent lines of oxidation and reduction of water, demonstrating the stability domain, it does not represent the stability domain of electrolyte selected for the evaluation. The stability domain obtained through the oxyreduction curve of the electrolyte in addition to the Pourbaix diagram is an advisable way to initially characterize the combination of electrolyte and material to be evaluated in tribocorrosion assessments. The oxyreduction curves can be obtained through a potentiodynamic polarization in a three-cell, with a RE, a platinum CE, and an inert platinum work electrode in the selected electrolyte and pH. The potentiodynamic polarization must be performed from cathodic potentials to anodic potentials, to cover the entire domain of solution stability. In the obtained potential–current densities, the range between the higher limit anodic potential from which there is an oxidation of the solution and the lower limit cathodic potential from which there is a reduction of the solution comprises the stability domain of the solution. As a practical example, the oxyreduction curves (redox curves) of the solutions selected for the evaluations cited in the previous example are reproduced in Figure 7.18, and the parameter of domain stability is obtained from the curves in Table 7.4. The combination of fluoride concentration and pH affected the redox potential and the solution stability domain. The lower pH reduced the range of stability domain of the solutions with a higher cathodic limit. The lower pH also increased the redox potential of the solution.

Returning to the selection mentioned above of Ti6Al4V in solution with 227 ppm F⁻ pH 5.5, in addition to the already discussed polarization of one-volt cathodic lead the material to the corrosion domain region (Figure 7.18), the solution would be in a process of reduction, since the lower stability limit was −743 mV (Table 7.4). The solution reduction would increase the amount of hydrogen, for the alloy in the corrosion domain, and it could facilitate the process of hydrogen embrittlement. The risk of hydrogen embrittlement for passive alloys in cathodic polarizations recommended by ASTM G 119-09 was already highlighted in the literature [54].

Another drawback of the standards is the indication of polarization tests to obtain Tafel constants and calculate the corrosion rate. Tafel law is applicable for uniform corrosion, thus, it is not directly applicable for passive alloys or for alloys susceptible to localized corrosion.

Electrochemical Techniques Applied to the Tribocorrosion Tests

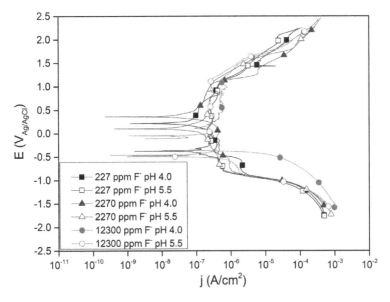

FIGURE 7.18 Oxyreduction curves (redox curves) of NaCl solutions with different combined concentrations of fluoride and pH to determine the domain stability of each solution.

TABLE 7.4
Parameters of Stability Domain Obtained from the Redox Curves

NaCl 0.9% + [x] F⁻ ppm	pH	Redox Potential ($V_{Ag/AgCl}$)	Domain Stability ($V_{Ag/AgCl}$)
227	4.0	0.215	1.04 to −0.390
	5.5	−0.376	1.01 to −0.743
2270	4.0	0.364	1.07 to −0.556
	5.5	0.099	1.06 to −0.714
12,300	4.0	−0.381	1.11 to −0.383
	5.5	−0.473	1.13 to −0.544

Some works in literature recommend an alternative protocol to identify the contribution of the active and repassivate areas of the wear track in the degradation, with equations to calculate each contribution [3, 54]. According to the authors, this new protocol would be more suitable for passive alloys than the standard ASTM G 119-09. This new protocol was a basis for a new standard, UNE 112086: 2016 [56]. The new protocol includes the electrochemical assessments of evolution of OCP during sliding instead of the cathodic polarization preconized in ASTM G 119-09, the galvanic corrosion between the passive and active areas, and the assessment of electrochemical impedance spectroscopy (EIS) to obtain the polarization resistance (Rp) instead of the corrosion rates. The choice movement type in this new protocol is the unidirectional sliding ball-on-disk or pin-on-disk.

7.5 TRIBOCORROSION RESULTS

Some recent results of tribocorrosion tests are summarized on this topic. Silva et al. [57], tested an austenitic ferritic stainless steel, using a pin and ball tribometer, and equipped with DC polarization, EIS- and ZRA-based methods, under load and non-load conditions. The CE was a large platinum grid. The authors pointed out one drawback of the ZRA technique since the entire current produced between worn and unworn areas was not registered by the instrument. A significant part of the current flows directly on WE. The increment of the anodic current under potentiostatic control of the loaded surface is clear, followed by the corresponding OCP decay. One correlation between the COF and the anodic potential was also identified. Lissajous figures were used to express in real time the correlation between potential and current during sliding at different contact forces. In summary, the link between the contact force and the electrochemical response was clearly demonstrated. Abolusoro and Akinlabi [14] tested aluminum alloys using in situ measurements and ZRA. The interpretation is based on the analysis transient of current signals. Faraday's law is used to convert current to volume loss due to corrosion.

Berradja et al. [4] present the results of an extensive investigation of tribocorrosion of an AISI 304 steel in the presence of Ringer solution. Unidirectional continuous and intermittent sliding methods of the test were used. Three-electrode cell and low noise potentiostat were used. The focus was on the effect of contact pressure and rotating speed. Potential and current fluctuations, electrochemical potential noise (EPN) and electrochemical current noise (ECN), respectively, were recorded and pos processed. The signals were digitalized using anti-aliasing protection and the assistance of a low pass filter. EPN and ECN were analyzed on the frequency domain, via power spectral density (PSD), calculated within 10 and 100 Hz, averaged 10 times.

The OCP decay commonly registered right after the sliding start and its recovery, when wear was interrupted, was informed. Time records of potential and current during continuous sliding were used. An attempt to identify elementary transients associated with depassivation and repassivation events was made. Correlation between the PSD of the electrochemical signals – produced by ECN and EPN – and PSD of mechanical parameters were observed.

Dalbert et al. [16] studied the galvanic coupling of ferritic stainless steels and graphite in sulfate solutions. Previous cathodic polarization of the WE technique was used to produce a uniform passive film on the surface. Anodic and cathodic polarization were used and OCP and current were registered during the tribocorrosion test. The analysis of elementary transients was carried out, but the detailed instrumentation used was not described in detail. Consequently, the accuracy of global and high-frequency data was not evident. The concept of galvanic coupling is not clear, since the coupling was between graphite and ferritic stainless steel.

Silva et al. [20], using the same standard electrochemical setup containing three electrodes and potentiostat, studied the previously modified Ti alloy surface by the incidence of the laser beam. Conventional methods, OCP, polarization, and impedance from 10 KHz to 10 MHz were used. Potential decay and oscillation after the onset of sliding was registered. Polarization curves exhibited the same OCP shift to lower potentials and oscillations of the anodic current under polarization. Current densities and OCP were influenced by wear, but the major difference was on OCP obtained at different surface conditions. The OCP of the laser-treated alloy was lower and less influenced by wear. Polarization resistance, defined as the limit of the electrochemical impedance at quasi zero frequency, is two orders of magnitude lower during wear than the same parameter obtained from the unworn surface. The passivation ability after wear of the laser modified alloy was higher, based on this parameter. Sun et al. [58] report another example of attenuation of the current under sliding promoted by protein adsorption on the surface of CoCrMo alloy used in hip joints.

Kappel et al. [21] observe that potential and current registered during tribocorrosion are commonly transient, due to complex overlapped processes of stochastic nature. Analytical interpretation based on averaged parameters, such as anodic current density, polarization resistance, OCP, and PSD is based on assumed quasi-stationary conditions. However, the complex nature of the electrochemical processes occurring at the metallic surface under wear can be obscured by the signal processing technique used. Current and potential spikes can be observed, without the possibility of identification of a deterministic law. These events are related to the more intense events of passive film rupture and repassivation. Non-stationary conditions can be approached by statistics analyses of the electrochemical parameters represented in the time domain. ZRA is used attached to identical titanium electrodes. Polynomial fit to remove the DC component of the signals.

Pejaković et al. [40] considered a slightly more aggressive corrosion condition, Ti6Al4V in artificial seawater, using constant potential, OCP, cathodic, and anodic polarization. Classic configuration using a three electrodes setup was used. The potentiostatic control under cathodic polarization permitted the elimination of the influence of anodic reactions by suppressing the dissolution. The apparatus used was the reciprocating sliding test system. The influence of the contact pressure on depassivation was informed. It was observed that low contact pressures were not able to promote depassivation and the material remained intact. At higher contact forces, the anodic current during sliding was unstable, exhibiting spikes achieving the magnitude of 10^{-5}A.

Dalmau Borrás et al. [38] tested titanium in artificial saliva, a less aggressive condition. Potentiostatic control during sliding was used, at low and high passive conditions, depending on the anodic potential. Cathodic removal of air-formed passive films were used, by application of -1.5 V. Different patterns of OCP versus time during sliding were observed. The positive slope of potential during sliding was attributed to the predominance of progressive repassivation during sliding. Alves et al. [41] investigated the influence of surface treatment of Ti on the improvement of wear resistance. Only OCP and COF were used. Corne et al. [37] used OCP and EIS during sliding using ordinary instrumentation. These authors bring another report of OCP increase during fretting in human saliva. Passivation recovery during fretting was considered as the advantage of modified surfaces of titanium alloys.

Dimah et al. [44] used a standard three-electrode cell, polarization, and the parameters extracted from the curves. The corrosion rate was calculated from Tafel and Faraday laws. Fully passive titanium alloys were observed without an indication of localized corrosion susceptibility. Phosphate buffer saline (PBS) was the environment used, but the preliminary assessment of its electrochemical stability was not carried out. A significant increase of the anodic current density measured during sliding at a constant anodic overpotential was registered, expressed in average numbers. Espallargas et al. [30] present an example of negative slope of OCP during sliding due to the decreasing repassivation ability induced by the cumulative wear/corrosion damage. Increasing average current during sliding was registered, coherent with the potential evolution. The use of ZRA and one CE of the same material, stainless steel, was adopted. It was demonstrated that the coating could mitigate the tribocorrosion degradation, as demonstrated by the opposite variations of OCP and current measured by the ZRA.

Ferreira et al. [8] present an attempt to separate mechanical and electrochemical contributions to tribocorrosion of Ti in Ringer solution. Highly oscillating anodic currents were achieved during wear. Very low cathodic currents were recorded on the same test carried out at cathodic potentials, which means a negligible contribution of hydrogen reduction within the thermodynamic immunity domain of Ti. However, it was unclear if there was a link between anodic current densities and the corrosion rate. Very high current amplitudes were achieved under anodic polarization, as commonly reported by titanium.

Geringer et al. [59] investigated the fretting corrosion process of one stainless steel/polymer contact interface, such as used on hip joints. Cyclic fretting at 1 Hz frequency in Ringer solution was the basic condition. Dissipated energy and anodic current density were the parameters of reference. It was concluded that both polymer and metal undergo mass loss, being higher for the 316 stainless steel tested.

Holmes et al. [11] used a micro-abrasion apparatus to test stainless steel in artificial saliva, using anodic and cathodic polarization curves, with and without abrasion. Electrochemical standard three-electrode cell instrumentation was the commonly used.

Jemmely et al. [60] report tribocorrosion results of ferritic stainless steel in sulfuric acid, using a reciprocating movement system. The same attempt to identify and separate the elementary steps of the mechanically assisted degradation was made. The setup used to acquire the electrochemical data was conventional, with constant anodic potential applied within the passive range. A numerical simulation of the transient currents was made. Experimental and simulated data were compared. Ohmic effects were taken into account for modeling, but not the impedance of the interface.

Fretting corrosion of Ti c.p. in Ringer solution was investigated by Kumar et al. [26] using a conventional setup. The build-up of passivation was observed by OCP vs. time measurements, followed by the abrupt decay of these parameters when fretting starts. Continuous decay of the average value during fretting and oscillations were registered, probably indicative of cumulative tribocorrosion damage. Passive condition is recovered right after the interruption of fretting. Oscillating current during wear was observed, with spikes at the beginning. Analysis of both parameters was carried out in the time domain. Results of surface analyses were not presented, however, and the electrochemical results could not be compared with volume loss, for instance.

Landolt et al. [6] addressed the tribocorrosion of ferritic stainless steels in 0.5 M sulfuric acid. Inert or active counter bodies were used. Galvanic interactions are out of the question for inert counter bodies. Current spikes were registered and the wear volume was lower at higher applied potentials.

Titanium in PBS-containing bovine serum albumin was the environment selected by Liamas et al. [49]. A pin-on-disk rotating system and conventional three-electrode electrochemical setup and potentiostat was used. OCP, anodic, and cathodic potentials were the techniques used. It was observed that the mechanical wear was higher at anodic potentials. This effect was explained by the influence of third bodies. AFM was used to support the surface analysis after the tribocorrosion tests. The effect of bovine serum albumin (BSA) was pointed out, increasing the passivation rate and the mechanical wear by the adhesion of debris into the wear track. The same pattern for OCP and current under sliding was reported, however, attenuated by the presence of BSA. However, volume loss was not measured by the authors.

Licausi et al. [61], using the traditional three electrodes cell configuration and potentiostat, studied the tribocorrosion of Ti6Al4V in fluoride environments. Potentiostatic polarization and parameters extracted from the curves were used to assess the corrosion resistance. Cast and sintered samples were used. Tafel and anodic current density on the passive range were calculated. The detrimental effect of fluoride concentration and pH were identified. Coulometric charge, Q, was also considered in the analysis. The performance of sintered alloy was considered as promising.

Licausi et al. [42] tested on a ball and flat reciprocating tribometer Ti6Al4V in artificial saliva using ZRA. The WE and the CE were made of Ti6Al4V. A conventional RE was used to follow the potential of the pair. Polarization curves were used. The main conclusion was the significant increment of anodic current and higher potential decay when the contact pressure excels the yield strength of the alloy. In conclusion, the governing factor of tribocorrosion was the contact pressure.

Mathew et al. [25] investigated the tribocorrosion of Ti c.p. in artificial saliva using a ball and flat apparatus. The effect of pH was the focus. EIS was used. The capacitance of the double layer or the passive film was calculated. It was concluded that, even at lower pH, 3.0, Ti c.p. remains passive. The anodic current density measured within the passive range was about 10^{-5} A/cm^2. Parameters derived from polarization and EIS are used to express the corrosion resistance. Tribocorrosion was more intense in pH 6.0. This conclusion was based on the magnitude of the anodic current achieved during sliding. An increment of the polarization resistance after sliding in more acid conditions – pH 3.0 – was observed. This result suggests that a more protective passive film is formed by the repassivation of the interface. The capacitance was also higher after sliding in pH 3.0. Both parameters before and after sliding were not influenced by pH 6.0 and 9.0. Remarkable was the lower polarization resistance measured in the more alkaline condition, pH 9.0.

Radice et al. [31] present experimental results using a biotribometer. CoCrMo alloy was tested in a CO_2 environment under controlled electrochemical potential. The possibility of controlling the formation of corrosion products and debris was assumed and the impact of these products on cells was assessed. The charge density,

Q, obtained from the integration of the anodic current measured, was used to quantify the mass loss related to corrosion in mg. Cell culture environments were used as the electrolyte. Fully faradaic process assumed.

Simsek and Ozyurek [39] report the higher tribocorrosion resistance of modified Ti alloy. Ti6Al4V was compared to Ti5Al2.5Fe. A pin-on-disk system was used to test sintered alloys. Polarization was used to assess the corrosion resistance. Icorr values in order of magnitude of mA/cm^2 are informed. This value was lower for the modified alloy. Pitting corrosion was identified as the corrosion morphology.

Mathew et al. [25] were able to make a clear demonstration of the benefits of the presence of bioabsorbable polymer through the reduction of the anodic current and COF during sliding of Ti c.p. A similar methodology for electrochemical measurements was used, three electrodes cell and potentiostat.

Vieira et al. [28] tested titanium grade 2 under fretting corrosion in artificial saliva. Citric acid and two inhibitors were added, but only the cathodic inhibitor had a significant effect on fretting corrosion. Conventional electrochemical setup was used. Repassivation trend during fretting was suggested by the positive shift of the potential. Anodic current confirms this passivation recovery trend, exhibiting a shift to lower values reaching almost zero during fretting.

Work presented by Wimmer et al. [24] report the behavior of CoCrMo alloy in bovine serum, pH 7.6. Alumina ball in contact with the WE and three electrodes configuration was the apparatus used. EIS and Rp were used to express the corrosion resistance. Polarization resistance was higher after wear, especially at higher contact forces. This result is explained by the formation of a tribofilm, containing the components of the environment. Total mass loss was estimated by interferometry and corrosion contribution was estimated by Faraday law. The parameter used on faradaic assumption was the total charge, Q.

Zhao et al. [50] demonstrated that diamond-like carbon is used to mitigate tribocorrosion. A reciprocating ball and plate tribometer was used and PBS, pH 7.4, selected as the environment at room temperature. Diamond-like carbon (DLC) coating was deposited by physical vapor deposition (PVD) on Ti, CoCr, and stainless-steel surfaces. Polarization was used before the tribocorrosion tests. OCP during sliding was registered. SEM after the tests. It was concluded that DLC was able to reduce the wear loss.

Yan et al. [34] investigated metal-on-metal biotribocorrosion – MoM – emulating one hip prostheses. Co and Cr release are a major concern. Debris and ions can be produced at the metal/metal interface. The phenomenon is defined as biotribocorrosion. Open circuit potential and polarization experiments in serum were used. A potential drop at the start of wear, followed by a positive shift during sliding was registered. The positive effect of organic molecules was concluded, based on both electrochemical parameters. Attenuation of anodic current spikes with time, coherent with the potential evolution.

7.6 METHODOLOGY PROPOSAL

Based on the content of the previous topics, it can be concluded that the experimental assessment of the tribocorrosion resistance of one specific material/environment system must be carried out by an integrated methodology, where the tribocorrosion

TABLE 7.5
Flowsheet Proposal with Experimental and Sequential Steps Supported by the Continuous Analysis of the Output Data

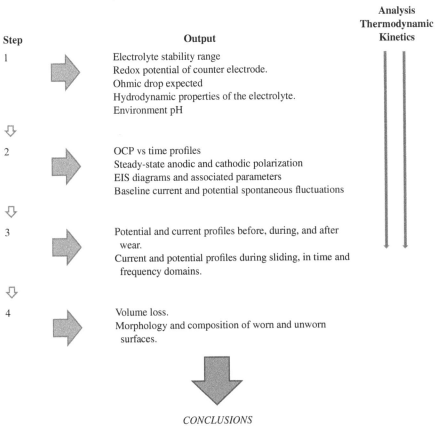

test is assisted by complementary but essential steps. The following proposal contains four experimental and sequential steps supported by the continuous analysis of the output data. Please refer to the flowsheet in Table 7.5.

One assumption made is the use of a linearly reciprocating ball-on–flat or rotational pin-on-disk considering the use of an inert material as counterbody, to avoid galvanic interaction between this component and the flat specimen. Consequently, the electrochemical measurements carried out corresponds to the global surface of the WE. Another assumption made is the use of similar materials as WE1 and WE2 for ZRA measurements. The area ratio is 1, which means twin flat samples of the same geometry and dimensions connected to the ZRA (Figures 7.19 and 7.20).

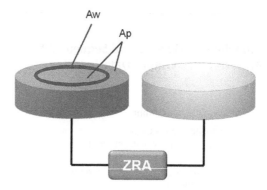

FIGURE 7.19 WE and CE electrodes connected by ZRA, being the CE made of platinum.

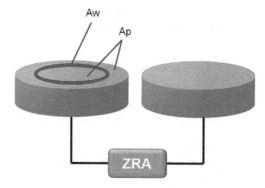

FIGURE 7.20 WE and CE electrodes connected by ZRA, being the CE made of the same material of WE.

7.6.1 Step 1 – Physicochemical Characterization of the Environment/Solution

Consistent knowledge about the right environment to be used in tribocorrosion tests is essential. As already pointed out, electrolytes can be electrochemically unstable beyond critical anodic and cathodic potentials. The stability range of the solutions can be assessed by redox curves using potentiostat and three electrodes cell. The results support the correct interpretation of anodic and cathodic polarization of the material under investigation carried out to assess its corrosion resistance. Increment of anodic currents, for instance, can be related to the oxidation of the electrolyte and not to corrosion. Titanium in chloride solutions with different fluoride contents is one example of a false indication of localized corrosion at very high anodic overpotentials. Redox curves are shown in Figure 7.18. The methodology is the same used to perform polarization curves, except for the use of flat platinum as the WE. The electrochemical stability of PBS environments, for instance, is not commonly informed in the literature. Volume loss would enhance the interpretation.

Another set of preliminary data, necessary to support the experimental assessment of tribocorrosion test results, is composed of the physicochemical characteristics of the same environment. Electrochemical conductivity, pH, and viscosity are basic parameters. The electrochemical conductivity, for instance, will affect all the electrochemical measurements done. Low conductivity implies a significant ohmic drop and errors in terms of the applied potential under polarization. The correct interpretation of galvanic interactions depends on the precise knowledge of the conductivity. Viscosity will have a strong influence on the COF and the corrosion mechanisms. The pH will be essential for the continuous thermodynamic analyses of the corrosion process.

The output of Step 1 will provide answers to the following points:

- The potential range where anodic and cathodic polarization methods can be applied without the interference of the electrolyte decomposition.
- Redox potential of material used as a CE.
- Ohmic drop expected using polarization methods and feasibility of correction.
- Estimation of the lubricant and hydrodynamic properties of the electrolyte.
- pH information is necessary to equilibrium thermodynamic assessments.

7.6.2 Step 2 – Preliminary Electrochemical Assessment

The main objective of this preliminary step is to provide a better understanding of the corrosion behavior of the material without the influence of wear. All the electrochemical techniques can be used, especially under steady-state conditions that can be achieved at the unworn surface. Anodic and cathodic polarization, OCP, EIS, amperometry, and even electrochemical noise can be used. The information will be the baseline for the interpretation of the system under wear conditions. Considering passive conditions, the results will inform the characteristics of the interface containing a protective film. The evolution with time of the passive state can be followed by OCP vs. time, polarization resistance – extracted from EIS data – and the profile of the anodic and cathodic polarization curves.

At this step, the assessment of localized corrosion susceptibility of the unworn surface is essential. Pitting corrosion is likely to occur even without the mechanical influence of wear. Consequently, during tribocorrosion tests, part of the electrochemical data registered could be produced by metastable and stable pits occurring at the unworn area. The transition from active to passive conditions at the potential referred to as Flade potential can also be observed. This process is likely to occur, for example, in the case system ferritic stainless steel in sulfuric acid, where the existence of this Flade potential could explain the improvement of the tribocorrosion resistance at higher anodic potential and the repassivation kinetics.

Another information possible to collect is about fluid-induced corrosion that can add value to the experimental work based on tribocorrosion and fretting tests. The test can be carried out on the tribometer with the WE under rotating movement, but without using the ball or pin. In other words, only under the influence of the solution flow.

The output of Step 1 will provide answers to the following points:

- OCP vs. time profiles indicative of the evolution of active or passive conditions at the interface, confirmed by equilibrium thermodynamic analysis.
- Steady-state anodic and cathodic polarization curves with the precise definition of the current vs. profile curves under anodic and cathodic conditions. Passive range and corrosion rate, in case of active dissolution in compliance with Stern and Geary equation and Faraday law.
- EIS diagrams and associated parameters like polarization resistance, Rp, capacitance, electrolyte resistance, Re. These parameters will be defined for dielectric properties of the passive film, in case of stable passivation or by the corrosion mechanism and kinetics in case of active dissolution.
- Baseline current and potential spontaneous fluctuations between identical electrochemical interfaces, using a ZRA.

Step 2 can be performed using the tribometer or another electrochemical cell of a second setup. The use of the tribometer implies on the imposition of the static condition and rotating without contact. The advantage of using the tribometer is the possibility of imposing very close conditions to the tests to be carried out under wear on Step 3.

7.6.3 Step 3 – Tribocorrosion Tests

Tribocorrosion tests are the core of the experimental investigation designed to assess the wear resistance of metallic materials in corrosive environments. The more adequate electrochemical techniques to be used during the tests are:

1. OCP vs. time before, during, and after sliding.
2. Current vs. time under constant potential before, during, and after sliding.
3. Potential and current oscillations vs time before, during, and after sliding.

The record of simple parameters – OCP and current vs time under constant potential before, during, and after sliding – permitted the identification of the higher repassivation ability of titanium in human saliva under fretting during sliding. The analysis of the slope of potential and current during sliding is important. Express the ability to recover protection or the opposite trend, cumulative damage. The positive slope of potential and negative slope of current are indicative of repassivation. Cumulative damage corresponds to opposite slopes. Positive results of surface modification can be identified by the same electrochemical measurements. The persistence of these modified layers can also be assessed. The same simple methodology, based on the analysis in the time domain, identifies the attenuation of anodic current spikes with time, coherent with the potential evolution. The efficiency of surface coating can be assessed by DC electrochemical parameters (Figures 7.9 through 7.12)

Current vs. time under constant potential before, during, and after sliding, are indicated to test the material under cathodic polarization at a constant potential within the immunity domain. Cathodic polarization is an efficient resource to determine the wear volume removed without the influence of anodic dissolution or corrosion. The optimum polarization condition is the imposition of potential into the immunity thermodynamic domain of the material, above the hydrogen reduction equilibrium potential. This value can be obtained from E × pH and redox curves. For titanium, e.g., the most adequate cathodic potential to be selected to perform the tribocorrosion tests should be within the Ti/Ti^{+++} and H/H$^+$ equilibrium potentials. titanium in Ringer solution is fully passive and is not susceptible to localized corrosion, despite the high magnitude of the anodic current transients recorded during tribocorrosion. Another use of cathodic polarization is the removal of air formed passive films.

The other electrochemical method is based on the measurements of current and potential fluctuations using ZRA instruments connecting similar materials as WE and CE. The use of the same materials can be a relevant contribution to support the interpretation of the ZRA data. Besides that, the same areas should be used for each electrode, since the area ratio will affect the ZRA response. The use of platinum as CE, as commonly reported, implies on a potential gap between CE and WE. This gap depends on the redox potential of the solution used, determined in the previous steps. Using the same tested material as CE can reduce this gap to zero under steady-state conditions. EIS data analysis is important to assess the contribution of the impedance of both interfaces and electrolyte conductivity, another determining factor to be taken into account for the consistency of the interpretation of ZRA measurements.

Galvanic interactions between worn and unworn surfaces are considered as the root causes of enhanced dissolution of metals during tribocorrosion and other mechanically assisted corrosion processes. The design of the experimental setup is a determining factor of the electrochemical response obtained, as already mentioned. On the present experimental work plan, for example, the use of stainless steel must be supported by the determination of anodic polarization tests to assess the localized corrosion susceptibility without the contribution of wear. Localized corrosion susceptibility implies on the possible occurrence of pitting on the passive area of the WE during tribocorrosion tests. This event brings another component to the electrochemical signals and must be considered on interpretation.

Preliminary electrochemical assessment will permit the best interpretation of the response of the unworn area during tribocorrosion tests. As already mentioned, the method used to obtain ZRA data is essential. The response will depend on the potential gap, impedance of the connected materials, and electrolyte conductivity. The definition of the rate of materials removed due to corrosion is a complex issue. The magnitude and time constants of the transients registered are governed by several parameters.

Moreover, part of the electrochemical response is non-faradaic, and the use of Faraday law and Stearn Geary equation is not fully consistent. In the case of passive biomaterials and corrosion resistant alloys, the correlation between anodic current and mass loss is not direct. Other parameters can be used to express the corrosion resistance, all of which are related to a mixed type of electrochemical interface.

The elementary transients contain components related to the relaxation of the double layer and passive films. The faradaic component related to the metal dissolution is embedded in the same signal. The amplitude and frequency of the signals will depend on the electrochemical processes occurring during sliding, and also on the design of the experimental apparatus, the type of CE, and geometric parameters. At the same time, the data acquisition protocols and instrumentation must comply with the expected amplitude and time constants of the electrochemical signals. Additionally, spurious noise rejection deserves special attention.

Complementary analytical methods for signal processing in the time domain can be more adequate to achieve a better understanding of tribocorrosion. Incidence of localized corrosion – pitting – is randomized and likely to occur on worn and unworn areas. The influence of this event is relevant for stainless steels, NiCr, and CoCr alloys, for instance. Not so relevant for Ti-based alloys in chloride environments. Besides the mechanical removal of the passive film by wear, followed by repassivation, is non-stationary *strictu sensu*.

Current spikes produced by randomized events are detectable on the time domain but can be attenuated or suppressed on the frequency domain after averaged calculations of PSD, for instance.

The Step 3 will provide the following outputs:

- Potential and current profiles before, during and after wear, with all parameters associated, such as wear induced potential drop, current and potential slopes during sliding, current and potential recover after wear.
- Current and potential profiles during sliding, in time and frequency domains.

7.6.4 Step 4 – Surface Analysis

The final result of tribocorrosion is the wear volume loss, physically reproduced during Step 3. Wear volume can be calculated by using different surface analysis techniques, like interferometry and confocal laser. Bidimensional profiles of the wear track can be obtained and integrated to reach the total volume loss after tribocorrosion. This value is converted to normalized information, considered the total wear length during the tests, calculated from the test duration.

Step 4 will provide the following outputs:

- Volume loss.
- Morphology and composition of worn an unworn surface.

Other surface analysis techniques must be used to characterize the morphology of the material after tribocorrosion, using as reference the same surface before the tribocorrosion tests. Optical microscopy, scanning electron microscope (SEM), rugosimeters, and AFM can be used. The characterization of the morphology of the wear track – in terms of plastic deformation, presence of third corps and debris, presence of corrosion products and cracks – is essential to clarify the degradation mechanism. Analytical techniques used together with SEM, like Energy dispersive spectroscopy (EDS), permit the identification of the semi-quantitative composition of elements found on the surface. Raman spectroscopy or XRD can also be used with the same objective. Analysis of the unworn surface using the same resources is important to detect localized corrosion or other damaged points.

In summary, the four steps methodology here outlined permit the achievement of a consistent set of information capable to support the quantification of the tribocorrosion damage and, in some extent, the understanding of the mechanism behind it. One point under discussion is the possibility of identification of the contribution of corrosion, mechanical wear, and synergic components. Guidelines to be followed toward this objective can be found in standards and other documents. However, it is important to point out that the assessment of the electrochemical dissolution rate is based on Faraday law and Stern Geary equation. Tribocorrosion of biomaterials and of other materials, like stainless steels, occurs under passive conditions. The corrosion rate, consequently, cannot be directly estimated by concepts appliable active dissolution conditions. Despite this limitation, empirical correlations can be stablished between electrochemical parameters here described and the intensity and morphology of corrosion under wear. This possibility depends on consistent knowledge obtained from physicochemical, electrochemical, and tribocorrosion analysis and tests. Each system metal/electrolyte of interest must be approached by tailored work plan supported by an integrated methodology, where the tribocorrosion tests play the major role, but are not sufficient to provide the information required to understand the phenomenon.

REFERENCES

1. American Society for Testing and Materials. ASTM G 119-09. *Standard Guide for Determining Synergism between Wear and Corrosion*. ASTM International West Conshohocken, PA: 2009.
2. American Society for Testing and Materials. ASTM G 40-17. *Standard terminology relating to wear and erosion*. ASTM International West Conshohocken, PA: 2017.
3. López-Ortega A, Arana JL, Bayón R. Tribocorrosion of passive materials: a review on test procedures and standards. *International Journal of Corrosion*. 2018; 18: 7345346.
4. Berradja A, Déforge D, Nogueira RP, Ponthiaux P, Wenger F, Celis JP. An electrochemical noise study of tribocorrosion processes of AISI 304 L in Cl– and media. *Journal of Physics D: Applied Physics*. 2006; 39 (15): 3184.
5. Mathew MT, Uth T, Hallab NJ, Pourzal R, Fischer A, Wimmer MA. Construction of a tribocorrosion test apparatus for the hip joint: validation, test methodology and analysis. *Wear*. 2011; 271 (9–10): 2651–2659.
6. Landolt D, Mischler S, Stemp M, Barril S. Third body effects and material fluxes in tribocorrosion systems involving a sliding contact. *Wear*. 2004; 256 (5): 517–524.
7. Jiang J, Stack MM, Neville A. Modelling the tribo-corrosion interaction in aqueous sliding conditions. *Tribology International*. 2002; 35 (10): 669–679.
8. Ferreira DF, Almeida SMA, Soares RB, Juliani L, Bracarense AQ, Lins VDFC, Junqueira RMR. Synergism between mechanical wear and corrosion on tribocorrosion of a titanium alloy in a Ringer solution. *Journal of Materials Research and Technology*. 2019; 8 (2): 1593–1600.
9. Rasool G, Y. El Shafei and M.M. Stack. Mapping tribo-corrosion behaviour of TI-6AL-4V Eli in laboratory simulated hip joint environments. *Lubricants*. 2020; 8 (7): 69.
10. Sampaio M, Buciumeanu M., Henriques B, Silva FS, Souza JCM, Gomes JR. Comparison between PEEK and Ti6Al4V concerning micro-scale abrasion wear on dental applications. *Journal of the Mechanical Behavior of Biomedical Materials*. 2016; 60: 212–219.

11. Holmes D, Sharifi S, Stack MM. Tribo-corrosion of steel in artificial saliva. *Tribology International*. 2014; 75: 80–86.
12. American Society for Testing and Materials. ASTM G133-05. *Standard Test Method for Linearly Reciprocating Ball-on-Flat Sliding Wear*. ASTM International West Conshohocken, PA: 2005a.
13. American Society for Testing and Materials. ASTM G 99-05. *Standard test method for wear testing with a pin-on-disk apparatus*. ASTM International West Conshohocken, PA: 2005b.
14. Abolusoro OP, Akinlabi ET. Tribocorrosion Measurements and Behaviour in Aluminium Alloys: An Overview. *Journal of Bio- and Tribo-Corrosion*. 2020; 6 (4): 1–13.
15. Barros CDR, Rocha JC, Bastos IN, Ponciano Gomes JAC. Tribocorrosion of Ti6Al4V and NiCr Implant Alloys: Effect of Galvanic Interaction. *Journal of Bio- and Tribo-Corrosion*. 2020a; 6: 117.
16. Dalbert V, Mary N, Normand B, Verdu C, Saedlou S. In situ determinations of the wear surfaces, volumes and kinetics of repassivation: Contribution in the understanding of the tribocorrosion behaviour of a ferritic stainless steel in various pH. *Tribology International*. 2010; 150: 106374.
17. López-Ortega A, Arana JL, Bayón R. On the comparison of the tribocorrosion behavior of passive and non-passivating materials and assessment of the influence of agitation. *Wear*. 2020; 456: 203388.
18. Voutat C, Nohava J, Wandel J, Zysset P. The dynamic friction coefficient of the wet bone-implant interface: influence of load, speed, material and surface finish. *Biotribology*. 2019; 17: 64–74.
19. Sivakumar B, Pathak LC, Singh R. Role of surface roughness on corrosion and fretting corrosion behaviour of commercially pure titanium in Ringer's solution for bio-implant application. *Applied Surface Science*. 2017; 401: 385–398.
20. Silva DP, Churiaque C, Bastos IN, Sánchez-Amaya JM. Tribocorrosion study of ordinary and laser-melted Ti6Al4V alloy. *Metals*. 2016; 6 (10): 253.
21. Kappel MAA, Silva DP, Sánchez-Amaya JM, Domingos RP, Bastos IN. Análise não Estacionária Aplicada a Sinais de Tribocorrosão. *Revista Virtual de Química* 2015; 7 (5): 1651–1662.
22. Li DG, Wang JD, Chen DR, Liang P. Influence of molybdenum on tribo-corrosion behavior of 316L stainless steel in artificial saliva. *Journal of Bio-and Tribo-Corrosion*. 2015;1(2): 14.
23. Souza JCM, Tajiri HA, Morsch CS, Buciumeanu M, Mathew MT, Silva FS, Henriques B. Tribocorrosion behavior of Ti6Al4V coated with a bio-absorbable polymer for biomedical applications. *Journal of Bio-and Tribo-Corrosion*. 2015; 1 (4): 27.
24. Wimmer MA, Laurent MP, Mathew MT, Nagelli C, Liao Y, Marks LD, Jacobs DD, Fischer A. The effect of contact load on CoCrMo wear and the formation and retention of tribofilms. *Wear*. 2015; 332: 643–649.
25. Mathew MT, Abbey S, Hallab NJ, Hall DJ, Sukotjo C, Wimmer MA. Influence of pH on the tribocorrosion behavior of CpTi in the oral environment: synergistic interactions of wear and corrosion. *Journal of Biomedical Materials Research Part B: Applied Biomaterials*. 2012; 100 (6): 1662–1671.
26. Kumar S, Narayanan TS, Raman SGS, Seshadri SK. Evaluation of fretting corrosion behaviour of CP-Ti for orthopaedic implant applications. *Tribology International*. 2010; 43 (7): 1245–1252.
27. Yan Y, Neville A, Dowson D, Williams S, Fisher J. Tribo-corrosion analysis of wear and metal ion release interactions from metal-on-metal and ceramic-on-metal contacts for the application in artificial hip prostheses. *Proceedings of the Institution of Mechanical Engineers, Part J: Journal of Engineering Tribology*. 2008; 222 (3): 483–492.

28. Vieira AC, Ribeiro AR, Rocha LA, Celis JP. Influence of pH and corrosion inhibitors on the tribocorrosion of titanium in artificial saliva. *Wear.* 2006; 261 (9): 994–1001.
29. Déforge D, Huet F, Nogueira RP, Ponthiaux P, Wenger F. Electrochemical noise analysis of tribocorrosion processes under steady-state friction regime. *Corrosion.* 2006; 62 (6): 514–521.
30. Espallargas N, Johnsen R, Torres C, Muñoz AI. A new experimental technique for quantifying the galvanic coupling effects on stainless steel during tribocorrosion under equilibrium conditions. *Wear.* 2013; 307 (1–2): 190–197.
31. Radice S, Holcomb T, Pourzal R, Hallab NJ, Laurent MP, Wimmer MA. Investigation of CoCrMo material loss in a novel bio-tribometer designed to study direct cell reaction to wear and corrosion products. *Biotribology.* 2019; 18: 100090.
32. Puppulin L, Leto A, Wenliang Z, Sugano N. and Pezzotti G. Innovative tribometer for in situ spectroscopic analyses of wear mechanisms and phase transformation in ceramic femoral heads. *Journal of the Mechanical Behavior of Biomedical Materials.* 2014; 31: 45–54.
33. Bruschi S, Bertolini R, Medeossi F, Ghiotti A, Savio E, Shivpuri R. Case study: The application of machining-conditioning to improve the wear resistance of Ti6Al4V surfaces for human hip implants. *Wear.* 2018; 394: 134–142.
34. Yan Y, Neville A, Hesketh J, Dowson D. Real-time corrosion measurements to assess biotribocorrosion mechanisms with a hip simulator. *Tribology International.* 2013; 63: 115–122.
35. Hua Z, Dou P, Jia H, Tang F, Wang X, Xiong X, Gao L, Huang X, Jin Z. Wear test apparatus for friction and wear evaluation hip prostheses. *Frontiers in Mechanical Engineering.* 2019; 5: 12.
36. Yan Y, Neville A, Dowson D, Williams S, Fisher J. The influence of swing phase load on the electrochemical response, friction, and ion release of metal-on-metal hip prostheses in a friction simulator. *Proceedings of the Institution of Mechanical Engineers, Part J: Journal of Engineering Tribology.* 2009; 223 (3): 303–309.
37. Corne P, De March P, Cleymand F, Geringer J. Fretting-corrosion behavior on dental implant connection in human saliva. *Journal of the Mechanical Behavior of Biomedical Materials.* 2019; 94: 86–92.
38. Dalmau Borrás A, Buch AR, Cardete AR, Navarro-Laboulais J, Munoz AI. Chemomechanical effects on the tribocorrosion behavior of titanium/ceramic dental implant pairs in artificial saliva. *Wear.* 2019; 426: 162–170.
39. Simsek I, Ozyurek D. Investigation of the wear and corrosion behaviors of Ti5Al2. 5Fe and Ti6Al4V alloys produced by mechanical alloying method in simulated body fluid environment. *Materials Science and Engineering: C.* 2019; 94: 357–363.
40. Pejaković V, Totolin V, Ripoll MR. Tribocorrosion behaviour of Ti6Al4V in artificial seawater at low contact pressures. *Tribology International.* 2018; 119: 55–65.
41. Alves SA, Bayón R, de Viteri VS, Garcia MP, Igartua A, Fernandes MH, Rocha LA. Tribocorrosion behavior of calcium-and phosphorous-enriched titanium oxide films and study of osteoblast interactions for dental implants. *Journal of Bio- and Tribo-Corrosion.* 2015; 1 (3): 23.
42. Licausi MP, Muñoz AI, Borrás VA, Espallargas N. Tribocorrosion mechanisms of Ti6Al4V in artificial saliva by zero-resistance ammetry (ZRA) technique. *Journal of Bio-and Tribo-Corrosion.* 2015; 1 (1): 8.
43. Swaminathan V, Gilbert JL. Potential and frequency effects on fretting corrosion of Ti6Al4V and CoCrMo surfaces. *Journal of Biomedical Materials Research Part A.* 2013; 101 (9): 2602–2612.
44. Dimah MK, Albeza FD, Borrás VA, Muñoz IA. Study of the biotribocorrosion behaviour of titanium biomedical alloys in simulated body fluids by electrochemical techniques. *Wear.* 2012; 294: 409–418.

45. Tekin KC, Malayoglu U. Assessing the tribocorrosion performance of three different nickel-based superalloys. *Tribology Letters.* 2010; 37 (3): 563–572.
46. International Organization for Standardization. ISO 4287:1997(en). *Geometrical Product Specifications (GPS) — Surface texture: Profile method — Terms, definitions and surface texture parameters.* ISO;1997.
47. International Organization for Standardization. ISO 25178-2 :2012(en).*Geometrical product specifications (GPS) — surface texture: areal — part 2: terms, definitions and surface texture parameters.* ISO; 2012.
48. Alves SA, Rossi AL, Ribeiro AR, Toptan F, Pinto AM, Shokuhfar T, Cellis JP, Rocha LA. Improved tribocorrosion performance of bio-functionalized TiO2 nanotubes under two-cycle sliding actions in artificial saliva. *Journal of the Mechanical Behavior of Biomedical Materials.* 2018; 80: 143–154.
49. Liamas E, Thomas OR, Muñoz AI, Zhang ZJ. Tribocorrosion behaviour of pure titanium in bovine serum albumin solution: A multiscale study. *Journal of the Mechanical Behavior of Biomedical Materials.* 2020; 102: 103511.
50. Zhao GH, Aune RE, Espallargas N. Tribocorrosion studies of metallic biomaterials: The effect of plasma nitriding and DLC surface modifications. *Journal of the Mechanical Behavior of Biomedical Materials.* 2016; 63: 100–114.
51. Butt A, Lucchiari NB, Royhman D, Runa MJ, Mathew MT, Sukotjo C, Takoudis CG. Design, development, and testing of a compact tribocorrosion apparatus for biomedical applications. *Journal of Bio- and Tribo-Corrosion.* 2015; 1: 4.
52. Stack MM, Corlett N, Zhou S. A methodology for the construction of the erosion-corrosion map in aqueous environments. *Wear.* 1997; 203: 474–488.
53. Stack MM. Mapping tribo-corrosion processes in dry and in aqueous conditions: some new directions for the new millennium. *Tribology International.* 2002; 35 (10): 681–689.
54. Diomidis N, Celis JP, Ponthiaux P, Wenger F. A methodology for the assessment of the tribocorrosion of passivating metallic materials. *Lubrication Science.* 2009; 21 (2): 53–67.
55. Barros CDR, Rocha JC, Braz BF, Santelli RE, Gomes JACP. Galvanic Corrosion of Ti6Al4V Coupled with NiCr as a Dental Implant Alloy in Fluoride Solutions. *International Journal of Electrochemical Science.* 2020b; 15: 394–411.
56. European Standards. UNE 112086: 2016. *Tribocorrosion testing procedure for passivating materials.* UNE (Normalización Española); 2016.
57. Silva RCC, Nogueira RO, Bastos IN. Tribocorrosion of UNS S32750 in chloride medium: Effect of the load level. *Electrochimica Acta.* 2011; 56 (24): 8839–8845.
58. Sun D, Wharton JA, Wood RJK. Effects of proteins and pH on tribocorrosion performance of cast CoCrMo—a combined electrochemical and tribological study. *Tribology-Materials, Surfaces & Interfaces.* 2008; 2 (3): 150–160.
59. Geringer J, Forest B, Combrade P. Fretting-corrosion of materials used as orthopaedic implants. *Wear.* 2005; 259 (7–12): 943–951.
60. Jemmely P, Mischler S, Landolt D. Electrochemical modeling of passivation phenomena in tribocorrosion. *Wear.* 2000; 237 (1): 63–76.
61. Licausi MP, Muñoz AI, Borrás VA. Influence of the fabrication process and fluoride content on the tribocorrosion behaviour of Ti6Al4V biomedical alloy in artificial saliva. *Journal of the Mechanical Behavior of Biomedical Materials.* 2013; 20: 137–148.

8 Future Outlooks in Biotribology

T. V. V. L. N. Rao
Madanapalle Institute of Technology & Science, Madanapalle, India

Salmiah Kasolang
Universiti Teknologi MARA, Shah Alam, Malaysia

Guoxin Xie
Tsinghua University, Beijing, China

Jitendra Kumar Katiyar
SRM Institute of Science and Technology, Chennai, India

Ahmad Majdi Abdul Rani
Universiti Teknologi PETRONAS, Seri Iskandar, Malaysia

CONTENTS

8.1 Introduction 231
8.2 Lubrication Characteristics of Artificial Joints 233
8.3 Biotribological Characteristics of Textured Surfaces 233
8.4 Tribological Characteristics of Implants 234
8.5 Conclusions and Further Outlook 234
References 234

8.1 INTRODUCTION

The future researches in lubrication characteristics of artificial joints are devoted mainly to (Ruggiero and Sicilia [1]): (i) mathematical models in a mixed lubrication regime, (ii) elastohydrodynamic lubrication solutions in conjunction with roughness together with wear phenomenon and various surface boundary conditions, (iii) establishing a link between lubrication models with finite element method based deformations of metal, polymer and composite implants, (iv) use of accurate synovial rheological fluid behavior based on non-Newtonian fluid models.

The biotribological characteristics of textured surfaces and nanofunctionalized bioinspired surfaces are rapidly emerging significant areas of research that has fascinated much attentiveness in recent years (Xie [2]). The nanofunctionalized bioinspired surfaces enhance the biomaterial surface interactions and physiological environment. The development of nanofunctionalized bioinspired surfaces most preferred by cells with tailored physical morphology and chemical composition will be effective for biosurface designs in future. Textured implant surfaces that inhibit the formation of biofilms and retard the bacterial adherence have a significant potential in the design of futuristic implants (Vadakkumpurath et al. [3]). Textured implant surfaces are a potential method for endowing implants with antibacterial properties, reducing the risk of implant-associated infections. The bacterial adhesion and growth are reduced in textured specimens in comparison with a polished specimen, which is attributed to its surface topography and the micro-dimples.

The future research on tribological characteristics of implants of artificial joints devoted mainly to (Shu et al. [4]): (a) computational modeling, (b) specific material properties, (c) experimental design and sensitivity, (d) comprehensive evaluation. The substantial attention in preclinical prosthesis design creates an effective platform to step up the design and optimization. Computational modeling for preclinical prosthesis design and testing has enticed great attention owing to features such as configurability, high efficiency, high precision, and low cost. Challenges continue in employing these computational models to commercial purposes, but technological developments in preclinical prosthesis design identification, model generation, and implant manufacturing lead to the rise of this implant technology.

The latest progressions in biotribology may lead to a robust foundation of future developments on sustainable long-life considerations. The principles of biotribological design can appreciably increase impact on future developments for health, durability, and sustainable long life of implants. An overview of future outlooks in biotribology is presented in Figure 8.1. The future outlooks in lubrication characteristics of artificial joints, biotribological characteristics of textured surfaces, and tribological characteristics of implants will establish the progress in biotribology. Following the brief overview based on the recent developments on biotribology with emphasis on health, durability, and long life, the following sections provide further explicit directions for future outlooks in biotribology.

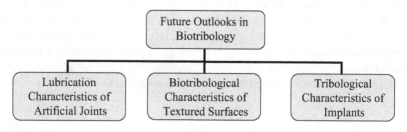

FIGURE 8.1 An overview of future outlooks in biotribology.

Future Outlooks in Biotribology

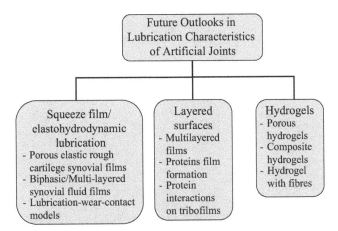

FIGURE 8.2 An overview of future outlooks in biotribology on lubrication of artificial joints.

8.2 LUBRICATION CHARACTERISTICS OF ARTIFICIAL JOINTS

An overview of future outlooks in biotribology on lubrication characteristics of artificial joints is presented in Figure 8.2. Following the recent developments on lubrication characteristics of artificial joints, the explicit directions for future outlooks are: (i) porous elastic rough cartilage and multi-layered synovial fluid films, and lubrication-wear-contact models, (ii) multi-layered and proteins films and protein interactions on tribofilms, and (iii) porous and composite hydrogels, and hydrogel with fibers.

8.3 BIOTRIBOLOGICAL CHARACTERISTICS OF TEXTURED SURFACES

An overview of future outlooks in biotribology on characteristics of textured surfaces is presented in Figure 8.3. Following the recent developments in textured surfaces,

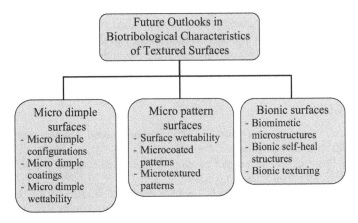

FIGURE 8.3 An overview of future outlooks in biotribology of textured surfaces.

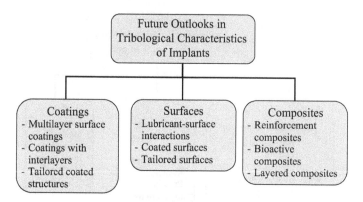

FIGURE 8.4 An overview of future outlooks in the biotribology of implants.

the explicit directions for future outlooks are: (i) micro-dimple configurations, coatings, and wettability, (ii) surface wettability, microcoated and microtextured patterns, and (iii) biomimetic microstructures, bionic self-heal structures, and textures.

8.4 TRIBOLOGICAL CHARACTERISTICS OF IMPLANTS

An overview of future outlooks in biotribology on texture surfaces is presented in Figure 8.4. Based on the recent status of investigations in the area on texture surfaces, the explicit directions for future outlooks are: (i) multilayer surface coatings, coatings with interlayers and tailored coated structures, (ii) lubricant-surface interactions, coated and tailored surfaces, and (iii) reinforcement, bioactive, and layered composites.

8.5 CONCLUSIONS AND FURTHER OUTLOOK

The future outlooks and prospects of biotribology for health and sustainable living are highlighted in the lubrication characteristics of artificial joints, biotribological characteristics of textured surfaces, and tribological characteristics of implants. The detailed directions in the future outlooks are established based on the recent developments in biotribology. The emphasis on biotribology in the areas of artificial joints, textured surfaces, and implants will greatly affect the endurance, durability, and sustainable long life of implants.

REFERENCES

1. Alessandro Ruggiero, Alessandro Sicilia. Lubrication modeling and wear calculation in artificial hip joint during the gait, *Tribol. Int.*, 2020, Vol. 142, p. 105993.
2. C Xie. Bio-inspired nanofunctionalisation of biomaterial surfaces: A review, *Biosurf. Biotribol.*, 2019, Vol. 5, Iss. 3, pp. 83–92.
3. Shiju Vadakkumpurath, Abhijith Njarakkadu Venugopal, Sudeep Ullattil. Influence of micro-textures on antibacterial behaviour of titanium-based implant surfaces: In vitro studies, *Biosurf. Biotribol.*, 2019, Vol. 5, Iss. 1, pp. 20–23.
4. Liming Shu, Shihao Li, Naohiko Sugita. Systematic review of computational modelling for biomechanics analysis of total knee replacement, *Biosurf. Biotribol.*, Vol. 6, Iss. 1, 2020, pp. 3–11.

Index

A

albumin, 5–9, 38, 40–44, 67
amperometry, 193
anodic and cathodic polarization, 193–196
Archard's law, 68, 71–72, 209
arthroplasty, 130
artificial hip joints, 16
artiflex chondro (AC), 165–167
atomic microscope (AFM), 203, 205–207

B

Barrett–Joyner–Halenda (BJH), 152
Berkovich indenter, 162
bioceramic coatings, 17
bioceramics, 135
bioinspired surfaces, 232
biomechanics, 91–92
biomimetic, 8, 11, 15, 233
bionic surfaces, 2, 11, 15, 233
biphasic lubrication, 9
boundary lubrication, 2–3, 9, 12, 35, 49, 66–67, 128–130, 139
bovine bone hydroxyapatite (BHA), 21
bovine serum albumin (BSA), 14
bovine serum (BS), 19, 37

C

calf serum (CS), 38
carbon nanodots, 132
ceramic-on-ceramic, 20, 36, 49
ceramic-on-metal, 49
ceramic-on-UHMWPE, 23
charge couple-device (CDD) camera, 185
chondroitin sulfate, 165
coatings, 2, 234
composites, 2, 234
computational biotribology, 64
computed tomography (CT), 79, 131
crosslinked polyethylene (XLPE), 135
cytotoxicity, 133

D

diamond-like carbon coatings, 11
diamond-like carbon (DLC), 12–19
dispersive energy spectroscopy (EDX), 203, 205–207

E

elastohydrodynamic lubrication, 2–6, 12–14, 36, 39, 43, 45, 50–51, 67, 74, 80, 231–233
elbow limb joint reactions, 118
elbow residual actuators, 117
elbow revolute joint, 97
elbow wrapping, 112
electrochemical assessment, 223
electrochemical cell, 180, 183–185
electrochemical current noise (ECN), 216
electrochemical impedance spectroscopy (EIS), 193–196
electrochemical noise (EN), 193, 197
electrochemical potential noise (EPN), 216
endoprosthesis, 147–149, 164
extracellular matrix (ECM), 132

F

femoral heads, 154
field emission scanning electron microscopic (FE-SEM), 203, 205–207
free lapping, 150–152

G

gait analysis, 92
gait cycle, 5, 75
γ-globulin, 5–9, 38, 40–44, 67
gemini hydrogel, 10
geodesics, 104–105

H

HA, *see* hyaluronan, *see* hyaluronic acid
hard-on-hard hip replacements, 34–36, 45–47, 53
hard-on-soft hip replacements, 34, 45–47, 53
Hill muscle model, 101
hip replacements, 35–36, 46–47
human synovial fluid (HSF), 19
hyaluronan (HA), 128
hyaluronic acid (HA), 3–7, 38, 40–44, 67
hyaluronic acid-nanoMOF, 134
hydration, 9
hydrodynamic lubrication, 5–6, 9, 37, 45, 66, 128–130, 138–139
hydrogels, 2, 8–11, 44, 134, 138, 233
hydroxyapatite (HAp), 10, 17, 19, 22, 135

Index

I
inverse dynamics, 93, 100, 114
ionic liquid crystals (ILCs), 137

K
knee joint prostheses, 3, 77
knee joint replacements, 16
knee replacements, 35, 43, 46, 51

L
laser confocal microscopy, 203, 205–207
layered surfaces, 2, 8, 233
light interferometer, 203, 205–207
liquid-crystalline components (LC), 164
lubricin, 7, 128, 138

M
magnetic resonance imaging (MRI), 79, 131
metal-on-metal (MOM), 18–20, 49
micro dimples, 2, 12–13, 233
micro patterns, 2, 13–14, 233
microtextures, 11–13
mixed lubrication, 3, 9, 35, 47–49, 66, 74, 138, 231
mucin, 7
multi-body dynamics (MBD), 78
multibody models, 92
multiscale modeling, 78–80
muscle activations, 115–116
muscle forces, 115–116
muscles' fiber deformation, 113
muscles' fiber length, 113

N
nanoscale coordination polymers (NCPs), 130
nanoscale metal-organic frameworks (NMOFs), 130, 134
natural coral (NC), 21
nitriding, 156–163, 167
numerical wear simulator, 70

O
open circuit potential (OCP), 193–194, 197, 216–219
OpenSim arm26 model, 94, 110, 115–116
optical microscopy, 203, 205–207
osteoarthritis-oriented synovial fluid (OASF), 12
osteochondral defects, 126
oxyreduction curves (redox curves), 214

P
pendulum tribometer, 163–166
phospholipids (PLs), 3, 6–10, 40–44, 128
physicochemical characterization, 222
polyacrylamide (PAAm), 10–11
polyethylene glycol (PEG), 138
poly(2-hydroxyethyl) methacrylate, 11
polyhydroxyethylmethacrylate (pHEMA), 11
polymer tribology, 124
poly (vinyl alcohol) (PVA), 9–11
potentiodynamic polarization, 212
Pourbaix diagram, 212–214
profilometer, 203, 205–207
proteoglycan, 128

R
Raman spectroscopy, 202
reciprocating ball-on-flat, 181
ring-on-plane tribosystem, 163–166
rotational ball-on-disk, 182
rugosimeter, 203, 205–207

S
scanning electron microscopy (SEM), 203, 205–207
shape memory alloys (SMAs), 134
shape memory polymers (SMP), 134
shoulder joint reactions, 117
shoulder residual actuators, 117
shoulder wrapping, 112
single-photon emission computed tomography (SPECT), 131
squeeze film lubrication, 2–6, 233
static optimization, 93, 106, 110, 113
surface analysis, 226
surface texturing, 11, 14, 40

T
textured surfaces, 2, 11–15, 232–234
thermodiffusion, 156, 160
thermodiffusion nitriding (TDN), 149, 163, 167
total hip arthroplasties (THAs), 33–35, 43, 53
total knee arthroplasties (TKAs), 33–35, 43–44, 51, 53
total knee replacement (TKR), 64–68, 74–81
tribocharging, 127
tribocorrosion damage, 227
tribocorrosion systems, 180
tribocorrosion tests, 224
triboluminescence, 127

Index

tribometers, 186–192
tribometry, 126
tribotesting, 126
T-24 stand-simulator, 171

V

vacuum annealing, 162
van der Waals interactions, 128
vascular smooth muscle cells (VSMCs), 130

W

wear modeling, 74–75, 81
wear simulator, 64, 69, 76, 80
wrapped muscle, 104

X

X-ray diffraction (XRD), 203, 205–207
X-ray excited photoelectron spectroscopy (XPS), 202

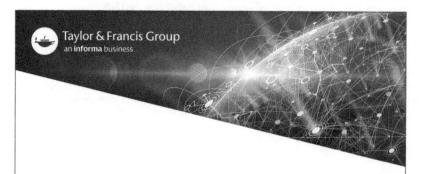